Trends in Hepatology

Trends in Hepatology

A Symposium in Honour of
Dr. Dr. Herbert Falk on the Occasion
of his 60th Birthday

Edited by
L. Bianchi; University of Basel, Switzerland
W. Gerok; University Medical Clinic, University of Freiburg, West Germany
H. Popper; Mount Sinai School of Medicine
of the City University of New York, USA

MTP PRESS LIMITED
a member of the KLUWER ACADEMIC PUBLISHERS GROUP
LANCASTER / BOSTON / THE HAGUE / DORDRECHT

Published in the UK and Europe by
MTP Press Limited
Falcon House
Lancaster, England

British Library Cataloguing in Publication Data

Trends in hepatology: a symposium in honour of
Dr Herbert Falk on the occasion of his 60th
birthday
1. Blood—Diseases
I. Falk, Herbert   II. Bianchi, L.
III. Popper, Hans   IV. Gerok, W.
616.1'5   RC636

ISBN-13: 978-94-010-8672-1

Published in the USA by
MTP Press
A division of Kluwer Boston Inc
190 Old Derby Street
Hingham, MA 02043, USA

Library of Congress Cataloging in Publication Data

Main entry under title:

Trends in hepatology.

  Includes bibliographies and index.
  1. Liver—Diseases—Congresses. 2. Falk,
Herbert, 1925-   —Congresses. I. Falk, Herbert.
II. Bianchi, Leonardo. III. Popper, Hans, 1903–
IV. Gerok, W. (Wolfgang), 1926-   . [DNLM: 1. Bile
Acids and Salts—congresses. 2. Biliary Tract
Diseases—congresses. 3. Liver Diseases—congresses.
WI 700 T794]
RC845.T74   1985   616.3'6   85-7279
ISBN-13: 978-94-010-8672-1   e-ISBN-13: 978-94-009-4904-1
DOI: 10.1007/978-94-009-4904-1

Phototypesetting by Blackpool Typesetting Services Ltd, Blackpool

Contents

Section 2

Section 3

CONTENTS

CONTENTS

Preface

This volume comprises a series of original articles, updates and reviews on relevant topics in hepatology which were presented at a meeting in Freiburg im Breisgau to honour the 60th anniversary of Dr. Herbert Falk. Since 1967, Dr. Falk and the Falk Foundation have generously sponsored more than 40 congresses and symposia on liver diseases, held mostly in Freiburg, The Black Forest or in Basel, which have become milestones in the exchange of scientific information in hepatology (see 'To Herbert Falk on his Sixtieth Birthday' in this volume). Many of these congresses and symposia have been published in the 'Falk Symposia' series by MTP Press.

We asked hepatologists who took part in former Falk liver meetings to contribute to a one day symposium to celebrate Dr. Falk's anniversary. We were greatly gladdened by the spontaneous and unrestrained acceptance that we received from all sides. We wish to express our deep appreciation to all the speakers and moderators who travelled, at their own expense, from all parts of the world to Freiburg and who with their presentations, made the meeting a stimulating and refreshing event. The editors' thanks are also addressed to Mr. D. G. T. Bloomer and Mr. P. M. Lister from MTP Press for their valuable cooperation in preparing this volume for publication. This book testifies to the worldwide appreciation and gratitude held for Dr. Falk by the community of hepatologists.

The Editors

List of Contributors

P. BACK
Medizinische Klinik
Universität Freiburg
Hugstetterstrasse 55
D-7800 Freiburg
West Germany

P. D. BERK
Polly Annenberg Levee Hematology Center
Department of Medicine
Mt Sinai School of Medicine
1 Gustave Levy Place
New York, NY 10029
USA

L. BIANCHI
Department of Pathology
University of Basel
Schöbeinstrasse 40
CH-4056 Basel
Switzerland

M. CLASSEN
II Medizinische Klinik rechts d. Isar
Techn. Universität München
Ismaninger Strasse 22
D-8000 München 80
West Germany

W. CREUTZFELDT
Medizinische Universitätsklinik
Rober-Koch-Strasse 40
D-3400 Göttingen
West Germany

P. DAYER
Department of Pharmacology
Biocenter of the University of Basel
Klingelbergstrasse 70
CH 4056 Basel
Switzerland

K. F. A. DECKER
Biochemisches Institut
Universität Freiburg
Hermann-Herder-Strasse 7
D-78000 Freiburg im Breisgau
West Germany

E. DEML
Department of Toxicology
Gesellschaft für Strahlen und
  Umweltforschung
Ingolstädter Landstrasse 1
D-8042 Neuherberg
West Germany

H. DENK
Department of Pathology
University of Graz
School of Medicine
Auenbruggerplatz 25
A-8036 Graz
Austria

C. DENZLINGER
Biochemisches Institut
Universität Freiburg im Breisgau
Hermann Herder Strasse 7
D-7800 Freiburg im Breisgau
West Germany

V. J. DESMET
Department of Pathology
Universitair Zeikenhuis Sint Rafael
Kaltolieke Universiteit Leuven
Leuven, Belgium

R. H. DOWLING
Gastroenterology Unit
Department of Medicine
Guy's Hospital and Medical School
London SE1 9RT
UK

O. EPSTEIN
Department of Medicine
Royal Free Hospital School of Medicine
London NW3 2QG
UK

G. T. EVERSON
Department of Medicine
Division of Gastroenterology
University of Colorado School of Medicine
4200 East Ninth Avenue B158
Denver, CO 80262
USA

C. FORSTHOVE
Biochemisches Institut
Universität Freiburg im Breisgau
Hermann Herder Strasse 7
D-7800 Freiburg im Breisgau
West Germany

W. W. FRANKE
Division of Membrane Biology and
  Biochemistry
Institute of Cell and Tumor Biology
German Cancer Research Center
Im Neuenheimer Feld 280
D-6900 Heidelberg 1
West Germany

H. GREIM
Department of Toxicology
Gesellschaft für Strahlen und
  Umweltforschung
Ingolstadter Landstrasse 1
D-8042 Neuherberg
West Germany

J. GUT
Department of Pharmacology
Biocenter of the University of Basel
Klingelbergstrasse 70
CH 4056 Basel
Switzerland

F. HAGENMÜLLER
Department of Gastroenterology
Centre for Internal Medicine
Johann Wolfgang Goethe University
Frankfurt am Main
West Germany

W. HAGMANN
Biochemisches Institut
Universität Freiburg im Breisgau
Hermann Herder Strasse 7
D-7800 Freiburg im Breisgau
West Germany

R. HAZAN
Division of Membrane Biology and
  Biochemistry
Institute of Cell and Tumor Biology
German Cancer Research Center
Im Neuenheimer Feld 280
D-6900 Heidelberg 1
West Germany

A. F. HOFMANN
Department of Medicine
UCSD Medical Center
225 Dickinson Street
San Diego, CA 92103
USA

E. A. JONES
Liver Diseases Section, NIADDK
National Institutes of Health
Building 10, Room 4D-52
Bethesda, MD 20205
USA

D. KEPPLER
Biochemisches Institut
Universität Freiburg im Breisgau
Hermann Herder Strasse 7
D-7800 Freiburg im Breisgau
West Germany

F. KERN
Department of Medicine
Division of Gastroenterology
University of Colorado School of Medicine
4200 East Ninth Avenue B158
Denver, CO 80262
USA

H. K. KOCH
Pathologisches Institut
Universität Freiburg im Breisgau
Albert Strasse 19
D-7800 Freiburg im Breisgau
West Germany

T. KRONBACH
Department of Pharmacology
Biocenter of the University of Basel
Klingelbergstrasse 70
CH-4056 Basel
Switzerland

W. KURTZ
Department of Gastroenterology
Centre for Internal Medicine
Johann Wolfgang Goethe University
Frankfurt am Main
West Germany

LIST OF CONTRIBUTORS

E. LACKINGER
Department of Pathology
University of Graz
School of Medicine
Auenbruggerplatz 25
A-8036 Graz
Austria

L. LANDMANN
Department of Anatomy
University of Basel
Pestalozzistrasse 20
CH-4056 Basel
Switzerland

K. P. MAIER
Department of Gastroenterology
Medical Clinic Esslingen
Academic Department, University of
  Tübingen
Tübingen
West Germany

W. R. MAYR
Institut für Blutgruppenserologie
Universität Wien
Spitalgasse 4
A-1090 Wien
Austria

U. A. MEYER
Department of Pharmacology
Biocenter of the University of Basel
Klingelbergstrasse 70
CH-4056 Basel
Switzerland

R. NUNES
Polly Annenberg Levee Hematology Center
Department of Medicine
Mt Sinai School of Medicine
1 Gustave L Levy Place
New York, NY 10029
USA

D. OESTERLE
Department of Toxicology
Gesellschaft für Strahlen und
  Umweltforschung
Ingolstadter Landstrasse 1
D-8042 Neuherberg
West Germany

H. OKUDA
Polly Annenberg Levee Hematology Center
Department of Medicine
Mt Sinai School of Medine
1 Gustave L Levy Place
New York, NY 10029
USA

H. POPPER
Mount Sinai School of Medicine
New York, NY 10029
USA

B. POTTER
Polly Annenberg Levee Hematology Center
Department of Medicine
Mt Sinai School of Medicine
1 Gustave L Levy Place
New York, NY 10029
USA

S. RAPP
Biochemisches Institut
Universität Freiburg im Breisgau
Hermann Herder Strasse 7
D-7800 Freiburg im Breisgau
West Germany

J. REGLI
Medizinische Abteilung
Stadspital Weid
Tièche Strasse 99
CH-8037 Zurich
Switzerland

W. REUTTER
Institut für Molekularbiologie und
  Biochemie der Freien Universität Berlin
D-1000 Berlin 33 (Dahlem)
West Germany

F. SCHAFFNER
Department of Medicine –
  Division of Liver Diseases
Mount Sinai School of Medicine
1 Gustave L Levy Place
New York, NY 10029
USA

D. L. SCHILLER
Division of Membrane Biology and
  Biochemistry
Institute of Cell and Tumor Biology
German Cancer Research Center
Im Neueheimer Feld 280
D-6900 Heidelberg 1
West Germany

M. SCHMID
Medizinische Abteilung
Stadspital Weid
Tièche Strasse 99
CH-8037 Zurich
Switzerland

S. SHERLOCK
Department of Surgery
Royal Free Hospital School of Medicine
London NW3 2QG
UK

I. STERNLIEB
Medicine and Liver Research Center
Albert Einstein College of Medicine
1300 Morris Park Avenue
Suite 517 – Ullman Building
Bronx, NY 10461
USA

A. STIEHL
Department of Internal Medicine
University of Heidelberg
D-6900 Heidelberg
Bergheimerstrasse 58
West Germany

W. STREMMEL
Polly Annenberg Levee Hematology Center
Department of Medicine
1 Gustave L Levy Place
New York, NY 10029
USA

N. TAVOLONI
Polly Annenberg Levee Hematology Center
Department of Medicine
Mt Sinai School of Medicine
1 Gustave L Levy Place
New York, NY 10029
USA

H. THALER and H. THALER
4 Medizinische Abteilung
Wilhelminenspital 37
A-1171 Wien
Austria

D. VALEER
Pathologische Ontleedkunde II
Universitair Ziekenhuis St Rafaël
B-3000 Leuven
Belgium

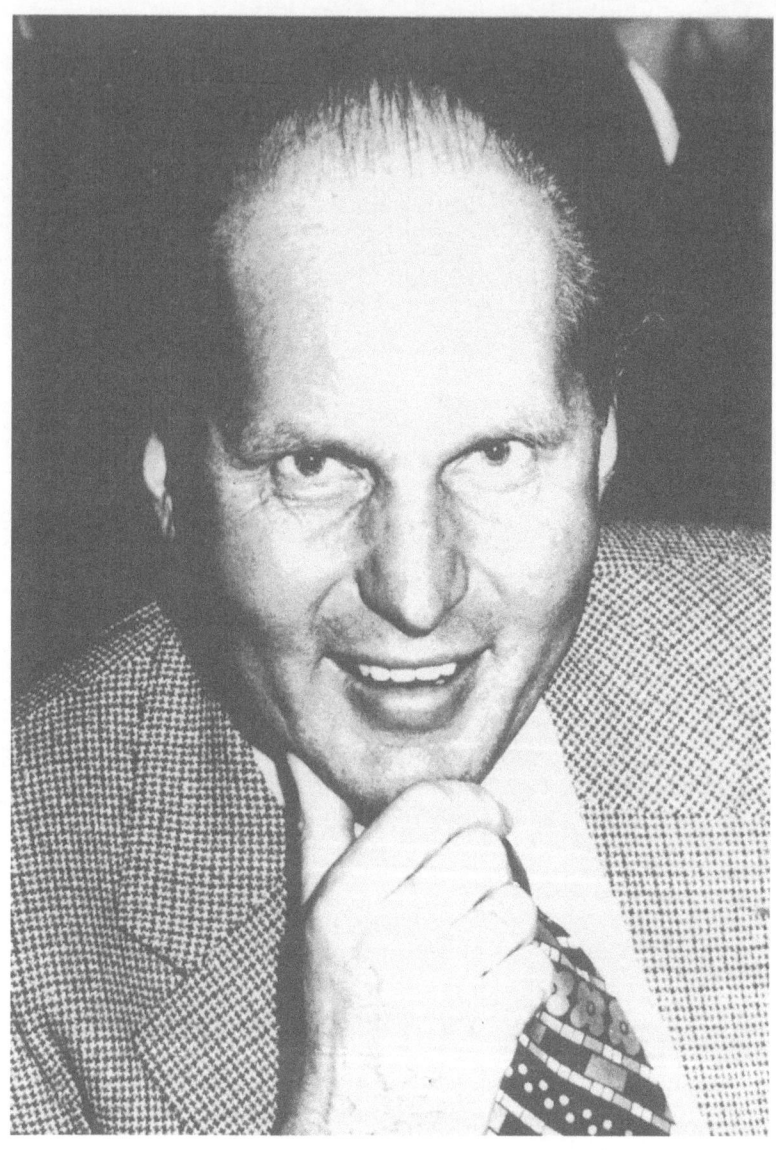

Dr. Dr. Herbert Falk

To Herbert Falk on his sixtieth birthday

H. POPPER

To pay tribute to an unusual person on his sixtieth birthday is a challenge. It is even more so if he is a member of the biomedical community who has distinguished himself by his deeds and actions rather than by his own scientific discoveries and writings. A tribute to this jubilarian is particularly interesting because it illuminates the infrastructure of biomedical sciences, which is less obvious and less frequently described, but essential to the performance of all three aspects - medical research, teaching and patient care.

Tributes to people who have contributed to medical knowledge and practice essentially serve three purposes. The first is to give credit to the individual and at the same time thank them for their contributions. The second is to describe her/him as an example, and thus to inspire others. And the third is an exercise in the sociology of biomedical science, because it illuminates the inner workings of the scientific enterprise. This tribute deals with both the personality responsible for these activities and particularly for their progress, and the motivation which fashioned the currents in the bio-medical sciences, including the importance of business activities. Regardless of the personal data and achievements in such a tribute, the information presented should be a valuable source to enable the sociologist to trace the development of biomedicine or one of its branches and thus improve its conduct.

Thus, a tribute for a good friend, Dr Herbert Falk of Freiburg, Germany, is written not only to wish him well on his birthday and to thank him, but also to explore his societal role, especially important and instructive because of his various activities. They are varied because, with a background of thorough education and training in biomedicine, he is essentially founder, owner and director (*Geschaeftsfuehrer*) of a pharmaceutical company, is also a publisher of medical literature, both directly and indirectly, and an organizer *par excellence* of medical meetings of different types. Having known him for about 19 years I still don't know to which of these three endeavours he devotes most of his time and most of his efforts. These three activities are interwoven, particularly since the conduct of his pharmaceutical business provides the funds necessary for the other two. Herbert Falk will be the last to deny that the other two activities, medical publishing and the organization of meetings, favour his pharmaceutical business by providing advance information capable of being applied to the development of drugs, by bringing him into contact with experts, and last, but not least, by bringing prestige to his drug manufacturing house. Like many other, usually much larger and presumably richer drug companies, the non-commercial activities are guided by an independent foundation, and any advertising of drugs is carefully avoided, at least at the major meetings and in books and serial publications brought out by the foundation. Both lack of concern and also of knowledge prevent me from dealing any further with Falk's drug house. Successful as it apparently is, it is dwarfed, in the minds of his friends, by the unique accomplishments of the Falk Foundation for which the drug house seems to provide quite impressive financial support.

The role of Dr Falk and his foundation is best appreciated by the emphasis placed on medical communication, and by considering the status of hepatology as a discipline at a time when his influence became noticeable in this field. It is usually said that before World War II the biology of the liver was of foremost interest in the Anglo-Saxon and Germanic countries, with various Latin countries placing the emphasis on the clinical symptomatology of liver diseases; while in what we now call the 'developing countries' liver diseases, particularly hepatocellular cancer with or without cirrhosis, and parasitic diseases, especially schistosomiasis, were serious public health problems causing morbidity and mortality in many people during their most productive years. The word 'hepatology' was mainly used, if at all, in Latin languages. After World War II the improvement of global communications led to a merging of interest and ideas in various parts of the world. This was reflected in the formation of national and international associations for the study of the liver, which are greatly credited with the development of hepatology as a defined discipline. The result of this endeavour was the widespread application of biology of the liver at the bedside, this markedly improved the management of those patients with liver disease. More recently, a series of disciplines previously barely applied to liver disease have become important, such as epidemiology, immunology and toxicology. Most recently, molecular biology has come to the foreground. The result of all these trends has been the acceptance of the term 'hepatology' in every language. Communication in verbal and written form became the mainstay in the creation of hepatology as an independent discipline.

In the area of communication the activities of Herbert Falk and his Foundation are original, indeed most innovative, and barely matched by any other person or organization. The emphasis on this uniqueness is the key message of this tribute.

To first describe the meetings Herbert Falk organizes, there are regional postgraduate symposia (*Fortbildungsveranstaltungen*) dealing with all aspects of hepatology and gastroenterology. Authorities, mainly from Germany but also from Austria and Switzerland, are invited as speakers. The increasing popularity of the meetings is reflected in that from 1974 to 1981 their yearly number had risen from 9 to 90, and of total participants, from less than 1000 to more than 10 000 per year. These *'Veranstaltungen'*, mostly attended by physicians in private practice, serve to bring recent information and particularly new diagnostic and therapeutic procedures of increasing complexity to the attention of the physicians, both specialists and generalists. The quality of the presentations in the past has been most effective in persuading physicians to remain lifelong students. These seminars organized by the Falk Foundation have been most successful particularly in Germany, but recently in other parts of the world, where they are usually scheduled at times of international meetings when experts are available. However, they are in intent and principle no different from those organized by medical schools, research institutes, medical societies, foundations and pharmaceutical houses.

Such a similarity does not hold true for a second type of Falk Foundation meeting – triennial gatherings which started in Freiburg in 1967 with an attendance which could be accommodated in the amphitheatre of the medical clinic. They continued 3 and 6 years later in the Aula Maxima in Freiburg. Subsequently they had, however, to be moved to facilities only available at the Mustermesse, Basel. They thus became known as the world-famous Basel Liver Week. These large assemblies, attended by more than 2000 participants, many accompanied by family or friends, have become the grand international gatherings of hepatology. The recent addition of poster sessions has not only increased the number of presentations, but also the opportunity for informal scientific exchange, frequently by people coming from different continents and also from different disciplines. The success and the considerable international participation from almost every country in the world results in the quality and variety of the presentations.

The main symposium is devoted to a major current topic in hepatology, which is discussed by world authorities in the specific field. Simultaneous translation into four languages is available. The characteristic of the presentations is the combination of review of the state of the art with frequently new unpublished observations. Part of the triennial meeting is also the award of the Eppinger Prize donated by the Falk Foundation for the outstanding contribution to hepatology. It has been distributed five times to renowned authorities, and has been called the 'Nobel Prize of Hepatology'. This was also justified by the subsequent award of the Nobel Prize to Baruch Blumberg following his receipt of the Eppinger Prize. More recently, a Hans Popper Prize is given to a scientist under 35 years of age from a German speaking country.

While the major meeting is attended both by physicians in general and specialized practice as well as by academic physicians, the participants of the accompanying meetings, held in English, are probably mostly academic physicians and biologic scientists (*Naturwissenschaftler*). One type of these associated meetings, which have been held four times so far, always deals with a basic science subject which is in the process of making an impact on hepatology, although most of the practising hepatologists have not yet been acquainted with this subject in any depth. These meetings, also of several days duration, bring together, as speakers, basic scientists who have usually not before been concerned with hepatic problems, with some hepatologists doing research in the specific area. The purpose is less the presentation of newly discovered information, but rather, mutual stimulation, often carried over successfully from research in other organ and cell systems. The result has been that basic scientists have learned to use the liver as a model for their studies, and the hepatologists are employing, on the liver, concepts and methods which had previously been used in other systems. The increase in the number of participants through the years, last time exceeding 500, bespeaks the success of these high specialized meetings. Furthermore, the Falk Foundation organizes biennial meetings dealing with bile acid metabolism in health and disease. The *7th International Bile Acid Meeting* was held at the Basel Liver Week in 1982 with more than 1000 people in attendance, and an Adolf Windaus Prize was given for the first time. Finally, the Basel Liver Week in 1982 again concluded with a *Seminar on Histopathological Alterations in the Liver*, where 700 participants listened to the histologic and clinical discussion of the individual problems of liver patients.

All these varied one-week-long stimulating activities carry the impact of Herbert Falk's genius of organization, both scientifically and technically. Although obviously speakers are selected and invited by the scientific organizers in cooperation with the president of each symposium, all of them feel the spirit and enthusiasm of Herbert and are aware that their selection is made possible by the generosity of the Foundation. Although the Liver Week consists of a series of different symposia, many of the participants, including biologic scientists, stay for parts of the Liver Week which, at first sight, are of lesser concern to them. This permits important cross fertilization. The rather rich and varied social programme is worked out exceedingly well by the Falk Foundation, and demonstrates not only Herbert Falk's meticulous interest for organizational detail but also his pleasure in showing his visitors that part of the world where he grew up. Moreover, the stimulating social programme provides an additional benefit, namely, physicians or biologic scientists, not particularly interested in hepatic problems, may be more ready to come to Basel to present their specialized work because of the interesting social activities and the many excursions.

I have described the Basel Liver Week in such detail not only to do justice to its importance in hepatology, but to point out how Herbert Falk's intelligence, diligence, inventiveness, hospitality and friendliness are a key factor in its success.

Somewhat in between the *'Fortbildungsveranstaltungen'* and the Basel Liver Week are additional scientific symposia held every year, dealing with various topics in hepatology and gastroenterology; they present a spectrum of varying emphasis from basic science to clinical application.

Herbert Falk's role as publisher consists of the initiation and financial support of the books containing the papers presented at the various symposia, which have now reached number 39 and cover all of hepatology and a significant part of gastroenterology. The international contacts of the Falk Foundation increase the popularity of this, probably the largest series of hepatologic books in existence. Nevertheless, of far greater importance to the growth and identification of hepatology as a discipline, and even exceeding the impact of the Basel Liver Week, is the series called HEPATOLOGY Rapid Literature Review, now entering its 14th year. It consists of the monthly publication of reproduced titles and original abstracts of virtually every paper dealing with hepatologic problems. They originate from journals all over the world, in any language, as long as an English summary is available. This ingenious idea of reproducing the original abstracts, and the monthly appearance of the volumes make rapid publication possible. Indeed in the United States the reader, if he subscribes to airmail delivery of the Review, becomes acquainted with the contents of, for instance, British journals before the original journal reaches him by surface mail. This rapid communication is, at least to the knowledge of this writer, not shared by hepatology with any other discipline. It has become an irreplaceable tool for any hepatologist who wishes to remain up-to-date with the literature, without personally surveying hundreds of different journals or depending only on titles available in *Current Contents*. The selection includes many journals publishing only the occasional paper on hepatology. Many of them are often rather highly specialized in clinical and, particularly, basic science problems and even the academic hepatologist may be barely aware of their existence. In addition, the monthly HEPATOLOGY Review contains statements, editorials and abstracts of meetings not only dealing with hepatology itself but also with other subjects in which hepatologic problems are presented. As hepatology as a discipline grew, so the monthly volumes increased in size, exceeding, as a rule, 400 pages, with each page containing several articles. To this main body of the volumes are added a few original scientific letters and recently Hepatitis Memoranda previously published by the National Institutes of Health (USA), as well as tables of contents of relevant books just published. Every year, an Abstract of Abstracts appears, reviewing the new information in all the twelve volumes of the year. A shortened German edition of the volumes is made available quarterly.

The listed achievements are augmented by Dr Falk's intense desire to bring scientists in contact not only at the meetings but in between: by correspondence, provision of literature, and often by financial support of research work and of other activities in many parts of the world. Surely no other person who is not themself conducting clinical or laboratory research work in hepatology has done so much for the field. The enumeration of all these feats teaches us what one person can do and the mechanisms available in enhancing scientific communication. This is the lesson to medical sociology referred to in the introduction. It may apply to other disciplines in the future, but today they are a blessing to hepatology.

Herbert's vital statistics deserve brief comment. Born 60 years ago in a small village, Müllheim in Baden, not far from Freiburg, he became, quite young, a soldier in the German Army during World War II. Serving in Rommel's Africa Corps he was taken prisoner by the British, and was shortly afterwards shipped to the United States, where he worked for several years on various farms in Texas, Utah and Iowa. He describes these, apparently not too unpleasant, years as an opportunity to learn English and to get acquainted with the American 'know-how'. After the war he worked for

2 years in the pharmacy (*Apotheke*) owned by his parents in Freiburg, studied pharmacy at the University of Freiburg, where he eventually graduated as *Doktor der Naturwissenschaften*. But simultaneously he studied medicine and obtained his second doctorate degree, namely, in medicine. During all this time, he acquired experience in the pharmacy, and for a while was active in research in the Division of Experimental Therapy of the University of Freiburg. Continuing to this day the supervision and ownership of the pharmacy. 20 years ago, he founded the pharmaceutical house which carries his name. Very soon after he engaged in the various activities just described and developed them, essentially supported by the income of his pharmaceutical house, with increasing skill and on an enlarging scale. Seven years ago these activities were taken over by the Falk Foundation, dedicated to the support of research in hepatic and biliary tract diseases. His academic interest in hepatology and gastroenterology has been recognized by membership in prestigious societies representing these fields.

The personal attributes of Herbert Falk, complex as they are, are the basis of his success. Outstanding are his restless drive, curiosity, generosity and loyalty to his friends. Despite his obvious abilities as a businessman, he is a serious student of biomedicine, at least of its hepatologic and gastroenterologic aspects, with surprising knowledge of the literature, old and new, and personal acquaintanceship with scientists all over the world.

He is highly intelligent, has a superb memory, and has a perfectionist interest in details as well as in broad organizational problems. His innovative spirit and inquisitiveness extend to a variety of other fields and to his recreational activities. He is interested in art and history, he loves nature and is a fanatic wanderer; this is reflected in another type of literature which he distributes, namely the yearly calendars, of Falk's firm, which are illustrated with pictures of many sites and objects in the vicinity of his beloved Freiburg. He is a gourmet who has investigated the restaurants and inns around Freiburg and has published a guide describing them. On his extensive travels all over the world he carefully consults guide and reference books before he selects a hotel or a place for a meal. He is a connoisseur of wines but really prefers cold beer. Last but not least he is an amusing raconteur with whom it is a pleasure to spend an evening. He enjoys being with his family, his daughter and son, as well as with Ursula, his gracious and charming wife, a thoughtful adviser in all aspects of his work.

All of his friends, joined by hepatologists all over the world, wish him many happy returns on this signal birthday, and hope he will continue his activities for a long time to come.

Section 1

1
Bile acid research: some major themes during the past 60 years

A. F. HOFMANN

INTRODUCTION

The occasion of the 60th birthday celebration of Dr Herbert Falk, sponsor of the biennial Bile Acid Meetings, is a stimulus to look back at the major themes in bile acid research during the past 60 years. To construct an accurate history of bile acid research during the past 60 years is an impossible task, and even the attempt to review developments in some major themes bespeaks more energy than wisdom. One approach, a 'cliometric' approach, would collate and organize every scientific article dealing with bile acids published during these six decades[1]. Such an approach would require an enormous amount of time and might not reflect the dominance of certain laboratory groups; in addition, it would also omit much of the industrial research which has never been documented by a formal scientific paper. The second approach, which will be taken in this brief paper, is to use review articles written by leaders in the field of bile acid research, and also to rely on the author's own contacts and experience during some 25 years of research largely focussed on these intriguing molecules. I shall use the word 'cholanology' to mean the body of knowledge relating to bile acids or bile salts. The suggestion that 'cholan-' was the appropriate combining form for bile acids (and bile salts) was made some years ago by the late American physiologist, Andrew C. Ivy.

Cholanology is not one discipline, but an 'enterprise' of disciplines; cholanology has a true universality, since it spans such a variety of scientific activities (Figure 1.1). At its most basic level, it is the chemistry of bile acid-like molecules (cholanoids). This involves organic chemistry, analytical chemistry and medicinal chemistry. (Activity in each of these areas will be discussed later.) At the next level, it involves aggregates of molecules in solvents or the behaviour of these molecules at interfaces - this is physical or colloid chemistry. The next level of complexity involves the interactions of these molecules with macromolecules such as albumin or macromolecular

3

THE MULTIPLE DISCIPLINES OF BILE ACID RESEARCH

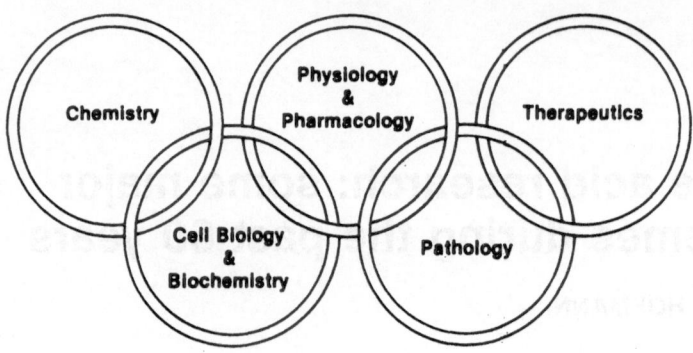

Figure 1.1 Some of the interrelated disciplines of bile acid research are illustrated using the logo of the Olympic games

assemblies, such as membranes (Figure 1.2). When molecules traverse membranes, the subject becomes that of epithelial cell transport and the active research areas of carrier molecules and receptors. The control of receptors is in the realm of cell regulation, which is termed cell biology. Passive transport of bile acids across molecules also involves membrane biology. Bile acid biosynthesis involves a multi-enzyme, multi-organelle pathway, whose understanding crosses the fields of genetics, enzymology, cell biology, and biochemistry. As bile acids move through the enterocyte or hepatocyte, they may be biotransformed – hydroxylated, amidated, sulphated, dehydrogenated or glucuronidated. Such biotransformations lie in the realm of pharmacology.

As the bile acid molecules pass through and out of the hepatocyte, they manifest biological activity: they induce bile flow; they induce biliary lipid

THE UNIVERSALITY OF BILE ACID RESEARCH

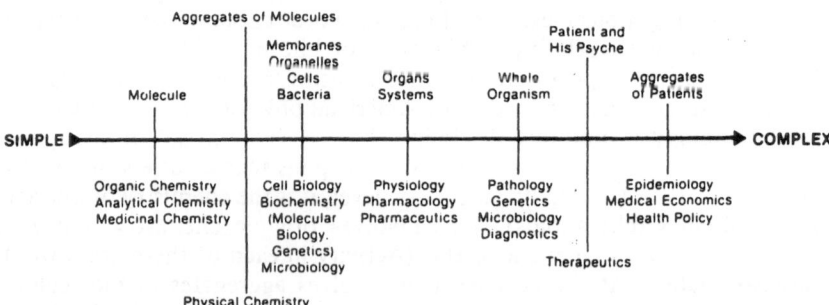

Figure 1.2 Bile acid research involves increasing levels of complexity of molecular organization ranging from single molecules to aggregates of patients

secretion; and they may modulate cholesterol synthesis, albeit indirectly. These 'activities' of bile acids belong to the physiologist or perhaps to the endocrinologist (or 'lipidologist') concerned with cell metabolism.

In the small intestine, the bile acids form mixed micelles with the products of fat digestion and accelerate their transport through the unstirred layer of water coating the intestine. The role of bile acids in fat absorption is of interest to the physical chemist, the enzymologist, the gastroenterologist and the nutritionist.

The movement of bile acid molecules out of the hepatocyte, into bile, into the intestine, through the enterocyte, and back to the liver is termed the enterohepatic circulation. This flux of molecules may be described in traditional pharmacological terms – absorption, distribution, metabolism and excretion. To the extent that its time-dependent movements can be quantified, it falls into the area of pharmacokinetics.

During their enterohepatic circulation, the bile acid molecules are exposed to and biotransformed by the enteric bacteria. The effect of bacteria on bile acids – and even the effect of bile acids on bacterial growth – lies in the domain of the microbiologist.

Certain bile acids such as lithocholate induce cirrhosis by unknown mechanisms[2,3]. To the extent that such pathology is purposefully induced, this property of bile acids may be considered to represent 'toxicology'.

Bile acids are involved in disease in two ways. There are primary cholanopathies – that is diseases caused by defective biosynthesis, transport or biotransformation of bile acids. And there are secondary cholanopathies – that is diseases that influence the synthesis, transport, flow, distribution or biotransformation of bile acids.

Assessment of the efficiency of bile acid transport has an emerging role in diagnostics. The level of bile acids in the blood is now known to be an enterohepatic quality – determined by the instantaneous balance between intestinal input and hepatic uptake[4]. Decreased postprandial levels may indicate ileal dysfunction; increased fasting-state levels may indicate liver disease. Recently a bile acid analogue with a gamma-particle emitting selenium atom in the side chain has been introduced onto the market[5]. This compound is termed 'SeHCAT' (seleno-homo-cholyltaurine), and it is clear that it can be used by the nuclear medicine specialist to detect bile acid malabsorption in patients with ileal dysfunction[6].

The most important new area of cholanology is in therapeutics. Bile acids have long been used as laxatives, and during the recent past, as choleretics. But with the discovery that chenodeoxycholic acid (CDCA) induced cholesterol desaturation of bile and cholesterol gallstone dissolution, bile acids became the first agents in a new class of drugs – 'cholelitholytic agents'[7,8]. In addition, bile acids are now widely used in certain countries as antidyspeptic agents. A related aspect of therapeutics is the use of bile acid sequestrants to lower serum cholesterol; the efficacy of such agents in reducing coronary events has recently been established in the Coronary Primary Prevention Trial of the National Heart Institute[9].

In the remainder of this article, each of these themes will be mentioned in more detail, as they have evolved during the past 60 years.

CHEMISTRY

Sixty years ago, much was understood about bile acid chemistry; yet there was much left to do. The major bile acids had been named – cholic, chenodeoxycholic, deoxycholic, ursodeoxycholic and lithocholic acids, and their approximate structure had been deciphered. It was known that bile acids were C_{24} steroids with an acidic side chain, and the concept of A/B ring stereoisomerism was also known. However, the correct molecular arrangement of the steroid nucleus was not known, as is clear from the Nobel Prize lectures of Windaus and Wieland[10, 11]. The correct structural assignments had to await the X-ray diffraction studies of Bernal[12] which stimulated Rosenheim and King to decipher the correct structure of the steroid nucleus[13]. When this was done, the extraordinary body of knowledge produced by the schools of Wieland and Windaus could be re-interpreted, and the structures of the major bile acids assigned with certainty and accuracy.

An important event in the history of bile acid chemistry occurred just 60 years ago. Wieland, working in Freiburg, decided to reinvestigate the bile acids of human bile. Together with his co-worker, Reverey, he isolated a dihydroxy bile acid with a melting point of about 136°C, and named it 'anthropodeoxycholic acid'[14]. At the same time, Windaus, working in Göttingen, decided to reinvestigate the major bile acid of goose bile, which had been described nearly a century before by Marsson[15]. He isolated the major bile acid and named it 'chenodeoxycholic acid'[16]. Somehow, Windaus discussed his work with Wieland, and the the two great chemists realized that they had the identical compound. Their two articles were accepted for publication in *Biochemische Zeitschrift* on August 7, 1924[14, 16].

Since then, the isolation and characterization of novel bile acids from natural sources have continued to be important themes in cholanology. E. A. Doisy, Sr., W. H. Elliott and their colleagues isolated and established the structure of the three muricholates[17]. G. A. D. Haslewood carried out a large body of investigation isolating, characterizing and naming the bile acids (and alcohols) of primitive vertebrates[18]. In Japan, Iwaski established the structure of ursodeoxycholic acid[19]. Kazuno and his colleagues carried out a superb body of work on the bile alcohols[20]. The group of Sjovall has continued the tradition of isolation, identification and synthesis of novel bile acids and bile alcohols[21, 22]. The final proof of the structure of any complex organic molecule is the total synthesis. Kametani and his colleagues have recently reported the total synthesis of chenodeoxycholic acid, thus establishing definitively its exact steric configuration and structure[23].

This line of endeavour may be termed 'natural product chemistry', and the task of the organic chemist has been greatly aided by the development of powerful analytical techniques such as nuclear magnetic resonance[24] and mass spectroscopy[25]. Of special value for bile acid chemistry will be the newer techniques of mass spectroscopy such as FABS (fast atom bombardment spectroscopy) which permit the spectrum to be obtained on the intact molecule, even when it is quite non-volatile, such as the bile amidates[26].

Of equal importance in bile acid chemistry has been the spectacular improvement in separation techniques. The group of Sjovall has made many remarkable contributions, including early studies on paper chromatography, gas chromatography, thin layer chromatography, ion exchange chromatography, reversed phase chromatography and coupled gas chromatography–mass spectroscopy[27]. The continuing improvement in reversed phase (high pressure) liquid chromatography means that it will be possible to analyse the complex mixtures of bile acid conjugates in bile without, in all likelihood, any isolation or derivitization procedures.

The availability of bile acid conjugates in high purity and gram amounts continues to be a problem today. The number of investigators interested in cholanology is so few that the biochemical supply houses (with one or two exceptions) have not thought it profitable to offer conjugated bile acids in high purity and at moderate cost. Improvements in counter-current distribution and preparative reversed phase chromatography may eventually alleviate this problem.

The discovery at the Mayo Clinic of the potent anti-inflammatory properties of cortisone led to an international competition for the best route to prepare 11-hydroxy steroids. Initially, cortisone was prepared from deoxycholic acid, since the 12-hydroxy group could be removed by dehydration to prepare the Δ^{11} cholenate, which could then be converted to the 11-hydroxy compound[28]. In 1949, the Research Corporation convened a meeting of the leading chemists to discuss how the impending global shortage of cholic acid could be dealt with. At that meeting, Louis Fieser, of Harvard University, suggested that a natural product could be found which would serve equally well as a precursor[28]. Within a few years, it was found that fungi could 11-hydroxylate plant saponogenins, and the route to cortisone from cholic acid was no longer cost effective[29]. Since that time, cholic acid has continued to be isolated from ox bile, but there has been little major use of bile acids by the pharmaceutical industry.

The discovery of the cholelitholytic properties of CDCA and ursodeoxycholic acid (UDCA), both of which are natural products and devoid of patent protection (except for use patents), might have served as a stimulus to the pharmaceutical industry to synthesize novel bile acids with improved therapeutic ratios. This does not appear to have happened because of scepticism that there was a large market for cholelitholytic agents. Pellicciari and his colleagues have begun a program aimed at synthesizing bile acids with modified side chains[30], and it is clear that modification of the bile acid nucleus or side chain, or both, could give rise to thousands of novel bile acids, each of whose physicochemical, pharmacological and physiological properties might differ. This field, which is just beginning, may be termed 'neocholanology'.

Analytical chemistry

Accurate measurement of bile acids is essential in many areas of cholanology. Early, non-specific, and insensitive methods of bile acid measurement were soon superseded by combined separation–measurement techniques such as gas chromatography. An important advance was made by Iwata and Yamasaki, who introduced the first method for enzymatic analysis of bile acids[31]. These workers showed that the 3-hydroxy steroid dehydrogenase (HSD) of *Pseudomonas testosteroni* could be used in an endpoint enzymatic method to measure 3-hydroxy bile acids with accuracy and moderate sensitivity. Since then, the enzyme has been purified and marketed. The sensitivity of the technique has been greatly improved by coupling the reduced NADH to tetrazolium dyes[32]. A remarkably sensitive modification of the technique features immobilized HSD, a diaphorase, and luciferase to generate light in direct relation to bile acid concentration[33, 34].

Some 10 years ago, Simmonds and his colleagues developed antibodies to bile acids[35], and since then, a large number of radioimmunoassays have been described[36]. Most RIA techniques work well, but production of satisfactory antibodies in extremely high titre continues to be a problem. Enzyme immunoassays, both heterogeneous[37, 38] and homogeneous (EMIT) assays[39], have been reported. HPLC offers excellent resolution of bile acid conjugates, but detection continues to be a problem, since the amide bond can only be detected at 200 nm. Improved detectors based on immobilized enzymes have been described[40]. Gas chromatography is a moderately sensitive but specific and useful technique. Coupled gas chromatography–mass spectroscopy with inverse isotope dilution offers exquisite sensitivity and acceptable accuracy[41], but the methodology is complex and the required instrumentation is formidably expensive.

Thus, during the past 60 years, spectacular progress has been made in developing methods of bile acid analysis. A great variety of analytical techniques are available, and most cholanologists should be able to use one of the existing methods and obtain satisfactory results.

Physical chemistry

Sixty years ago, virtually nothing was known about the physicochemical properties of bile acids. Wieland and Sorge had shown that bile acid solutions have solvent properties, and they proposed that bile acids form complexes with molecules in solution[42], just as deoxycholic acid can co-crystallize with other molecules to form inclusion compounds termed 'choleic acids'. Within a few years, it was recognized that soap molecules aggregate above a certain concentration to form micelles; but micelle formation had not been related to bile acids, except for a few suggestions in the literature[43].

After the war, Ekwall and his colleagues (Norman, Danielsson, Mandel, Setala and others) in Abo, Finland, began a systematic study on bile acid solutions, defining the critical micellar concentration of bile acids, their pK_a values, their surface properties, and even their interactions with polar additives[44, 45]. Similar work was conducted a few years later in Lund by Hofmann and Borgstrom[46, 47]. By the mid 1960s, it became generally recognized that bile contained mixed micelles of bile acids, phospholipids and cholesterol, and that the small intestinal contents contained mixed micelles of bile acids, fatty acids and monoglycerides[48]. Small, working with Dervichian at the Institut Pasteur, defined the equilibria phase present in model systems simulating human gallbladder bile[49]. He then showed that the rules for cholesterol solubility in such systems could be applied directly to gallbladder bile, and that patients with cholesterol gallstones had supersaturated bile[50]. This work stimulated the gastroenterologist to consider digestive disease in physicochemical terms – a minor intellectual revolution. Carey, working with Small, began an extensive study of the physicochemical properties of bile acids, which defined the phase equilibria present in bile in more detail[51], distinguished the physicochemical properties of individual bile acids[52], and proposed that vesicles, rather than micelles, would be present in dilute bile[53]. At the same time, physical chemists began to take an interest in the properties of bile acid solutions, the uncommon pattern of self-association of bile acid molecules, and the relationship between bile acid structure and self-association patterns[54, 55]. It has become clear that the low CMC of the natural bile acids results from not only the pattern of nuclear substituents, but also the length of the side chain. The CMC increases if hydroxy groups are not restricted to one side of the molecule, or if the side chain is shortened.

A recent symposium summarizes in considerable detail the relationship between the physicochemical properties of bile acids and the pathogenesis of gallstone disease[56]. Recent studies have also suggested that bile acids modulate Ca^{2+} activity in bile[57], so that the function of bile acids in bile is not only to transport cholesterol, but also to buffer calcium ions. Studies of the interaction of bile acids and Ca^{2+} can be expected to expand greatly in the next decade.

The emphasis on relating physiological properties of bile acids to their physicochemical properties has sometimes been premature because the biological process was not understood. Our group has recently attempted to classify model systems involving bile acids, and to suggest when these can be related to physiological processes – and when they cannot be[58].

CELL BIOLOGY AND BIOCHEMISTRY

Bile acid transport

Modern work on bile acid transport could only begin when the concept of active transport was developed. Active transport of bile acids into bile was always thought likely, but the magnitude of the concentration gradient could not be even guessed until accurate analytical methods became available. The mystery of efficient intestinal conservation was solved by Lack and Weiner's discovery, in 1961, of active ileal transport of conjugated bile acids[59]. Since that time, Lack and his colleagues have developed a body of knowledge defining the structural requirements for active ileal transport[60].

Current approaches to active transport are to isolate a carrier molecule, reconstitute the transport system by adding the molecule to vesicles, and then to sequence the carrier molecule (and perhaps define its interaction with its ligand by X-ray diffraction). For hepatic and ileal bile acid transport, this field is just beginning. Considerable progress has been made by synthesizing photoaffinity-labelled bile acids, and to use these compounds to isolate a putative carrier molecule from the hepatic sinusoidal membrane[61, 62]. These approaches are complemented by improved methods for isolating hepatic membrane fractions[63, 64]. Satisfactory preparative methods are now available for cell membrane fractions enriched in sinusoidal or canalicular domains.

At the same time, the binding of bile acids to cytosolic transport proteins is being explored, and putative carrier molecules are being isolated and characterized[65].

The passive transport of bile acids into cells has been described using *in vitro* preparations[66, 67], but true membrane permeation coefficients have not yet been defined, except in preliminary studies[68].

Bile acid biotransformation

Modern concepts of bile acid biotransformation awaited the development of radioactively labelled bile acids and chromatography. Much of our knowledge was developed by Bergstrom and his colleagues such as Sjovall, Lindstedt, Norman, Danielsson, Tryding and Samuelsson[69] (before his epochal achievements in prostanoids). Subsequent work by Bjorkhem, Einarsson, Hellstrom, Johansson, and Gustafsson have extended the early studies[70]. This work showed that cholic and CDCA were primary bile acids, that bacteria carried out 7-dehydroxylation, and that the liver could rehydroxylate, and could reduce oxo groups to hydroxy groups. It was shown that unconjugated bile acids were amidated with glycine or taurine. Subsequently Palmer showed that lithocholate was sulphated[71], and this work was extended to man by Cowen *et al.*[72, 73]. Later, Makino[74] and Stiehl[75] carried out a large number of studies showing that bile acid sulphation was a major novel biotransformation in cholestasis, and that sulphated bile acids were excreted in urine. Alme, Bremmelgaard, Sjovall, and Thomassen developed improved methods for bile acid separation, identifying bile acid glucuronides[76], and the Materns and their colleagues showed that microsomes from human liver formed three glucuronides from lithocholate as well as the other primary bile acids[77]. Recently, Tephly and his colleagues have purified a 3-androstane glucuronoyl transferase and have shown that this enzyme can form three-ethereal glucuronides of primary bile acids[78].

Thus, with the discovery of sulphation and glucuronidation pathways, the pattern of bile acid biotransformation has come to resemble that of many other steroids and xenobiotics. Indeed, the hydroxylation of cholesterol to form bile acids can be considered a phase I step, and the subsequent conjugation (amidation, sulphation or glucuronidation) is a phase II step[79]. Despite these advances, the enzymology of bile acid biotransformation is still in its early stages.

REGULATORY EFFECTS

It would seem most astonishing if the large flux of bile acids passing through the hepatocyte and enterocyte did not influence the metabolic activity of these cells. To the extent that such modification of enzyme activity appears useful to the organism, it may be termed a 'regulatory' function, although the distinction between regulatory effects and physiological effects may well be artificial.

The following types of regulatory effects have been proposed for bile acids in the hepatocyte and are currently under study: (1) regulation of lipoprotein membrane receptors; (2) regulation of cholesterol biosynthesis; (3) regulation of bile acid biosynthesis; (4) regulation of bile secretion; and (5) regulation of biliary lipid secretion. There is also considerable evidence that bile acids regulate triglyceride synthesis in the hepatocyte, and directly or indirectly, they must also regulate cholesterol synthesis. To date, bile acids have not been proposed to influence drug biotransformation, protein biosynthesis, the urea cycle, glucose homeostasis or fatty acid oxidation.

Evidence that bile acids modulate low density lipoprotein (LDL) receptors has been published[80], but there continues to be controversy in this area. The observation that chronic CDCA ingestion caused a modest but consistent elevation of serum LDL cholesterol levels has been interpreted to indicate that bile acids down-regulate the LDL receptors on the hepatocyte[81], and bile acids may modify the rate of lipoprotein uptake using the isolated perfused rat liver[82]. It is certainly well accepted that increased cholesterol synthesis occurring in response to an interruption of the enterohepatic circulation of bile acids by bile acid sequestrant administration is likely to cause an increase in the activity of LDL receptors, which in turn leads to a decrease in serum LDL cholesterol levels[83].

Whether bile acids influence cholesterol synthesis directly continues to be a matter of controversy. There is little doubt that bile acid feeding can lower HMG CoA-reductase activity, and that interruption of the enterohepatic circulation of bile acids can cause increased HMG-CoA reductase activity[84]. These effects can be dissociated from any effect on cholesterol input into the hepatocyte[85], but there remains the possibility that the effect of bile acids is mediated through changes in an intracellular pool of hepatocyte cholesterol.

It seems well established that CDCA, cholic and deoxycholic acids influence their own biosynthesis from cholesterol. The effect is not large, since bile acid synthesis is generally quite low; but the effect has been demonstrated in several species[86, 87]. Recently it has been observed that UDCA does not suppress the biosynthesis of other bile acids[88, 89]. Presumably this effect is mediated by a change in the activity of the rate limiting enzyme, cholesterol-7α-hydroxylase.

Bile acids induce bile secretion, and this effect is known as 'bile acid dependent flow' (BADF)[90, 91]. The BADF is measured in $\mu l/\mu mol$ and for many species this value is in the range of 8–20 $\mu l/\mu mol$, being greater for unconjugated bile acids or bile acids which have high CMC values[92]. The mechanism of the BADF is considered to be a flow of water and electrolytes from plasma through the 'tight junctions' lining the canaliculus, and the stimulus for this flow is the osmotic effect of the secreted bile acid anions. There are, however, certain species, such as the guinea pig and rabbit, in whom the value of the BADF, at least for some bile acids, is far higher – 40–60 $\mu l/\mu mol$[93]. Whether this strikingly high value for BADF indicates a direct effect of bile acids on ion secretion by the hepatocyte remains unknown.

Bile acids also induce biliary lipid secretion. The biliary secretion of phospholipid and cholesterol is coupled to bile acid secretion in a curvilinear manner – nearly linear at low bile acid outputs, but displaying a plateau at high bile acid outputs (reviewed in Reference 94). The relationship between secretion of biliary phospholipid or biliary cholesterol and that of bile acids may be expressed as a coupling coefficient, i.e. the ratio of the phospholipid secretion to the bile acid secretion, but use of such a coupling coefficient appears justifiable only at low bile acid concentrations where the coupling is linear[95]. There are moderate differences between individual bile acids, and marked differences between species[92]. The biochemical mechanism of biliary lipid secretion is poorly understood.

PHARMACOLOGY OF BILE ACIDS

The pharmacology of bile acids may be considered to be limited to a description of the movement of the bile acid molecules in the enterohepatic circulation. Older work on the enterohepatic circulation has been summarized in delightful, historical reviews by Heaton[96] and Hislop[97], and several recent reviews are available[98, 99].

The overall principles of the enterohepatic circulation of bile acids were well understood some decades ago, as indicated in Sobotka's monograph[100]. The three new qualitative contributions of the past three decades have been the discovery of the negative feedback control of bile acid biosynthesis by Bergstrom and Danielsson and their colleagues[101], the identification of the ileal transport system by Lack and Weiner[59], and the recognition by the Mayo group that the level of serum bile acids is an enterohepatic quality, determined by the moment-to-moment balance between intestinal input and hepatic uptake[4].

There has been a great effort in attempting to quantify the enterohepatic circulation of individual bile acids in man. Lindstedt showed that the exchangeable mass of bile acids in the enterohepatic circulation could be measured by the technique of isotope dilution[102], and this technique has been widely applied to measure the synthesis and exchangeable mass of primary and secondary bile acids in the enterohepatic circulation[103]. In addition, the method has been used to measure the hepatic synthesis rate of primary bile acids and the input from the large intestine of secondary bile acids. Indicator dilution techniques were developed by Grundy and Metzger[104] and the Mayo group[105] which permitted the measurement of bile acid secretion rates into the intestine, as well as rates of intestinal absorption along the intestine. Isotope dilution techniques were also used to quantify the degree of deconjugation and reconjugation of bile acids during enterohepatic cycling[106].

These studies led to the accumulation of a vast body of physiological data for bile acid metabolism in man. Recently, these data have been used to model the enterohepatic circulation of cholic acid and its conjugates[107]. The model developed was a linear multicompartmental model, which can be classified as a physiological pharmacokinetic model. A minimum of three different classes of transfer coefficients were needed to describe bile acid metabolism completely – transport coefficients, which denote movements of molecules across boundary (unstirred water) layers, cell membranes and through cells; flow coefficients, which describe passive movements of groups

of bile acid molecules caused by convective flow such as gallbladder contraction or intestinal motility; and biotransformation coefficients, which
denote a change from one molecular species to another. The model has been
described and fully simulated for cholic acid and its conjugates in healthy
man; in the future, it should be possible to extend the model to the other
major primary and secondary bile acids.

The challenge for the future in bile acid pharmacology is to develop steady
state pharmacokinetic models of bile acid metabolism encompassing all bile
acids during bile acid feeding. It may also prove useful to model bile acid
metabolism in diseases of the enterohepatic circulation.

PHYSIOLOGY OF BILE ACIDS

By physiological effects of bile acids, one means the effects of bile acids on
various organs. In the liver, the effects of bile acids have been known for
many decades. The ability of bile acids to induce bile flow was discovered
by Schiff[108], who mistakenly believed that bile was being absorbed from the
intestine and resecreted by the liver. Recognition that bile acids had choleretic
effects probably occurred in the late 19th century, when reasonably pure bile
acid preparations became available for animal experimentation. In this
paper, the effect of bile acids on bile flow and biliary lipid secretion has been
considered a 'regulatory property' of bile acids, rather than a physiological
property.

In the intestine, bile acids have been known for decades to stimulate fat
absorption. Wieland and Sorge[42], and later Verzar[109] proposed that bile
acids formed colloidal complexes with fatty acid soaps. Moore and Parker[110]
noted that bile acids solubilize the digestion products of dietary lipids in the
form of a clear solution, from which intestinal absorption of the lipids occurs
rapidly. Subsequently, Mattson and Beck[111] discovered the positional specificity of pancreatic lipase, and workers in Lund showed that the two digestive
products, fatty acid and 2-monoglyceride, readily formed mixed micelles
with bile acids[47], that a micellar phase could be isolated from small intestinal
content during fat digestion[112], and that such lipolytic products were readily
absorbed from these micellar solutions[113]. Bile acids, especially conjugates
of cholate, stimulate cholesterol absorption in a manner that is not yet
understood[114-116].

An increasing number of 'functions' of bile acids have been identified
during the past decade. For example, bile acids appear to modulate intestinal
motility[117] and may also influence gastrointestinal hormone release[118]. High
concentrations of di-hydroxy bile acids may induce electrolyte and water
secretion by both the small[119] and large intestine[120, 121].

SPECIFIC EFFECTS OF INDIVIDUAL BILE ACIDS

As soon as they were isolated in pure form, bile acids were known to have
biological differences since they tasted different. Fischer isolated lithocholic
acid from ox gallstones[122] and must have thought that this bile acid had

different properties, since he named it for the stones, rather than for the species in which the stones occurred. Even the idea of naming the bile acids after the species from which they were isolated, e.g. chenocholic acid (the original name for CDCA), suggests that the early workers thought that individual bile acids must have distinguishing properties.

One of the earliest claims to the discovery of a specific physiological property of a bile acid was that of Neubauer, who in 1924, just 60 years ago, reported that dehydrocholate, which had been synthesized some 15 years before by Hammarsten, not only had striking choleretic properties but, in addition, had far less toxicity than the common bile acids[123]. Subsequently, Treadwell and his colleagues[114], and later Gallo-Torres et al.[115] found that cholate derivatives had a unique ability to enhance cholesterol absorption in the rat, an observation recently confirmed by Watt and Simmonds[116]. Mekhjian et al. showed that dihydroxy bile acids, but not trihydroxy bile acids, induce colonic secretion of electrolytes and water[120]. About 25 years ago, Holsti discovered the cirrhogenic effect of administered lithocholate[124], and a few years later, Javitt found that lithocholyltaurine was cholestatic when infused intravenously in the rat[125]. Later, the groups of Palmer[126] and the late James B. Carey[127] found that continuous feeding of lithocholate to the taurine-deficient rat induced the formation of gallstones, consisting of the insoluble calcium salt of lithocholylglycine and its 6β-hydroxy metabolite.

However, the most important example of specific physiological effects of bile acids is the desaturating effect of CDCA and UDCA, an effect which is not shared by cholate or deoxycholate. This work has led to the widespread use of CDCA and UDCA for the medical dissolution of gallstones.

DIAGNOSTICS

Digestive and hepatobiliary disease are among the most common ailments of man, and frequently these cause disturbances in bile acid metabolism. Accordingly, it is reasonable to predict that measurements of bile acid concentrations in body fluids might provide useful diagnostic information. In fact, bile acid measurements are still performed extremely infrequently in the diagnostic laboratory. The reasons for the failure of bile acid measurements to become important in clinical chemistry are multiple: (1) the recognition that altered bile acid metabolism is important in digestive disease has occurred only recently; (2) for diseases in which altered bile acid metabolism is important, it has not always been clear that measurements of bile acids provide important, clinically-useful information; (3) until recently, the chemical measurements for measuring bile acids have not been sufficiently sensitive or accurate, and even now, bile acid measurement methods cannot be performed by the most common automated procedures; (4) current widely-used tests are perceived to provide information of equal or superior value at lower cost; (5) for some diseases, no specific therapy is available, so that quantitation of the magnitude of hepatic injury or dysfunction has no therapeutic value.

Bile acid tests may be classified as follows:

(1) Measurement of bile acid concentrations in body fluids to distinguish clinical situations in which the usual concentration is altered – for example, the normal serum level is increased or decreased or the normally low gastric juice content is increased;
(2) Measurement of bile acid deconjugation during enterohepatic cycling;
(3) Measurement of bile acid retention in the enterohepatic circulation; and
(4) Detection of abnormal bile acids in the enterohepatic circulation.

Measurement of abnormal concentrations of bile acids in body fluids

In health, the serum concentration of bile acids is extremely low because of the efficiency of hepatic uptake. With meals, there is an increased input of bile acids into the portal blood during intestinal absorption; the hepatic first-pass clearance remains constant (as a fraction of the sinusoidal blood which is cleared) and systemic levels increase. Thus, an increased fasting-state serum level usually indicates decreased hepatic uptake, which in turn can indicate decreased blood flow to the liver, decreased hepatic uptake of bile acids, or portal–systemic venous blood shunting, or any combination of these[4]. Serum bile acid measurements have good specificity for the presence of liver disease, but their sensitivity is low compared to that of other liver tests[128, 129]. They are generally used to supplement information provided by the common liver tests. The only methods with acceptable sensitivity are competitive binding techniques or a recently described bioluminescence technique. Studies are continuing to define the correct place of bile acid measurements in the detection of hepatic disease. However, it should be noted that most hepatologists appear content with existing tests, and that the absence of specific therapy for liver disease means that diagnostic tests, which provide information on the magnitude of hepatic injury, may not have a satisfactory benefit/cost ratio.

Bile acid levels in gastric aspirates are used to detect duodeno–gastric reflux[130], and increased concentrations of bile acids in the aqueous phase of faeces suggest bile acid malabsorption which may cause a secretory diarrhoea[131].

Although the serum level of bile acids is always quite low in the person with normal hepatic function, the usual postprandial elevation of serum bile acids may be smaller or even absent in the patient with bile acid malabsorption because of ileal dysfunction[132]. Accordingly, the feasibility of using post-prandial serum bile acid levels to detect bile acid malabsorption is under active investigation.

Bile acid deconjugation

During their sojourn in the enteral ring of the enterohepatic loop, a small fraction of the bile acids are deconjugated by intestinal bacteria before intestinal absorption. In the patient with an abnormally elevated concentration

15

of bacteria in the small intestine, bile acid deconjugation is increased and may be detected by measuring $^{14}CO_2$ in breath after administration of cholyl-1-^{14}C-glycine[133, 134]. Increased bile acid deconjugation is also indicated by an increased concentration of unconjugated bile acids in the systemic circulation (see Reference 135).

The bile acid breath test appears to have acceptable specificity for detecting increased bile acid deconjugation, but it does not have specificity for the 'stagnant loop' syndrome, since bile acid malabsorption also causes increased bile acid deconjugation. In addition, for the test to be positive, the bacteria present must possess deconjugating activity. Accordingly, the test has stimulated the search for other substrates which are oxidized to CO_2 (or reduced to H_2) by bacteria. Some workers believe that other substrates, for example xylose, are superior to cholylglycine for the detection of bacterial overgrowth in the small intestine[136].

Bile acid retention in the enterohepatic circulation

In health, the efficiency of bile acid absorption from the intestine is extremely high – well above 95%. The efficiency of this 'conservation' is largely due to active ileal absorption, since the conjugated bile acids, especially those of the trihydroxy bile acids, are too hydrophilic to undergo extensive passive absorption. Active bile acid absorption occurs in the terminal ileum, and terminal ileal dysfunction causes bile acid malabsorption. Bile acid malabsorption is important clinically, since it may cause bile acid diarrhoea, fat malabsorption, or secondary hyperoxaluria[137].

Bile acid malabsorption may be detected by showing a decreased retention in (or increased loss of bile acids from) the enterohepatic circulation. This may be shown in a variety of ways: (1) increased faecal bile acid output (the rationale of this measurement is that increased bile acid loss is associated with a compensatory increase in bile acid synthesis); (2) increased faecal excretion of a tracer bile acid added to the enterohepatic circulation; (3) decreased postprandial serum bile acid levels; (4) increased bile acid deconjugation, as measured by the bile acid deconjugation breath test.

In the past few years, a bile acid analogue tagged with radioactive selenium has been introduced[6]. This molecule, termed SeHCAT, may be similar to homo-cholyl-taurine (the taurine conjugate of the C_{25} bile acid, homocholic acid, in which there is one additional methylene group in the side chain); in SeHCAT, the C_{23} carbon has been replaced by a ^{75}Se atom which emits gamma particles with a half life of about 90 days. SeHCAT can be used to label the enterohepatic circulation and then increased loss of SeHCAT may be detected by the finding of less retention in the body (detected by whole body counting), less retention in the gallbladder (detected using the gamma camera positioned to count the gallbladder region) or by determining the faecal output of ^{75}Se radioactivity. A number of groups are exploring the utility of this novel radionuclide; certainly the preliminary results suggest that it can be used to measure bile acid malabsorption, as well as to measure reflux of bile acids into the stomach. SeHCAT does not appear likely to be useful for hepatobiliary imaging, since the ^{75}Se-labelled bile acids offer less resolution than the [99]Tm iminodiacetic acid-based cholescintigraphic agents, which are widely available.

Uncommon bile acids in the EHC

Detection of abnormal bile acids in the EHC could not be considered until the chemistry of bile acid biosynthesis and biotransformation was well understood, and until chromatographic methods had been developed which permitted the separation and identification of individual bile acids. Bile acid biosynthesis and biotransformation are now rather well understood, and both GLC and HPLC afford excellent chromatographic separation of individual bile acids; bile acid structure is readily confirmed by mass spectroscopy.

Since the concentration of bile acids in bile is at least four orders of magnitude higher than that of serum, it is easier to search the bile for abnormal bile acids than to search serum. In all diseases where there are appreciable proportions of abnormal bile acids in the EHC, the abnormal bile acid has been found to be present in both bile and serum. In principle, abnormal bile acids in the EHC should reflect either defective bile acid biosynthesis (or subsequent hepatic biotransformation) or increased input from the intestine of an abnormal bile acid formed by the enteric flora. In fact, only defects in bile acid biosynthesis have been identified to date. Three defects have been identified:

(1) Zellweger's syndrome, a defect in peroxisome formation which results in a defective side chain of the bile acids; coprostanic acid appears in bile and serum in greatly increased amounts[138].

(2) Cerebrotendinous xanthomatosis, a defect in C_{26} hydroxylation[139], with decreased chenodeoxycholic acid biosynthesis and a greatly increased amount of C_{25} bile alcohols appearing in bile and urine[140].

(3) An unnamed defect in which large amounts of 6-substituted bile acids are present in bile in association with fat malabsorption[141]. Since the feeding of hyodeoxycholic acid does not induce any nutritional problems[142], it seems likely that this patient had defective bile acid synthesis.

In the healthy person, the profile of serum bile acids is about 50% cheno-deoxycholyl conjugates, about 25% cholyl conjugates, and about 25% deoxycholyl conjugates. With biliary obstruction, deoxycholyl conjugates disappear, and the proportion of cholyl conjugates increases[143]. The exact mechanisms responsible for this new steady state have not been elucidated, but a major factor is the preferential urinary excretion of chenodeoxycholyl conjugates in the form of their sulphated derivatives. In cirrhosis, the proportion of cholyl conjugates does not increase similarly, perhaps because capillarization of the hepatic sinusoids decreases the exposure of albumin-bound bile acids to the hepatocyte, and the fractional hepatic extraction of chenodeoxycholyl conjugates falls to a greater extent than that of cholyl conjugates. Thus, in cirrhosis, the dihydroxy/trihydroxy ratio is increased, but this change in the profile of serum bile acids does not have sufficient sensitivity or specificity to have diagnostic use for distinguishing cirrhosis from other types of chronic liver disease.

Thus, since disorders of bile acid biosynthesis are extremely uncommon, and serum bile acid profiles do not provide information of diagnostic use, in most patients with digestive disease there appears to be little value in measuring the composition of either serum or biliary bile acids solely for diagnostic purposes. The lack of useful information results from the profile being the end result of a large number of independent physiological factors.

BILE ACIDS IN THERAPEUTICS

Historical aspects

The idea of using bile as a therapeutic agent goes far back into antiquity, and long preceded the knowledge that bile acids were its major active ingredients. In 1871, Moritz Schiff, the discoverer of the enterohepatic circulation, proposed that sodium 'cholinate' might be useful in treating patients with cholesterol gallstones[144]. Probably bile acids were used as laxatives, in the form of dried animal bile, for several centuries in the Western World. In the Eastern World, dried bear bile was considered to have important curative properties for the treatment of liver and biliary disease.

Neubauer's demonstration of the choleretic properties of dehydrocholate led to the widespread use of this compound as a choleretic agent, although there is no evidence that controlled trials were performed to establish its efficacy or safety. It may well be that dehydrocholate was the first pure bile acid used for therapeutic purposes[145]. If so, 1984 marks not only the 60th birthday of our sponsor, but also the 60th anniversary of bile acid therapy. Dehydrocholate was also used to measure the circulation time, but this technique was gradually abandoned, as superior non-invasive and invasive techniques were developed for detecting congenitive heart failure.

Bile acids as cholelitholytic agents

The only pure bile acids that were available in bulk up to the mid 1950s were cholic acid and deoxycholic acid. Cholic acid was available because of the tradition of processing ox bile. Deoxycholic acid had become available because of its value as a precursor for the preparation of 11-hydroxy steroids. In the mid 1950s, Weddel Pharmaceuticals, a small division of the large conglomerate company named Union International, began the production of several less common bile acids, among them CDCA and lithocholic acid. A shipment of several kilograms of chendeoxycholic acid to the Mayo Clinic was arranged in 1968, and this material was subsequently used in an exploratory trial of several bile acids for the purpose of inducing bile desaturation and gallstone dissolution in women with radiolucent gallstones. The experiment was conducted by Johnson Thistle and Leslie J. Schoenfield, and their report that CDCA, but not cholic acid, induced bile desaturation in cholesterol was presented in November, 1969[146]. Subsequently controlled trials of CDC by the Mayo group showed convincingly, and for the first time, that cholesterol gallstones could be dissolved by CDC therapy[147]. In Europe, these trials led to the rapid development of CDC as a cholelitholytic agent[148]. In 1973, the National Cooperative Gallstone Study was inaugurated in the United States. Eight years later, results were published showing unequivocal dose-related efficacy of CDC, especially in patients with 'floatable' gallstones[149]. CDC was licensed on the American market about 2 years later.

In Japan, the chemical structure of UDC was established, and the Tokyo Tanabe company developed a procedure for synthesizing UDC from cholic acid. UDC was marketed as a drug for almost every kind of hepatic and biliary disease in the mid 1960s. Some years later, two patients with gallstones self-medicated themselves with high doses of UDC. Their gallstones were observed to dissolve[150], leading to trials of UDC which established its efficacy and safety[151]. The Japanese trials were quickly followed by European trials which confirmed the efficacy and safety of UDCA[152], and within a short time it was marketed in the major European countries. Double blind studies in Italy suggested that UDCA was also beneficial in dyspepsia of gallstone patients, so that the drug has been used for treating symptoms as well as radiolucent gallstones[153].

In the future we are likely to see the development of patented analogues which have superior efficacy and lower cost.

Work from several laboratories indicates that modification of the side chain of the bile acid can result in the appearance of striking choleretic properties far greater than have ever before been observed for bile acids[154]. Whether such novel choleretic bile acids will have important therapeutic properties remains to be seen.

Bile acid sequestration

Bile acids are also involved in therapy whose aim is to lower the concentration of bile acids. This approach to therapy is rather recent, and began with the historic studies of Tennent et al. who developed the first bile acid binding resins, and showed that they would lower the serum cholesterol levels in experimental animals[155]. In patients with ileal dysfunction causing bile acid diarrhoea (cholerrheic enteropathy), the administration of bile acid sequestrants such as cholestyramine causes symptomatic improvement[156].

Interruption of the enterohepatic circulation by bile acid sequestrant administration causes increased hepatic synthesis of cholesterol; this in turn induces the synthesis of LDL receptors which increases the removal rate of LDL and lowers serum LDL cholesterol levels[83]. In the Coronary Primary Prevention Trial, the lowering of serum cholesterol levels by cholestyramine was associated with a decreased number of coronary events[9]. In the past few years, agents that inhibit HMG-CoA reductase activity have been used together with sequestrants to cause a marked decrease in hepatocyte cholesterol[157]. This combination therapy causes a spectacular lowering of serum LDL cholesterol levels and should lead to the reversal of early atherosclerotic lesions.

EPIDEMIOLOGY AND BILE ACIDS

Abnormalities in bile formation and bile acid metabolism lead to disease. The disease may be silent and detectable only by diagnostic techniques or may be symptomatic requiring intervention. The incidence and prevalence of disease are the subject of the epidemiologist. Recently, prospective epidemiological studies using questionnaires and gallbladder imaging by ultrasound have given the first accurate data for the incidence and prevalence of gallbladder symptoms, gallstone disease and gallbladder surgery in several Italian communities[158].

These studies should lead to a better understanding of the cost of gallstone disease, permitting in time a comparison of the costs of disease with those of treating the disease by medicine or surgery (see Reference 159). Such studies will also provide badly needed information on the natural history of the disease, which may or may not provide a rationale for therapeutic intervention. What continues to be lacking is the epidemiology of biliary disease surgery, because it seems highly likely that the surgical literature has bias. Unfortunately, the conclusions of these epidemiological studies may not be able to be generalized outside of the population studied, since both the nature of the disease as well as the effect of the disease on the action of the patient and his interacton with the physician may be influenced by local cultural and economic factors.

SUMMARY

This overview of the past 60 years of bile acid research has indicated that some areas of bile acid research are very old – such as chemistry – and some areas are very young – such as the use of bile acids in diagnosis and therapy. It is clear that bile acid research is multi-disciplinary and must remain so to be healthy. It also seems that bile acid research is a bit old fashioned, and has not made use of many of the newer techniques of molecular biology such as gene cloning. The field has had little strong support from the larger pharmaceutical companies, probably because of their scepticism that the market for bile acid products is too small to justify research and development expenditures, and probably because the entire field of drugs for digestive disease had been neglected until the past decade. The enlighted support of the Falk Foundation (and also Gipharmex SpA), has permitted investigators in this field to communicate readily with each other, and to accelerate progress. Still, in my judgment, the field will only reach the early stages of maturity when patentable drugs based on the structure of the naturally-occurring bile acids are shown to be effective, safe and profitable.

Acknowledgement

The author's work is supported in part by NIH grants AM 21506 and AM 32130.

References

1. Durr, W. T. (1984). Humanistic science and the public. *The Public Historian*, **6**, 49–79
2. Palmer, R. H. (1972). Bile acids, liver injury, and liver disease. *Arch. Intern. Med.*, **130**, 606–17
3. Fischer, C. D., Cooper, N. S., Rothschild, M. A. and Mosbach, E. H. (1974). Effect of dietary chenodeoxycholic acid and lithocholic acid in the rabbit. *Am. J. Dig. Dis.*, **18**, 877–86
4. Gilmore, I. T. and Hofmann, A. F. (1980). Altered drug metabolism and elevated serum bile acids in liver disease: a unified pharmacokinetic explanation. *Gastroenterology*, **78**, 177–9
5. Boyd, G. S., Merrick, M. V., Monks, R. and Thomas, I. L. (1981). ^{75}Se-labeled bile acid analogues. New radiopharmaceuticals for investigating the enterohepatic circulation. *J. Nucl. Med.*, **22**, 720–5
6. Nyhlin, H., Merrick, M. V., Eastwood, M. A. and Brydon, W. G. (1983). Evaluation of ileal function using 23-selena-25-homotaurocholate, a γ-labeled conjugated bile acid. *Gastroenterology*, **84**, 63–8
7. Dowling, R. H. (1983). Cholelithiasis: medical treatment. *Clin. Gastroenterol.*, **12**, 125–77
8. Bachrach, W. H. and Hofmann, A. F. (1982). Ursodeoxycholic acid in the treatment of cholesterol cholelithiasis: a review. *Dig. Dis. Sci.*, **27**, 737–61 and 833–56
9. Lipid Research Clinics Program (1984). The lipid research clinics coronary primary prevention trial results. I. Reduction in incidence of coronary heart disease. II. The relationship of reduction in incidents of coronary heart disease to cholesterol lowering. *J. Am. Med. Assoc.*, **251**, 351–74
10. Windaus, A. (1928). Constitution of sterols and their connection with other substances in nature. In *Nobel Lectures in Chemistry*. pp. 105–21, 1966. (Amsterdam: Elsevier Publishing Co.)
11. Wieland, H. (1927). The chemistry of the bile acids. In *Nobel Lectures in Chemistry*. pp. 94–104, 1966. (Amsterdam: Elsevier Publishing Co.)
12. Bernal, J. D. (1932). Crystal structures of vitamin D and related compounds. *Nature*, **129**, 277–8
13. Rosenheim, O. and King, H. (1932). The ring system of sterols and bile acids. *Nature*, **130**, 315
14. Wieland, H. and Reverey, G. (1924). Untersuchungen ueber die Gallensaeuren. XXI. Zur Kenntnis der menschlichen Galle. *Z. Physiol. Chem.*, **140**, 186–202
15. Marsson, T. (1849). Ueber die Gaensegalle. *Annal. Chem.*, **72**, 317–18
16. Windaus, A., Bohne, A. and Schwarzkopf, E. (1924). Ueber die Chenodesoxycholsaeure. *Z. Physiol. Chem.*, **140**, 177–85
17. Hsia, S. L., Elliott, W. H., Matschiner, J. T., Doisy, E. A., Jr., Thayer, S. A. and Doisy, E. A. (1960). Bile acids. XIII. Further contributions to the constitution of muricholic acids. *J. Biol. Chem.*, **235**, 1963–7
18. Haslewood, G. A. D. (1978). *The Biological Importance of Bile Salts*. (Amsterdam: North-Holland Publishing Co.)
19. Iwasaki, T. (1936). Ueber die Konstitution der Urso-desoxycholsaeure. *Z. Physiol. Chem.*, **244**, 181–93
20. Hoshita, T. and Kazuno, T. (1968). Chemistry and metabolism of bile alcohols and higher bile acids. In Paoletti, R. and Kritchevsky, D. (eds.) *Advances in Lipid Research*. Volume 6, pp. 207–54. (New York: Academic Press)
21. Setchell, K. D. R., Lawson, A. M., Tanida, N. and Sjovall, J. (1983). General methods for the analysis of metabolic profiles of bile acids and related compounds in feces. *J. Lipid Res.*, **24**, 1085–100
22. Karlaganis, G. and Sjovall, J. (1984). Formation and metabolism of bile alcohols in man. *Hepatology*, **4**, 966–73
23. Kametani, T., Suzuki, K. and Nemoto, H. (1981). First total synthesis of (+)-chenodeoxycholic acid. *J. Am. Chem. Soc.*, **103**, 2891–2
24. Barnes, S. and Geckle, J. M. (1982). High resolution nuclear magnetic resonance spectroscopy of bile salts: individual proton assignments for sodium cholate in aqueous solution at 400 mHz. *J. Lipid Res.*, **23**, 161–70
25. Sjovall, J. (1983). Gas chromatography–mass spectrometry in studies of steroids, bile acids, and bile alcohols. *Proc. Jpn. Soc. Med. Mass Spectrom.*, **8**, 29–46

26. Burlingame, A. L., Whitney, J. O. and Russell, D. H. (1984). Mass spectrometry. *Anal. Chem.*, **56**, 417R–467R
27. Sjovall, J. and Axelson, M. (1982). Newer approaches to the isolation, identification, and quantitation of steroids in biological materials. *Vitam. Horm.*, **39**, 31–144
28. Fieser, L. F. and Fieser, M. (1963). *Topics in Organic Chemistry.* pp. 245–50. (New York: Reinhold Publishing Company)
29. Shoppee, C. W. (1966). *Chemistry of the Steroids.* 483 pp. (London: Butterworths)
30. Pellicciari, R., Cecchetti, S., Natalini, B., Roda, A., Grigolo, B. and Fini, A. (1984). Bile acids with a cyclopropyl-containing side chain. I. Preparation and properties of 3α,6β-dihydroxy-22,23-methylene-5β-cholan-24-oic acid. *J. Med. Chem.*, **27**, 746–9
31. Iwata, T. and Yamasaki, K. (1964). Enzymatic determination and thin-layer chromatography of bile acids in blood. *J. Biochem.* (Tokyo), **56**, 424–31
32. Mashige, F., Tanaka, N., Maki, A., Kamei, S. and Yamanata, M. (1981). Direct spectrophotometry of total bile acids in serum. *Clin. Chem.*, **27**, 1352–6
33. Roda, A., Kricka, L. J., DeLuca, M. and Hofmann, A. F. (1982). Bioluminescent measurement of primary bile acids using immobilized 7α-hydroxysteroid dehydrogenase: application to serum bile acids. *J. Lipid Res.*, **23**, 1354–61
34. Schoelmerich, J., van Berge Henegouwen, G. P., Hofmann, A. F. and DeLuca, M. (1984). A bioluminescence assay for total 3α-hydroxy bile acids in serum using immobilized enzymes. *Clin. Chim. Acta*, **137**, 21–32
35. Simmonds, W. J., Korman, M. G., Go, V. L. W. and Hofmann, A. F. (1973). Radioimmunoassay of conjugated cholyl bile acids in serum. *Gastroenterology*, **65**, 705–11
36. Roda, A. (1983). Sensitive methods for serum bile acid analysis. In Barbara, L., Dowling, R. H., Hofmann, A. F. and Roda, E. (eds.) *Bile Acids in Gastroenterology.* pp. 57–68. (Lancaster: MTP Press)
37. Ozaki, S., Tashiro, A., Makino, I., Nakagawa, S. and Yoshizawa, I. (1979). Enzyme-linked immunoassay of ursodeoxycholic acid in serum. *J. Lipid Res.*, **20**, 240–5
38. Matern, S., Tietjen, K., Matern, H. and Gerok, W. (1978). Enzyme labeled immunoassay for a bile acid in human serum. In Pal, S. B. (ed.) *Enzyme Labelled Immunoassay of Hormones and Drugs.* pp. 457. (Berlin: Walter De Gruyter and Co.)
39. Baqir, Y. A., Ross, P. E. and Bouchier, I. A. D. (1979). Homogeneous enzyme immunoassay of chenodeoxycholate conjugates in serum. *Anal. Biochem.*, **93**, 361–5
40. Okuyama, S., Kokubun, N., Higashidate, S. *et al.* (1979). A new analytical method of individual bile acids using high performance liquid chromatography and immobilized 3α-hydroxysteroid dehydrogenase in column form. *Chem. Lett.*, 1443–6
41. Angelin, B., Bjoerkhem, I. and Einarsson, K. (1978). Individual serum bile acid concentrations in normo- and hyperlipoproteinemia as determined by mass fragmentography: relation to bile acid pool size. *J. Lipid Res.*, **19**, 527–37
42. Wieland, H. and Sorge, H. (1916). Untersuchungen ueber die Gallensaeuren. *Hoppe Seylers Z. Physiol. Chem.*, **97**, 1–27
43. Hartley, G. S. (1936). Aqueous solutions of paraffin-chain salts. A study in micelle formation. In *Actualités Scientifiques et Industrielles.* (Paris: Hermann and Cie)
44. Ekwall, P. (1953). The solubilization of lipophilic substances by bile acid salts. In Ruyssen, R. (ed.) *Proceedings of the First International Conference on Biochemical Problems of Lipids.* pp. 103–119, Brussels
45. Ekwall, P., Ekholm, R. and Norman, A. (1957). Surface balance studies of bile acid monolayers. II. Monolayers of lithocholic and glycolithocholic acids. *Acta Chem. Scand.*, **11**, 703–9
46. Hofmann, A. F. and Borgstrom, B. (1962). Physico-chemical state of lipids in intestinal content during their digestion and absorption. *Fed. Proc.*, **21**, 43–50
47. Hofmann, A. F. (1963). The function of bile salts in fat absorption: the solvent properties of dilute micellar solutions of conjugated bile salts. *Biochem. J.*, **89**, 57–68
48. Hofmann, A. F. and Small, D. M. (1967). Detergent properties of bile salts: correlation with physiological function. *Ann. Rev. Med.*, **18**, 333–76
49. Small, D. M., Bourges, M. C. and Dervichian, D. G. (1966). Tertiary and quaternary aqueous systems containing bile salt, lecithin, and cholesterol. *Nature*, **211**, 816–18
50. Admirand, W. H. and Small, D. M. (1968). The physicochemical basis of cholesterol gallstone formation in man. *J. Clin. Invest.*, **47**, 1043–52

51. Carey, M. C. and Small, D. M. (1978). The physical chemistry of cholesterol solubility in bile. *J. Clin. Invest.*, **61**, 998-1026
52. Igimi, H. and Carey, M. C. (1980). pH-Solubility relations of chenodeoxycholic and ursodeoxycholic acids: physical-chemical basis for dissimilar solution and membrane phenomena. *J. Lipid Res.*, **21**, 72-89
53. Carey, M. C. and Mazer, N. A. (1984). Biliary lipid secretion in health and in cholesterol gallstone disease. *Hepatology (suppl)*, **4**, 31S-37S
54. Fini, A., Roda, A. and DeMaria, P. (1982). Chemical properties of bile acids. Part 2. pK_a values in water and aqueous methanol of some hydroxy bile acids. *Eur. J. Med. Chem.*, **17**, 467-70
55. Roda, A., Hofmann, A. F. and Mysels, K. J. (1983). The influence of bile salt structure on self-association in aqueous solutions. *J. Biol. Chem.*, **258**, 6362-70
56. Hofmann, A. F. (ed.) (1984). The physical chemistry of bile in health and disease. *Hepatology (suppl)*, **4**, 1S-252S
57. Moore, E. W., Celic, L. and Ostrow, J. D. (1982). Interactions between ionized calcium and sodium taurocholate: bile salts are important buffers for prevention of calcium-containing gallstones. *Gastroenterology*, **83**, 1079-89
58. Hofmann, A. F. and Roda, A. (1984). Physicochemical properties of bile acids and their relationship to biological properties: an overview of the problem. *J. Lipid Res.*, **25**, 1477-89
59. Lack, L. and Weiner, I. M. (1961). *In vitro* absorption of bile salts by small intestine of rats and guinea pigs. *Am. J. Physiol.*, **200**, 313-17
60. Lack, L. and Weiner, I. M. (1966). Intestinal bile salt transport: Structure–activity relationships and other properties. *Am. J. Physiol.*, **210**, 1142-52
61. Von Dippe, P. and Levy, D. (1983). Characterization of the bile acid transport system in normal and transformed hepatocytes. Photoaffinity labeling of the taurocholate carrier protein. *J. Biol. Chem.*, **258**, 8896-901
62. Kramer, W., Burckhardt, G., Wilson, F. A. and Kurz, G. (1983). Bile salt-binding polypeptides in brush-border membrane vesicles from rat small intestine revealed by photoaffinity labeling. *J. Biol. Chem.*, **258**, 3623-7
63. Meier, P., Meier-Abt, A., Barrett, C. and Boyer, J. L. (1984). Mechanism of taurocholate transport in canalicular and basolateral rat liver plasma membrane vesicles: evidence for an electrogenic canalicular organic ion carrier. *J. Biol. Chem.*, **98**, 991-1000
64. Blitzer, B. L. and Donovan, C. B. (1984). A new method for the rapid isolation of basolateral plasma membrane vesicles from rat liver: Characterization, validation and bile acid transport studies. *J. Biol. Chem.*, **259**, 9295-301
65. Kaplowitz, N., Stolz, A. and Sugiyama, Y. (1985). Bile acid binding proteins in hepatic cytosol. In *The Enterohepatic Circulation of Sterols and Bile Acids*. Falk Symposium 42. (Lancaster: MTP Press Limited). (In press)
66. Schiff, E. R., Small, N. C. and Dietschy, J. M. (1972). Characterization of the kinetics of the passive and active transport mechanisms for bile acid absorption in the small intestine and colon of the rat. *J. Clin. Invest.*, **51**, 1351-62
67. Wilson, F. A. (1981). Intestinal transport of bile acids. *Am. J. Physiol.*, **4**, G83-G92
68. Dupas, J.-L. and Hofmann, A. F. (1984). Passive jejunal absorption of bile acids *in vivo*: Structure–activity relationships and rate limiting steps. *Gastroenterology*, **86**, 1067 (abstract)
69. Bergstrom, S. and Danielsson, H. (1968). Formation and metabolism of bile acids. In Code, C. F. and Heidel, W. (eds.) *Handbook of Physiology, Section 6: Alimentary Canal*. Volume 5, pp. 2391. (Washington, D.C.: American Physiology Society)
70. Bjorkhem, I. and Danielsson, H. (1974). Hydroxylations in biosynthesis and metabolism of bile acids. *Mol. Cell. Biochem.*, **4**, 79-95
71. Palmer, R. H. (1967). The formation of bile acid sulfates: a new pathway of bile acid metabolism in humans. *Proc. Nat. Acad. Sci. USA*, **58**, 1047-50
72. Cowen, A. E., Korman, M. G., Hofmann, A. F. and Cass, O. W. (1975). Metabolism of lithocholate in healthy man. I. Biotransformation and biliary excretion of intravenously administered lithocholate, lithocholylglycine, and their sulfates. *Gastroenterology*, **69**, 59-66
73. Cowen, A. E., Korman, M. G., Hofmann, A. F., Cass, O. W. and Coffin, S. B. (1975). Metabolism of lithocholate in healthy man. II. Enterohepatic circulation. *Gastroenterology*, **69**, 67-76

74. Makino, I., Hashimoto, H., Shinozaki, K., Yoshino, K. and Nakagawa, S. (1975). Sulfated and nonsulfated bile acids in urine, serum, and bile of patients with hepatobiliary diseases. *Gastroenterology*, **68**, 545-53
75. Stiehl, A. (1974). Bile salt sulphates in cholestasis. *Eur. J. Clin. Invest.*, **4**, 59-63
76. Alme, B., Bremmelgaard, A., Sjovall, J. and Thomassen, P. (1977). Analysis of metabolic profiles of bile acids in urine using a lipophilic anion exchanger and computerized gas-liquid chromatography-mass spectrometry. *J. Lipid Res.*, **18**, 338-62
77. Matern, S., Matern, H., Farthmann, E. H. and Gerok, W. (1984). Hepatic and extrahepatic glucuronidation of bile acids in man. *J. Clin. Invest.*, **74**, 402-10
78. Kirkpatrick, R. B., Falany, C. N. and Tephly, T. R. (1984). Glucuronidation of bile acids by rat liver 3-OH androgen UDP-glucuronyltransferase. *J. Biol. Chem.*, **259**, 6176-80
79. Williams, R. T. (1975). Chemistry of detoxication. In Gerok, W. and Sickinger, K. (eds.) *Drugs and the Liver.* pp. 51-64 (Stuttgart: F. K. Schattauer Verlag)
80. Angelin, B., Einarsson, K., Leijd, B., Rudling, M., Hershon, K. and Brunzell, J. (1984). Enterohepatic circulation of bile acids and lipoprotein metabolism. *Abstract of VIII International Bile Acid Meeting.* p. 33, August 31-September 2, Berne
81. Marks, J., Lan, S.-P., The Steering Committee and The National Cooperative Gallstone Study Group (1984). Low-dose chenodiol to prevent gallstone recurrence after dissolution. *Ann. Intern. Med.*, **100**, 376-81
82. Takata, K., Kost, L. J. and LaRusso, N. F. (1984). Bile acids inhibit hepatic extraction of lipoproteins. *Hepatology*, **4**, 1056 (abstract)
83. Shepherd, J., Packard, C. J., Bicker, S., Lawrie, T. D. V. and Morgan, H. G. (1980). Cholestyramine promotes receptor-mediated low-density-lipoprotein catabolism. *N. Engl. J. Med.*, **302**, 1219-22
84. Rodwell, V. W., Nordstrom, J. L. and Mitschelen, J. J. (1976). Regulation of HMG-CoA reductase. *Adv. Lipid Res.*, **14**, 1-74
85. Barth, C. A. (1983). Regulation and interaction of cholesterol, bile salt and lipoprotein synthesis in liver. *Klin. Wochenschr.*, **61**, 1163-70
86. Duane, W. C. and Pries, J. M. (1983). Regulation of bile acid synthesis. In Paumgartner, G., Stiehl, A. and Gerok, W. (eds.) *Bile Acids and Cholesterol in Health and Disease.* pp. 73-5. (Lancaster: MTP Press)
87. LaRusso, N. F., Szczepanik, P. A., Hofmann, A. F. and Coffin, S. B. (1977). Effect of deoxycholic acid ingestion on bile acid metabolism and biliary lipid secretion in normal subjects. *Gastroenterology*, **72**, 132-40
88. Hardison, W. G. M. and Grundy, S. M. (1984). Effect of ursodeoxycholate and its taurine conjugate on bile acid synthesis and cholesterol absorption. *Gastroenterology*, **87**, 130-5
89. Einarsson, E., Nilsell, K., Angelin, B. and Leijd, B. (1983). Effects of ursodeoxycholic acid and chenodeoxycholic acid on bile acid kinetics and secretion rates of biliary lipids in man. In Paumgartner, G., Stiehl, A. and Gerok, W. (eds.) *Bile Acids and Cholesterol in Health and Disease.* pp. 267-8. (Lancaster: MTP Press)
90. Boyer, J. L. (1980). New concepts of mechanisms of hepatocyte bile formation. *Physiol. Rev.*, **60**, 303-20
91. Erlinger, S. (1981). Hepatocyte bile secretion: current views and controversies. *Hepatology*, **1**, 352-9
92. Gurantz, D. and Hofmann, A. F. (1984). Influence of bile acid structure on bile flow and biliary lipid secretion in the hamster. *Am. J. Physiol.*, **247**, 6736-48
93. Rutishauser, S. C. B., Burns, P. and Weil, S. C. (1980). Comparative effects of tauro-cholate, taurodeoxycholate and glycodeoxycholate on the flow and ionic composition of bile in guinea-pigs anaesthetized with urethane. *Comp. Biochem. Physiol.*, **66A**, 493-8
94. Mazer, N. A. and Carey, M. C. (1984). Mathematical model of biliary lipid secretion: a quantitative analysis of physiological and biochemical data from man and other species. *J. Lipid Res.*, **25**, 932-53
95. Danzinger, R. G., Nakagaki, M., Hofmann, A. F. and Ljungwe, E. B. (1984). Differing effects of hydroxy-7-oxotaurine-conjugated bile acids on bile flow and biliary lipid secretion in dogs. *Am. J. Physiol.*, **246**, G166-G172

96. Heaton, K. W. (1971). Bitter humour: the development of ideas about bile salts. *J. R. Coll. Physicians*, **6**, 83-97
97. Hislop, I. G. (1970). The absorption and entero-hepatic circulation of bile salts. An historical review. *Med. J. Austr.*, **1**, 1223-6
98. Hofmann, A. F. (1977). The enterohepatic circulation of bile acids in man. *Clin. Gastroenterol.*, **6**, 3-24
99. Carey, M. C. (1982). The enterohepatic circulation. In Arias, I., Popper, H., Schachter, D. and Shafritz, D. A. (eds.) *The Liver: Biology and Pathobiology*. pp. 429-465. (New York: Raven Press)
100. Sobotka, H. (1938). *Chemistry of the Steroids*. (Baltimore: Williams and Wilkins)
101. Bergstrom, S. and Danielsson, H. (1958). On the regulation of bile acid formation in the rat liver. *Acta Physiol. Scand.*, **43**, 1-7
102. Lindstedt, S. (1957). The turnover of cholic acid in man. Bile acids and steroids 51. *Acta Physiol. Scand.*, **40**, 1-9
103. Hofmann, A. F. and Cummings, S. A. (1983). Measurement of bile acid and cholesterol kinetics in man by isotope dilution: principles and applications. In Barbara, L., Dowling, R. H., Hofmann, A. F. and Roda, E. (eds.) *Bile Acids in Gastroenterology*. pp. 75-117. (Lancaster: MTP Press)
104. Grundy, S. M. and Metzger, A. L. (1972). A physiologic method for estimation of hepatic secretion of biliary lipids in man. *Gastroenterology*, **62**, 1200-17
105. Go, V. L. W., Hofmann, A. F. and Summerskill, W. H. J. (1970). Simultaneous measurements of total pancreatic, biliary, and gastric outputs in man using a perfusion technique. *Gastroenterology*, **58**, 321-8
106. Hepner, G. W., Hofmann, A. F. and Thomas, P. J. (1972). Metabolism of steroid and amino acid moieties of conjugated bile acids in man. II. Glycine-conjugated dihydroxy bile acids. *J. Clin. Invest.*, **51**, 1898-905
107. Hofmann, A. F., Molino, G., Milanese, M. and Belforte, G. (1983). Description and simulation of a physiological pharmacokinetic model for the metabolism and enterohepatic circulation of bile acids in man. Cholic acid in healthy man. *J. Clin. Invest.*, **71**, 1003-22
108. Schiff, M. (1870). Gallenbildung abhaengig von der Aufsaugung der Gallenstoffe. *Pfluegers Arch. Physiol.*, **3**, 598-613
109. Verzar, F. (1936). *Absorption from the Intestine*. pp. 1-294. (London: Longmans, Green and Co.)
110. Moore, B. and Parker, W. H. (1901). On the functions of the bile as a solvent. *Proc. R. Soc. B.*, **68**, 64-76
111. Mattson, F. H. and Beck, L. W. (1956). The specificity of pancreatic lipase for the primary hydroxyl groups of glycerides. *J. Biol. Chem.*, **219**, 735-40
112. Hofmann, A. F. and Borgstrom, B. (1964). The intraluminal phase of fat digestion in man: the lipid content of the micellar and oil phases of intestinal content obtained during fat digestion and absorption. *J. Clin. Invest.*, **43**, 247-57
113. Simmonds, W. J., Hofmann, A. F. and Theodor, E. (1967). Absorption of cholesterol from a micellar solution: intestinal perfusion studies in man. *J. Clin. Invest.*, **46**, 874-90
114. Swell, L., Trout, E. C. Jr., Hopper, J. R., Field, H. Jr. and Treadwell, C. R. (1958). Specific function of bile salts in cholesterol absorption. *Proc. Soc. Exp. Biol. Med.*, **98**, 174-6
115. Gallo-Torres, H. E., Miller, O. N. and Hamilton, J. G. (1971). Further studies on the role of bile salts in cholesterol esterification and absorption from the gut. *Arch. Biochem. Biophys.*, **143**, 22-36
116. Watt, S. M. and Simmonds, W. J. (1984). Effects of four taurine-conjugated bile acids on mucosal uptake and lymphatic absorption of cholesterol in the rat. *J. Lipid Res.*, **25**, 448-55
117. Flynn, M., Darby, C., Hyland, J., Hammond, P. and Taylor, I. (1979). The effect of bile acids on colonic myoelectrical activity. *Br. J. Surg.*, **66**, 776-9
118. Hanssen, L. E. (1980). Pure synthetic bile salts release immunoreactive secretin in man. *Scand. J. Gastroenterol.*, **15**, 461-3
119. Wingate, D. L., Phillips, S. F. and Hofmann, A. F. (1973). Effect of glycine-conjugated bile acids with and without lecithin on water and glucose absorption in perfused human jejunum. *J. Clin. Invest.*, **52**, 1230-6

120. Mekhjian, H. S., Phillips, S. F. and Hofmann, A. F. (1971). Colonic secretion of water and electrolytes induced by bile acids: perfusion studies in man. *J. Clin. Invest.*, **50**, 1569-77

121. Chadwick, V. S., Gaginella, T. S., Carlson, G. L., Debongnie, J.-C., Phillips, S. F. and Hofmann, A. F. (1979). Effect of molecular structure on bile acid-induced alterations in absorptive function, permeability and morphology in the perfused rabbit colon. *J. Lab. Clin. Med.*, **94**, 661-74

122. Fischer, H. (1911). Zur Kenntnis der Gallenfarbstoffe. *Z. Physiol. Ch.*, **73**, 204-39

123. Neubauer, E. (1924). Ueber die cholagoge Wirkung der Dehydrocholsaeure beim Menschen. *Klin. Wochenschr.*, **3**, 883

124. Holsti, P. (1962). Bile acids as a cause of liver injury: Cirrhogenic effect of chenodeoxycholic acid in rabbits. *Acta Path. Microbiol. Scand.*, **54**, 479

125. Javitt, N. B. and Emerman, S. (1968). Effect of sodium taurolithocholate on bile flow and bile acid excretion. *J. Clin. Invest.*, **47**, 1002-14

126. Palmer, R. H. and Hruban, Z. (1966). Production of bile duct hyperplasia and gallstones by lithocholic acid. *J. Clin. Invest.*, **45**, 1255-67

127. Zaki, F. G., Carey, J. B. Jr., Hoffbauer, F. W. and Nokolo, C. (1967). Biliary reaction and choledocholithiasis induced in the rat by lithocholic acid. *J. Lab. Clin. Med.*, **69**, 737-48

128. Ferraris, R., Colombatti, G., Fiorentini, M. T., Carosso, R., Arossa, W. and de la Pierre, M. (1983). Diagnostic value of serum bile acids and routine liver function tests in hepatobiliary diseases. *Dig. Dis. Sci.*, **28**, 129-36

129. Festi, D., Morselli Labate, A. M., Roda, A., Bazzoli, F., Frabboni, R., Rucci, P., Taroni, F., Aldini, R., Roda, E. and Barbara, L. (1983). Diagnostic effectiveness of serum bile acids in liver diseases as evaluated by multivariate statistical methods. *Hepatology*, **3**, 707-13

130. Ritchie, W. P. (1984). Alkaline reflux gastritis: a critical reappraisal. *Gut*, **25**, 975-87

131. Hofmann, A. F. and Poley, J. R. (1972). Role of bile acid malabsorption in pathogenesis of diarrhea and steatorrhea in patients with ileal resection. I. Response to cholestyramine or replacement of dietary long chain triglyceride by medium chain triglyceride. *Gastroenterology*, **62**, 918-34

132. Suchy, F. J. and Balistreri, W. F. (1981). Ileal dysfunction in Crohn's disease assessed by the postprandial serum bile acid response. *Gut*, **22**, 948-52

133. Fromm, H. and Hofmann, A. F. (1971). Breath test for altered bile acid metabolism. *Lancet*, **2**, 621-5

134. Hess-Thaysen, E. (1977). The ^{14}C-cholylglycine assay. *Clin. Gastroenterol.*, **6**, 227-45

135. Tabaqchali, S. and Booth, C. C. (1966). Jejunal bacteriology and bile-salt metabolism in patients with intestinal malabsorption. *Lancet*, **2**, 12-15

136. King, D. E., Toskes, P. P., Spivey, J. C., Lorenz, E. and Welkos, S. (1979). Detection of small intestine bacterial overgrowth by means of a ^{14}C-D-xylose breath test. *Gastroenterology*, **77**, 75-82

137. Hofmann, A. F. (1983). The enterohepatic circulation of bile acids in health and disease. In Sleisenger, M. H. and Fordtran, J. S. (eds.) *Gastrointestinal Disease*, 3rd Edn. pp. 115-31. (Philadelphia: W. B. Saunders)

138. Hanson, R. F., Szczepanik, P. A., Williams, G. C., Grabowski, G. and Sharp, H. L. (1979). Defects in bile acid synthesis in Zellweger's syndrome. *Science*, **203**, 1107-8

139. Oftebro, H., Bjorkhem, I., Skrede, S., Schreiner, A. and Pedersen, J. I. (1980). Cerebrotendinous xanthomatosis. A defect in mitochondrial 26-hydroxylation required for normal biosynthesis of cholic acid. *J. Clin. Invest.*, **65**, 1418-30

140. Hoshita, T., Yasuhara, M., Kihira, K. *et al.* (1976). Identification of (23S)-5β-cholestane-3α,7α,12α,23,25-pentol in cerebrotendinous xanthomatosis. *Steroids*, **27**, 657-64

141. Alme, B., Norden, A. and Sjovall, J. (1978). Glucuronides of unconjugated 6-hydroxylated bile acids in urine of a patient with malabsorption. *Clin. Chim. Acta*, **86**, 251-9

142. Thistle, J. L. and Schoenfield, L. J. (1971). Induced alterations in composition of bile of persons having cholelithiasis. *Gastroenterology*, **61**, 488-96

143. van Berge Henegouwen, G. P., Brandt, K.-H., Eyssen, H. and Parmentier, G. (1976). Sulfated and unsulfated bile acids in serum, bile, and urine of patients with cholestasis. *Gut*, **17**, 861-9

144. Schiff, M. (1873). Il coleinato di soda nella cura dei calcoli biliari. *L'Imparziale*, **13**, 97-9
145. Kosidowski, H. (1946). Zur Geschichte der Gallensaeuren. *Pharmazie*, **1**, 282-6 and 323-5
146. Thistle, J. L. and Schoenfield, L. J. (1969). Induced alterations of bile composition in humans with cholelithiasis. *J. Lab. Clin. Med.*, **74**, 1020-1 (abstract)
147. Thistle, J. L. and Hofmann, A. F. (1973). Efficacy and specificity of chenodeoxycholic acid therapy for dissolving gallstones. *N. Engl. J. Med.*, **289**, 655-9
148. Dowling, R. H. (1977). Chenodeoxycholic acid therapy of gallstones. *Clin. Gastroenterol.*, **6**, 141-63
149. Schoenfield, L. J., Lachin, J. M., the Steering Committee and the National Cooperative Gallstone Study Group (1981). Chenodiol (chenodeoxycholic acid) for dissolution of gallstones: The National Cooperative Gallstone Study. *Ann. Intern. Med.*, **95**, 257-82
150. Sugata, F. and Shimizu, M. (1974). Retrospective studies on gallstone disappearance. *Jpn. J. Gastroenterol.*, **71**, 75-80
151. Nakagawa, S., Makino, I., Ishizaki, T. and Dohi, I. (1977). Dissolution of cholesterol gallstones by ursodeoxycholic acid. *Lancet*, **2**, 367-9
152. Erlinger, S., Go, A. L., Husson, J.-M. and Fevery, J. (1984). Franco-Belgian cooperative study of ursodeoxycholic acid in the medical dissolution of gallstones: a double-blind, randomized dose-response study and comparison with chenodeoxycholic acid. *Hepatology*, **4**, 308-14
153. Frigerio, G. (1979). Ursodeoxycholic acid (UDCA) in the treatment of dyspepsia: report of a multicenter controlled trial. *Curr. Ther. Res.*, **26**, 214-24
154. Yoon, Y. B., Hagey, L. R., Gurantz, D., Cecchetti, S. and Hofmann, A. F. (1984). The unusual physiological properties of *nor*-ursodeoxycholate. *Hepatology*, **4**, 1086 (abstract)
155. Tennent, D. M., Siegel, H., Zanetti, M. E., Kuroh, G. W., Ott, W. H. and Wolf, F. J. (1960). Plasma cholesterol lowering action of bile acid binding polymers in experimental animals. *J. Lipid Res.*, **1**, 469-73
156. Hofmann, A. F. and Poley, J. R. (1969). Cholestyramine treatment of diarrhea associated with ileal resection. *N. Engl. J. Med.*, **281**, 397-402
157. Bilheimer, D. W., Grundy, S. M., Brown, M. S. and Goldstein, J. L. (1983). Mevinolin and colestipol stimulate receptor-mediated clearance of low density lipoprotein from plasma in familial hypercholesterolemic heterozygotes. *Proc. Natl. Acad. Sci. USA*, **80**, 4124-8
158. Capocaccia, L., Ricci, G., Angelico, F., Angelico, M. and Attili, A. F. (eds.) (1984). *Epidemiology and Prevention of Gallstone Disease*. pp. 1-240. (Lancaster: MTP Press)
159. von Sonnenberg, A., Leuschner, U. and Leuschner, M. (1982). Erwartungskosten bei der konservativen und chirurgischen Behandlung der unkomplizierten Cholezystolithiasis. *Z. Gastroenterol.*, **20**, 66-77

2
Bile acids in therapy – pre-1924, circa 1924 and in 1984

R. H. DOWLING

The theme – 'Bile Acids in Therapy' is far from new. For example, in the year when Dr Herbert Falk was born the French literature[1] included an article on *'La bile en thérapeutique digestive'* and in the same year, Adlersberg and Neubauer from Vienna[2] published a paper *'Ueber die therapeutische Verwendung der Dehydrocholsaure'*. A few years later, Vorhaus and Marks[3] described the use of *'Bile salts in the treatment of biliary tract disease'* and then in the American medical press, Pleasants[4] discusses *'Bile Salts Therapy'* – so much for the originality of the author's choice of title!

In fact bile, and its major constituents the bile acids, have been used in therapy for centuries but the scientific era of bile acid treatment has been a 20th century phenomenon – especially over the past 15 years. Herbert Falk, his pharmaceutical company and the Falk Foundation have played an important catalytic role in advancing our knowledge about bile acid treatment in this scientific era – not only by sponsoring major international conferences in bile acid research (and in many other fields) but also by supporting smaller workshops on chenodeoxycholic acid (CDCA) during the early days of its development as a treatment for gallstone dissolution[5, 6]. On the occasion of his 60th birthday, this chapter briefly reviews the uses of bile and bile acids in treatment before the year of his birth, then around 1924 and ends with a summary, or 'state-of-the-art', about bile acids in therapy today.

THE PRE-1924 HISTORY OF BILE ACIDS IN THERAPY

In the past, as now, the two main sources of bile acids were avian and mammalian bile. According to Carey (personal communication), the domestic and medicinal uses of ox and avian bile may have begun in Macedonia. The Greeks traded (and fought) continuously with Macedonia between 1200 B.C. and 100 A.D. and although they did not use soaps derived from saponification of animal fats, they did use ox and avian bile for washing garments. In turn, it seems likely that the wandering Celts (the Scots, Welsh, Bretons, Galacians and particularly the Irish) learned that "the dung of the goose is good for jaundice" from Greece when they travelled there to raid Delphi in the first millenium B.C. According to one theory, as the Irish then followed the silk routes to the East, they transported this therapeutic lore to China, Korea, India and Indonesia. According to another theory, however, the use of animal biles in therapy may have originated in China. The first officially commissioned pharmacopia in medical history – Su Kung's *Hsin Hsiu Pên Tshao* of 659 A.D. – records the medicinal use of dried *black* bear's bile (hsiung tan in Chinese or yûtan in Japanese) for the treatment of jaundice and abdominal pain. The equivalent of the prescribing notes or data sheets of that time would have gladdened the hearts (and indeed swollen the pockets) of any pharmaceutical company today since they stressed 'precaution – the treatment should be given for life'.

Dessicated bear bile

Although it is tempting to relate contemporary therapy with ursodeoxycholic acid to ancient medicinal uses of dried bear bile there is, in fact, considerable confusion about the bile acid composition of bile from different sub-species of bears. It is known that at certain times of the year, the bile of the black Himalayan bear may contain large amounts ($> 50\%$) of ursodeoxycholic acid. It has also been suggested that UDCA is found in the bile of Chinese white collar bears. However, the principle bile acid in gallbladder bile of most Japanese and American black bears is not UDCA but cholid acid (Haslewood 1978; Carey 1984). Furthermore, contrary to popular belief (and despite the fact that contemporary advertisements for therapeutic ursodeoxycholic acid frequently depict white or polar bears), the polar bear does not have appreciable amounts of UDCA in its bile. In fact, although Hammersten[7] claimed to have isolated ursocholic acid from polar bear bile in 1902, in all probability, this was CDCA (Shoda 1927; Takun 1949). Despite this confusion, in the blissful days before gas chromatography – mass spectrometry, the biles of many other species, such as the snake, lizard, carp, ox and sheep, was also used as treatment. In the days before prespective, random-allocation, cross-over, double-blind trials, history records little about the efficacy of these preparations.

Dried bear bile was almost certainly introduced into Japan as one of the 'secrets of life' or 'treasures', by the personal physicians to the Japanese Emperor. At that time, the tradition was that the Emperor's doctors should travel and acquire these 'treasures' of information which were then brought home and jealously guarded in the Emperor's temples.

Despite the influence of the Celts and their use of 'the dung of the goose', about 1000 years were to elapse before the therapeutic traditions of the Orient reached Europe. In 1650, William Harvey, the discoverer of the circulation, records for the first time in the *Pharmacopoeia Londoniensis*, the use of bile salts in therapy[8]. Then another century was to elapse before the paramedical use of bile appeared in Holland – the incorporation of bulls bile into soap which contained 3–5% bile salts. Indeed, in remote parts of Fresianland, this bulls bile soap may still be obtained today.

The idea that bile acids might be used as therapeutic agents to aid gallstone dissolution was also recorded in the middle of the last century by the famous German clinical scientist, Naunyn. Not only did he demonstrate that human cholesterol gallstones, when placed in the gallbladder of the dog, would dissolve[9] but he also suggested that bile acids, when given as choleretics, might promote gallstone dissolution in man[10].

As we approach 1924, however, there are many more detailed accounts of the use of bile in treatment. In Japan, for example, during the 19th and early 20th centuries the tradition for using bear bile (also known by the trade name *'Kumanoi'* from the Japanese *Kuma* = bear, *no* = of, *i* = the gallbladder*), were strong. Before enjoying their relatively recent industrial revolution and prosperity, Japanese people were comparatively poor. Doctors were few and besides, the majority of the population could not afford professional medical care. As an alternative, they took dried bear bile as a folk medicine, for a wide variety of abdominal disorders. In some parts of Japan, such as the Kansai/Kinki prefecture or district which is in the southern central part of the main island, Honshu, salesmen, *toyama no kusuriya*, so-called because they came from the main northern districts of Toyama, would travel from home to home around the country, bringing with them large quantities of the bear bile folk medicine, *Kumanoi*. They called at each household once or twice each year leaving supplies of a range of medical drugs, including *Kumanoi*, with the family and collected payment on a 'no sale/return' basis, the next visit.

The tradition of using dried animal bile as treatment still persists in Japan today and it is possible, at a price, to obtain dried bear pellets in Japan's North Island, Hokkaido, provided that one is willing to pay 600 US $ for 2 g. At the same time, the use of dried animal biles, with varying degrees of purity, was also developing in Europe, and dessicated ox or avian bile was marketed under various trade names such as Dessibyl (Parke Davis) and Decholin.

BILE ACIDS IN THERAPY – CIRCA 1924

Around the time of Herbert Falk's birth, there are several accounts of bile acids being advocated as therapeutic agents. In 1919, for example, Whipple[11] studied the effect of giving bile, bile acids or taurine plus cholic acid by stomach – of interest because the administration of the combination of bile acids plus taurine was hailed as one of the latest advances in gallstone dissolution therapy at the 8th International Bile Acid meeting in Berne[12] only one week before the 'Trends in Hepatology' symposium. In 1920, Wieland talked about pharmacological studies using deoxycholic and choleic acids[13] (choleic acid being a mixture of bile acids and fatty acids) and then, just

---

*I is normally translated as 'the stomach' but in this context, it is more correctly translated as 'the gallbladder'.

2 years into the Falk era, we find that Muller[14] has anticipated the use of trade names such as Chenofalk and Ursofalk, with 'a new bile acid preparation – Biligat'.

But apart from these general accounts of bile acids in treatment, around this time there were several studies describing more specific indications for bile acid therapy. Neubauer, for example, describes the use of dehydrocholic acid as a cholagogue in man[15] while, in the same year (1924), Brugsch and Horsters[16] discuss bile acid treatment under the title 'choleresis and choleretics'. Three years later in the French literature we read about the use of bile enemas in the treatment of constipation[17] – a forerunner, perhaps, of the idea that di-alpha hydroxy bile acids inhibit water and electrolyte transport in the colon[18], alter colonic motility[19] and indeed influence the interdigestive motor complex[20].

Influenced, perhaps, by Naunyn's studies in 1859, Moehle returns to the idea that dehydrocholic acid (or Decholin) might be used in the management of patients with gallstones[21], and in the same year (1928) Bignon, in a small monograph from Paris[22], talks about 'the prevention and curative treatment of biliary colic and jaundice by the dissolution of (gall)stones in the biliary tree'. Claims that bile acids might have more widespread therapeutic indications included the recommendation, in the Rumanian Medical Press, that dehydrocholic acid might be used in the treatment of acute cholecystitis[23].

BILE ACIDS IN THERAPY – 1984

There is, of course, a large chapter which has been written about the logarithmic increase in our knowledge of bile acid treatment between the 1920s and the present day, but this has been reviewed elsewhere and need not be restated here. Instead, the remainder of this chapter will deal with the use of bile acids in therapy today. Table 2.1 summarizes the many conditions for which bile acids have been, or are being, used in 1984.

Table 2.1 Summary of disorders for which bile acids are being, or have been, used

GALLSTONE DISSOLUTION	*REPLACEMENT THERAPY*
—oral therapy (alone or combined with other agents)	—in patients with defective bile acid synthesis
—T-tube infusion	—in patients with ileal disease/resection (UDCA)
Biliary pain/colic	
Non-specific dyspepsia	*GASTRO-TENDINOUS XANTHOMATOSIS* (CDCA)
—duodeno-gastric reflux with bile acid mediated gastritis	*DOUBTFUL/CONTROVERSIAL INDICATIONS*
—gallstone patients	—migraine
—patients with normal gastro-duodenal anatomy	—arthritis
—patients with previous gastro-duodenal surgery	—constipation
Irritable/Spastic Colon	—as choleretics, e.g., liver transplantation
Hypertriglyceridaemia	

Gallstone dissolution (oral therapy)

Without doubt, the principal indication for bile acid treatment is oral dissolution therapy for cholesterol-rich gallstones. The bile acids which have been used alone, or in combination with other bile acids, with or without amino acids, are listed in Table 2.2. It is beyond the scope of this brief chapter to review gallstone dissolution therapy in detail: this is done elsewhere[24]. However, the situation may be summarized as follows:

Table 2.2 Summary of the bile acids which have been or are being used/evaluated as oral dissolution therapy for cholesterol-rich gallstones

Chenodeoxycholic Acid (CDCA)	Tauroursodeoxycholic Acid (TUDCA)	Ursocholic Acid (UCA) Methyl Ursodeoxycholic
Ursodeoxycholic Acid (UCDA)	Taurine + UDCA	Acid (MUDCA)
CDCA + UDCA	7-ketolithocholic Acid (7-KLC)	Methyl Ursocholic Acid (MUCA)

Chenodeoxycholic acid (CDCA)

CDCA treatment, when given in an adequate dose (approximately 15 mg $kg^{-1} day^{-1}$) will lead to confirmed complete gallstone dissolution in approximately 40% of patients with radiolucent stones in functioning gallbladders, in 60% of non-obese patients with small or medium-sized stones and in a maximum of 80% of selected patients – provided that complications of stones and/or of treatment, or non-compliance, do not result in 'premature' withdrawal from therapy. However, CDCA causes dose-related, although often transient, diarrhoea, hypertransaminasaemia and, in the United States NCGS at least, electron microscopic changes in liver biopsies of a small percentage of patients, and 10–20 mg/dl rise in fasting serum cholesterol levels.

Ursodeoxycholic acid (UDCA)

UDCA, in contrast, is virtually free from these side-effects. However, its efficacy in producing complete gallstone dissolution is either comparable[25, 26], or inferior[27], to that of CDCA. In part (but only in part), this is due to acquired gallstone calcification. In one series[28], up to 25% (by life table analysis) of patients treated with UDCA developed acquired rim or surface opacification of their stones, which is thought to inhibit or prevent subsequent gallstone dissolution.

CDCA plus UDCA

Several reports[29, 30] suggest that the combination of these two bile acids may be at least as effective as either given alone – but without the side-effects. Since each bile acid is given in approximately half its normal dose, the absence of complications may simply mean that the threshold for dose-dependent side-effects has not been reached. Whether or not UDCA has a 'protective' effect against the diarrhoea and hypertransaminasaemia induced by CDCA, and whether CDCA can prevent the acquired gallstone calcification provoked by UDCA, is unknown.

Other bile acids

As shown in Table 2.2, 7-ketolithocholic acid (7-KLC), tauroursodeoxycholic acid (TUDCA), taurine plus UDCA, ursocholic acid (UCA)[31, 32] and other bile acid derivatives – such as the methyl esters of UDCA and UCA – have been or are now being tested, not only for their ability to desaturate bile but also for their capacity to solubilize cholesterol by non-micellar mechanisms (the formation of liquid crystalline vesicles), and ultimately for their capacity to dissolve cholesterol-rich gallstones completely.

Gallstone dissolution: T-tube infusion

Although sodium cholate[33] was one of the first 'solvents' to be infused for the dissolution of retained common bile duct stones in post-cholecystectomy T-tube patients, it is no longer widely used. Mono-octanoin[34], and newer solvents such as methyl tertiary butyl ether[35] and n-methyl pyrrolidone[36], are now being evaluated for T-tube infusions, for perfusion through endoscopically placed naso–biliary catheters and even for the dissolution of gallstones within the gallbladder by percutaneous transhepatic catheterisation[37]. It should be emphasised, however, that this latter technique is new and has not been fully evaluated. It is potentially dangerous and should not be attempted until the method has been more fully evaluated.

Bile acids still have a place, however, when combined with calcium-chelating agents such as EDTA, in the infusion treatment of mixed common bile duct stones containing both cholesterol and calcium salts[38].

Biliary pain and colic

The results of many uncontrolled studies and of a few, mainly short-term, double-blind trials, suggest that the frequency and/or severity of biliary pain may diminish during CDCA or UDCA therapy.

The mechanism for this putative 'side-benefit' of bile acid treatment is unknown, but may relate to the fact that during ursotherapy, gallbladder emptying in response to either a meal or to i.v. infusions of CCK, is prolonged[39]. In other words, if forceful expulsion of particulate matter from the gallbladder into the biliary tree with resultant obstruction and proximal dilatation, is the mechanism for the production of biliary pain, then the less 'aggressive' gallbladder contraction seen during bile acid treatment might explain the alleged reduction in biliary pain. This working hypothesis remains to be proven.

Non-specific dyspepsia

Even more controversial is the use of bile acids in the treatment of 'dyspepsia'. Dyspeptic symptoms are difficult to define: the mechanism for their production is unknown: they are non-specific in that they occur with approximately equal frequency in individuals with and without gallstones[40]. Despite this, many investigators have noted a reduction in these non-specific abdominal symptoms during bile acid treatment of gallstone patients.

One possible mechanism for the production of symptoms in such patients is alkaline reflux gastritis or duodeno–gastric reflux (DGR). DGR is said to occur more frequently in gallstone patients than in controls[41]. The candidate substances for the role of gastrotoxins in the refluxed duodenal contents include bile acids, either alone or in combination with hydrolysed biliary phospholipids (lysolecithin), and/or hydrolytic pancreatic enzymes. The results of recent studies suggest that during UDCA treatment, the glycine conjugated bile acids and particularly the 'benign' glycoursodeoxycholic acid predominate, rendering the refluxed bile acids less soluble in the gastric lumen and theoretically, therefore, less toxic. Based on this rationale, bile acids have also been successfully used in the treatment of bile reflux gastritis in post-gastric surgery patients[42].

The irritable/spastic colon

In some patients, gallstones are diagnosed fortuitously when upper abdominal symptoms, arising in the colon, are incorrectly attributed to disease in the gallbladder. The results of many uncontrolled, and often anecdotal, studies suggest that bile acid treatment in these patients may benefit the colonic symptoms in these patients. Could it be that bile acid treatment affects colonic smooth muscle motor function in much the same way that it affects the gallbladder[39] – thereby relieving the irritable colon symptoms? The results of double-blind trials are badly needed to prove or disprove this somewhat tenuous hypothesis.

The hypotriglyceridaemic effect of bile acid treatment

CDCA lowers fasting serum triglyceride levels by 10–30% both in normo- and hyper-triglyceridaemic patients with[43] or without[44] gallstones. This reduction affects mainly the very low density lipoprotein (VLDL) fraction of serum triglycerides, and is thought to be due to an inhibitory effect of CDCA therapy on hepatic triglyceride synthesis[45].

The effect of UDCA on serum triglycerides is controversial: some investigators have shown a similar hypotriglyceridaemic effect[46] to that seen with CDCA, while others found little or no change in serum triglyceride levels[47]. However, it is far from clear that the benefits of treating raised serum triglyceride levels outweigh the potential disadvantages. In those patients in whom it is considered justifiable and/or necessary, there are many powerful triglyceride lowering alternatives, to bile acid treatment.

Replacement therapy

In exceptionally rare situations of bile acid deficiency secondary to defective hepatic bile acid synthesis, the patients may be treated by bile acid replacement therapy. For example, a unique case has been described of a young woman with markedly reduced bile acid levels in her serum, bile, small intestinal lumen and faeces – apparently due to defective primary bile acid synthesis[48]. She had associated steatorrhoea and severe constipation. Treatment first with the dessicated ox bile preparation, Dessibyl[49], and then with CDCA[48] helped to alleviate these symptoms.

Replacement therapy for bile acid deficiency in patients with bile acid malabsorption secondary to ileal disease or resection or to putative defects in bile acid transport[50], however, is not satisfactory. In the presence of a compromised ileal active transport system, the oral administration of cholic acid and/or chenodeoxycholic acid simply compounds the pre-existing diarrhoea as the exogenous bile acids and/or their bacterial metabolites, spill into the colon[51]. However, UDCA does not cause diarrhoea. Initially, therefore, it seemed logical to try UDCA as replacement therapy in patients with steatorrhoea due to ileal dysfunction. Unfortunately, UDCA is a rather poor detergent and its capacity to solubilize hydrolysed dietary lipids in the intestinal lumen, is limited. Although treatment of such patients with large doses (up to 4 g/day) of UDCA does significantly reduce faecal fat excretion[52], this is not practical as longterm therapy.

Cerebrotendinous xanthomatosis

Cerebrotendinous xanthomatosis or CTX is an extremely rare metabolic disorder which is associated with raised plasma cholesterol levels, abnormal bile acid synthesis, tendon xanthomata, cataracts, dementia, pyramidal and cerebellar dysfunction and peripheral neuropathy. Beringer et al.[53] have recently shown that CDCA treatment may help these patients considerably.

Doubtful indications and/or unproven claims for bile acids in therapy

With the widespread use of CDCA and UDCA as treatment for gallstone patients who have, coincidentally, other disorders, and given the fact that the placebo influence of any drug is strong, it is not surprising that claims have been made suggesting that there may be other indications for bile acids in treatment, than just for gallstone dissolution.

Migraine

For example, Levy and colleagues from Paris[54] found that CDCA was of benefit in patients with migraine, and this subsequently led to a preliminary report of a double-blind trial of CDCA for the treatment of migraine[55].

Rheumatoid arthritis

Similarly, Bruusgaard and Andersen[56] claimed that CDCA was helpful in the treatment of rheumatoid arthritis.

It is far from clear how bile acids could influence the course of these diseases. Until more rigorous testing of these clinical observations has been made, preferably with longterm, double-blind trials, CDCA could not be recommended as a therapy for either migraine or rheumatoid arthritis.

Choleretics

As indicated above (*see* historical review) the choleretic properties of bile acids have been recognized for years. Based mainly on the results of studies in bile fistula animals, structure/activity relationships have now been defined and 'league tables' of the hydrophilic/choleretic properties of bile acids, determined. UCA, for example, is a potent choleretic as are the *nor*-bile acids which have a total of 23 carbon atoms (as opposed to the normal 24) with one carbon less in the side chain[57].

Despite the fact that in some parts of the world, bile acids are still widely prescribed as choleretics, there are few, if any, well documented clinical indications for the use of choleretics today.

Constipation

Despite the widespread use of dried animal biles and of crude bile salt preparations as purgatives in the past (*see* above), and although occasional contemporary clinical trials have confirmed the efficacy of bile acids as a treatment for constipation[58], there are so many simple effective dietary and drug alternatives that bile acid treatment has not become widely accepted as a treatment for constipation in the 1980s.

CONCLUSIONS

As stated above, the principle indication for bile acids in therapy in the 1980s is the treatment of patients with cholesterol-rich gallstones. With the advent of large epidemiologial studies in which ultrasound screening of the population has confirmed that the majority of gallstones is silent or asymptomatic, the question of whether either medical or surgical intervention is needed for the majority of gallstone patients is, quite rightly, being disputed. Before providing a rational answer, we now need longitudinal studies to learn more about the natural history of untreated *silent* gallstone disease. Until this information becomes available, the ultimate role of oral bile acid therapy (and indeed of surgery) in the treatment of gallstones remains uncertain. Undoubtedly bile acid treatment will have a place but how large a role it will play is, as yet, unclear. However, if the rapid expansion in our knowledge about bile acids and their use in therapy, progresses at the same rate over the next 60 years as it has done since 1924, the future will indeed be bright.

Acknowledgements

The author gratefully acknowledges valuable help from Dr Martin C. Carey with the historical information, and from Dr Motonobu Hosomi who kindly amplified the history of bile acids as therapeutic agents in Japan. Miss Cathy Weeks kindly typed the manuscript.

References

1. Bignon, L. (1924). La bile en thérapeutique digestif. *Rev. Gén. Thér.*, **38**, 393
2. Adlersberg, D. and Neubauer, E. (1924). Ueber die therapeutische Verwendung der Dehydrocholsäure. *Wein. Med. Wochrs*, **74**, 1716–18
3. Vorhaus, M. G. and Marks, J. A. (1930). Bile salts in the treatment of biliary tract disease. *Trans. Am. Ther. Soc.*, **29**, 107–14
4. Pleasants, H. Jr. (1935). Bile salts therapy. *Med. World*, **53**, 440
5. Hofmann, A. F. and Paumgartner, G. (1974). *Chenodeoxycholic Acid Therapy of Gallstones.* (Stuttgart, New York: FK Schattauer Verlag)
6. Hofmann, A. F. and Paumgartner, G. (1975). *Chenodeoxycholic Acid Therapy of Gallstones: Update 1975.* (Stuttgart, New York: FK Schattauer Verlag)
7. Hammersten, O. (1902) Hoppe Seylers Z. *Physiol. Chem.*, **36**, 525–55
8. Harvey, W. (1650.
9. Naunyn, B. (1882). *Klinik der Cholelithiasis.* (Leipzig: F. C. W. Vogel)
10. Franken (1968). *Die Leber Und Ihre Krankheiten. Zweihundert Jahre Hepatologie.* (Ferdinand Enke: Verlag, Stuttgart)
11. Whipple, G. H. (1919). The metabolism of bile acids: administration by stomach of bile, bile acids, taurine and cholic acid to show the influence upon bile acid elimination. *J. Biol. Chem.*, **38**, 379–92
12. Thistle, J. L., LaRusso, N. F., Tietz, P. S., Center, C. L. and Ott, B. J. (1982). Combination of taurine or chenodeoxycholate with ursodeoxycholate therapy: effects on biliary lipids, bile acids and gallstones. *Gastroenterology*, **84**, 1400 (Abst.)
13. Wieland, H. and Hilderbrand, T. (1920). Pharmakologische Untersuchungen uber Gallensauren: die Deoxycholsaure und die Choleinsauren. *Arch. Pharm. Exp. Path.*, **86**, 76–91
14. Muller, A. H. (1926). Ueber Biligat, ein neues gallensaurepraparat. *Wein. Med. Wochrs*, **76**, 529
15. Neubauer, E. (1924). Ueber die cholagoge Wirkung der Dehydrocholsaure beim menschen. *Klin. Wochrs*, **3**, 883
16. Brugsch, T. and Horsters, H. (1924). Cholerese und Choleretica; ein Beitrag zur Physiologie der Galle. *Zschr. Ges. Exp. Med.*, **43**, 517–38
17. Beaumont, A. R. (1927). Les lavements de bile dans la constipation. *Vie Med.*, **8**, 415
18. Chadwick, V. S., Gaginella, T., Carlson, G., Debongnie, J-C., Phillips, S. F. and Hofmann, A. F. (1979). Effect of molecular structure on bile acid induced alterations in absorptive function, permeability and morphology in the perfused rabbit colon. *J. Lab. Clin. Med.*, **94**, 661–74
19. Kirwan, W. D., Smith, A. N., Mitchell, W. D., Falconer, J. D. and Eastwood, M. A. (1975). Bile acids and colonic motility in the rabbit and the human. *Gut*, **16**, 894
20. Kruis, W., Haddad, A. and Phillips, S. F. (1985). Chenodeoxycholic and Ursodeoxycholic Acids alter motility and fluid transit in the canine ileum. *Gastroenterology*. (In press)
21. Moehle, H. (1928). Behandlung Gallensteinkranker mit Dehydrocholsaure (Decholin). *Med. Klin. Berl.*, **24**, 184
22. Bignon, L. (1928). *Traitement preventif et curatif des coliques hepatiques et de l'ictere par la dissolution des calculs dans voies biliaires.* (Paris: Vigo Freres)
23. Winkler, L. (1930). Dehydrocholeic acid in the treatment of acute cholecystitis. *Cluj Med.*, **11**, 184–8
24. Dowling, R. H. (1982). Cholelithiasis: medical treatment. *Clin. Gastroenterol.*, **12**, 125–78

25. Meredith, T., Williams, G. V., Maton, P. N., Saxton, H. M. and Dowling, R. H. (1982). Retrospective comparison of 'cheno' and 'urso' in the medical treatment of gallstones. *Gut*, **23**, 382-9
26. Roda, E., Bazzoli, F., Morselli Labate, A. M., Mazzella, G., Roda, A., Sama, C., Festi, D., Aldini, R., Taroni, F. and Barbara, L. (1982). Ursodeoxycholic acid *vs* chenodeoxycholic acid as cholesterol gallstone-dissolving agents: a comparative randomized study. *Hepatology*, **2**, 804-10
27. Gleeson, D., Ruppin, D. C., Murphy, G. M. and Dowling, R. H. (1983). Second look at ursodeoxycholic acid (UDCA): high efficacy for partial but low efficacy for compete gall-stone dissolution and a high rate of acquired stone opacification. *Gut*, **24**, A999 (Abstract)
28. Gleeson, D., Murphy, G. M. and Dowling, R. H. (1985). Calcium binding by bile acids *in vitro* studied using a calcium ion electrode. *Clin. Sci.*, **68**, 38 (Abstract)

29. Stiehl, A. (1981). Effects of chenodeoxycholic acid and ursodeoxycholic acid on bile acid and biliary lipid metabolism in patients with radiolucent gallstones. Correlation with efficacy and toxicity. In Paumgartner, G., Stiehl, A. and Gerok, W. (eds.) *Bile Acids and Lipids*. pp. 309-17. (Lancaster: MTP Press)
30. Thistle, J. L., LaRusso, N. F., Tietz, P. S., Center, C. L. and Ott, B. J. (1982). Combination of taurine or chenodeoxycholate with ursodeoxycholate therapy: effects on biliary lipids, bile acids and gallstones. *Gastroenterology*, **84**, 1400 (Abstr.)
31. Howard, P., Gleeson, D., Murphy, G. M. and Dowling, R. H. (1984). Ursocholic acid (UCA): a new cholesterol gallstone dissolving agent? Bile acid and bile lipid dose-response studies in man. *Clin. Sci.*, **67**, 35-6 (Abstr.)
32. Loria, P., Medici, G., Iori, R. and Carulli, N. (1984). Ursocholic acid (UCA): a new potential agent for dissolving cholesterol gall stones. *Gut*, **25**, A1172 (Abstract)
33. Way, L. W., Admirand, W. H. and Dunphy, J. E. (1972). Management of cholelithiasis. *Ann. Surg.*, **176**, 347-59
34. Palmer, K. R. and Hofmann, A. F. (1984). Mono-octanoin therapy – combined experience in 343 cases of retained biliary calculi. *Gut*, **25**, A1172 (Abstract)
35. Allen, M. J., Borody, T. J., Bugliosi, T. F., May, G. R., La Russo, N. F. and Thistle, J. L. (1985). Cholelitholysis using methyl tertiary butyl ether. *Gastroenterology*, **88**, 122-5
36. Corrigan, O. I., Kennelly, P. and Cleary, C. M. (1984). Physicochemical investigation of dipolar aprotic solvents as potential cholelitholytic agents. Abstracts of *VIII International Bile Acid Meeting*. p. 420. Berne, Switzerland
37. Allen, M. J., Borody, T. J., Bugliosi, T. F., May, G. R., La Russo, N. F. and Thistle, J. L. (1985). Rapid dissolution of gallstones by methyl tert-butyl ether. *N. Engl. J. Med.*, **312**, 217-20
38. Leuschner, U., Baumgartner, H. and Lang, S. (1983). Investigations of calcium binding capacity and toxicity of gallstone dissolution media. In *Bile Acids and Cholesterol in Health and Disease*. pp. 107 11. (Lancaster. MTP Press)
39. Forgacs, I. C., Maisey, M. N., Murphy, G. M. and Dowling, R. H. (1984). Influence of gallstones and ursodeoxycholic acid therapy on gallbladder emptying. *Gastroenterology*, **87**, 299-307
40. GREPCO. (1984). Prevalence of gallstone disease in an Italian adult female population. *Am. J. Epidemiol.*, **119**, 796-805
41. Johnson, A. G. (1972). Pyloric function and gall-stone dyspepsia. *Br. J. Surg.*, **59**, 449-54
42. Stefaninsky, A. B., Tint, G. S., Speck, J. and Salen, G. (1982). Ursodeoxycholic acid (UDCA) reduces pain, nausea and vomiting in patients with bile acid reflux gastritis. *Gastroenterology*, **82**, 1188 (Abstract)
43. Bell, G. D., Lewis, B., Petrie, A. and Dowling, R. H. (1973). Serum lipids in cholelithiasis: Effect of chenodeoxycholic acid therapy. *Br. Med. J.*, **3**, 520-3
44. Miller, N. E. and Nestel, P. J. (1974). Triglyceride-lowering effect of chenodeoxycholic acid in patients with endogenous hypertriglyceridaemia. *Lancet*, **ii**, 929-31
45. Begemann, F. (1978). Influence of chenodeoxycholic acid on the kinetics of endogenous triglyceride transport in man. *Eur. J. Clin. Invest.*, **8**, 283-8
46. Williams, G., Murphy, G. M. and Dowling, R. H. (1980). Effect of ursodeoxycholic acid (UDCA) on total and VLDL triglycerides in gallstone patients. *Clin. Sci.*, **58**, 15 (Abstract)

47. Nakagawa, S., Makino, I., Ishizaki, T. and Dohi, I. (1977). Dissolution of cholesterol gallstones by ursodeoxycholic acid. *Lancet*, **2**, 367-9
48. Iser, J. H., Dowling, R. H., Murphy, G. M., Ponz de Leon, M. and Mitropoulos, K. A. (1976). Congenital bile salt deficiency associated with 28 years of intractable constipation. In *Bile Acid Metabolism in Health and Disease*. pp. 231-4. (Lancaster: MTP Press)
49. Ross, C. A. C. and Frazer, A. C. (1955). Coeliac disease. The relative importance of wheat gluten. *Lancet*, **1**, 1087
50. Hess Thaysen, E. and Pedersen, L. (1973). Diarrhoea associated with idiopathic bile acid malabsorption. Fact or fantasy? *Dan. Med. Bull.*, **20**, 174-7
51. Hofmann, A. F. and Grundy, S. M. (1965). *Clin. Res.*, **13**, 254 (Abstract)
52. Huijbregts, A. W., Cox, T. M., van Berge Henegouwen, G. P., van Schaik, A. and Chadwick, V. S. (1981). Micellar solubilisation of intestinal lipids after ursodeoxycholic acid therapy in short bowel patients and healthy controls. *Neth. J. Med.*, **24**, 108-13
53. Beringer, V. M., Salen, G. and Shefer, S. (1984). Chenodeoxycholic acid reduces elevated plasma cholestanol levels and improves. In Paumgartner, G., Stiehl, A. and Gerok, W. (eds.) *Enterohepatic circulation of bile acids and sterol metabolism*. (In Press). (Lancaster: MTP Press)
54. Levy, V., Nusinovici, V., Rosner, D. and Darnis, F. (1978). Chenodeoxycholic acid in the prevention of migraine. *N. Engl. J. Med.*, **299**, 630 (letter to editor)
55. Pradalier, A., Dry, J. and Luce, H. (1981). Essai de prevention de la migraine commune par l'acide chenodesoxycholique. *Nouv. Presse Med.*, **10**, 180 (Abstr.)
56. Bruusgaard, A. and Andersen, R. B. (1976). Chenodeoxycholic acid treatment of rheumatoid arthritis. *Lancet*, **1**, 700 (letter to editor)
57. Palmer, K. R., Gurantz, D., Hofmann, A F. and Ljungwe, E. B. (1982). Novel choleretic properties of *nor*-chenodeoxycholate. *Hepatology*, **3**, 816 (Abstr.)
58. Hepner, G. W. and Hofmann, A. F. (1973). Cholic acid therapy for constipation: A controlled trial. *Mayo Clin. Proc.*, **48**, 356-8

3
Progress in understanding the mechanisms of organic anion uptake by the liver

P. D. BERK, W. STREMMEL, R. NUNES, B. J. POTTER,
H. OKUDA, N. TAVOLONI, S. KOCHWA, C.-L. KIANG,
M. SHEPARD, B. BLADES AND M.-J. T. JONES

INTRODUCTION

In order to elucidate the processes by which cells take up specific molecules it has to be established whether uptake occurs by simple diffusion or by some form of facilitated transport[1]. In the latter case, determination of the driving forces and of the specific membrane transport machinery at the molecular level is also essential. Bile acids[2, 3], non-bile acid cholephils such as sulpho-bromophthalein (BSP) and bilirubin[4-6], and free fatty acids[7] represent three classes of organic anions, the hepatocellular uptake of which has been extensively studied. In recent years it has become apparent that these three classes, which differ widely in both their physicochemical properties and their metabolic roles, nevertheless share a number of similarities with respect to their hepatocellular uptake[8]. Specifically (Table 3.1):

Table 3.1 Analogous features of the hepatocellular uptake of bile acids, BSP and bilirubin, and free fatty acids

Feature	Bile acids	BSP/ bilirubin	Free fatty acids
(1) Tight albumin binding	+	+	+
(2) 'Albumin receptor' effect	+	+	+
(3) Cytosolic binding protein	+	+	+
(4) Specific membrane binding protein	+	+	+
(a) evidence for transport function	+	?	?
(5) Uptake kinetics imply carrier mediated transport	+	+	?
(6) Driving forces known	+	?	?

41

(1) All are tightly bound to albumin in the circulation[9-12].
(2) All manifest some form of accelerated dissociation of their albumin complexes at the hepatocellular surface, the so-called 'albumin receptor' effect[13-16].
(3) For each, a unique integral membrane binding protein has been isolated from the hepatocellular sinusoidal plasma membrane[17-22].
(4) A cytosolic binding protein has been identified for each class of compound[23-25].

Some crucial information is still lacking. The uptake kinetics of BSP and bile acids are known to be compatible with carrier-mediated transport[2-6, 8] while those of free fatty acids are controversial[7, 26]. A biologic function for the bile acid membrane binding protein has been established in liposome reconstitution studies[18], while direct demonstration of the transport function of the BSP/bilirubin – and free fatty acid-binding proteins remains to be established. Finally, bile acid uptake is sodium coupled[3], while the driving forces for BSP and bilirubin uptake and for that of free fatty acids are unknown.

The aims of the current studies, therefore, are:

(1) To examine the nature of the hepatocellular uptake kinetics for free fatty acids in an isolated hepatocyte preparation;
(2) To study the effects of specific antibodies to the BSP/bilirubin and free fatty acid binding proteins on the hepatocellular uptake of the corresponding ligands; and
(3) To study the relationship of BSP and free fatty acid uptake to the transport of inorganic ions in isolated hepatocytes and isolated sinusoidal membrane vesicles.
(4) Finally, we will examine whether an 'albumin receptor' effect, previously demonstrated in the isolated perfused liver, also occurs with isolated single cell suspensions of hepatocytes.

METHODS

Rat hepatocyte suspensions were prepared by a modification of the collagenase perfusion technique of Berry and Friend[27]. Preparations used for transport studies met the following viability criteria: greater than 90% trypan blue exclusion; intracellular K^+ greater than 85 mmol/l; less than 15% loss of LDH; and less than 20% stimulation of respiration by succinate. Sinusoidal membrane vesicles were prepared from male Sprague-Dawley rat livers by the discontinuous Percoll–sucrose gradient technique of Inoue, Kinne, Tran and Arias[28]. Purity of the vesicles was established with multiple enzymatic markers, and their right side out orientation assessed using both biochemical and ultrastructural observations. Triton X-100 extracts of total sinusoidal liver plasma membrane protein, containing the BSP/bilirubin-, free fatty acid-, and bile acid-binding proteins, have been incorporated into liposomes consisting of phosphatidyl choline and cholesterol at ratios of 1:1 or 2:1, as initially described by Gerritsen et al.[29]. After incubation of radiolabelled organic anions with hepatocytes, vesicles, or liposomes, organic anion uptake was determined by a rapid vacuum filtration technique[30] after applying an appropriate correction for the radioactivity which was merely membrane bound.

RESULTS

Kinetics of hepatocellular oleate uptake

Because oleate is insoluble in aqueous solutions at concentrations in excess of 10^{-6} to 10^{-5} mol/l, isolated rat hepatocytes were incubated with [^{14}C]-oleate in the presence of varying concentrations of bovine serum albumin (BSA), such that the BSA:oleate ratio varied from 5:1 to 0.25:1. As this ratio decreases, the calculated free oleate concentration in the incubation mixture increases, while remaining within the range of solubility[22]. Figure 3.1

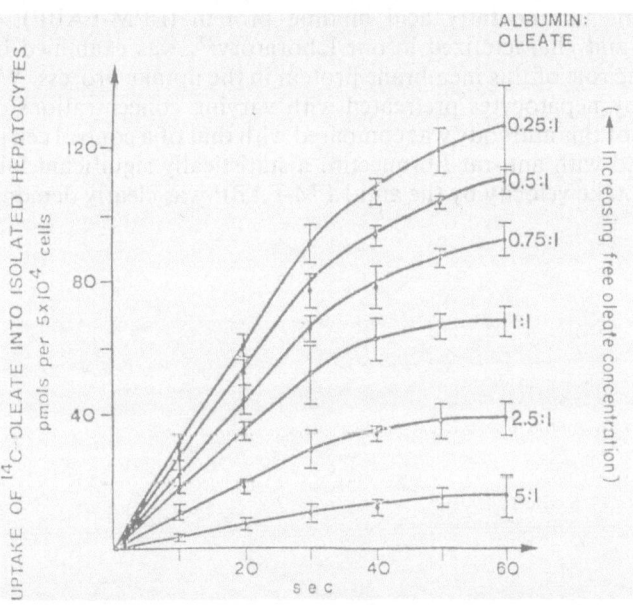

Figure 3.1   Uptake of [^{14}C]-oleate by isolated rat hepatocytes at various albumin:oleate molar ratios

illustrates the time course of hepatocellular oleate uptake over the initial 60 seconds in a series of experiments at different albumin:oleate molar ratios. For each ratio uptake was linear over the initial 30 seconds, gradually decreasing thereafter and remaining essentially constant between 1 and 7 minutes. The initial uptake velocity, V_0, was estimated from the slope of the initial 30 second portion of the curve. As evident from Figure 3.1, the initial uptake rates of [^{14}C]-oleate increased as the albumin:oleate molar ratio decreased. However, the magnitude of the progressive increments in V_0 declined at the highest concentrations of free oleate studied, indicative of saturation.

In other studies, the initial uptake velocity of [14C]-oleate was shown to be temperature and pH dependent, with maxima at 37°C and 7.4 respectively; and to be inhibited by coincubation with other free fatty acids but not by [14C]-taurocholate or [35S]-BSP. In addition, oleate uptake was inhibited by pre-incubating the cells with trypsin or by the inclusion in the incubation medium of calcium ions at concentrations in excess of 5 mmol/l. Hence the uptake kinetics of [14C]-oleate by isolated hepatocytes are compatible with a carrier mediated transport mechanism.

Role of liver plasma membrane fatty acid- and BSP/bilirubin- binding proteins

The effect on hepatocellular [14C]-oleate uptake of an antibody to the liver plasma membrane fatty acid binding protein (LPM-FABP), previously isolated and characterized in our laboratory[22], was examined in order to define the role of this membrane protein in the uptake process. When oleate uptake by hepatocytes pretreated with varying concentrations of the IgG fraction of this antibody was compared with that of a control cell population pretreated with anti-rat fibronectin, a statistically significant inhibition of initial uptake velocity by the anti LPM-FABP was clearly demonstrated. In

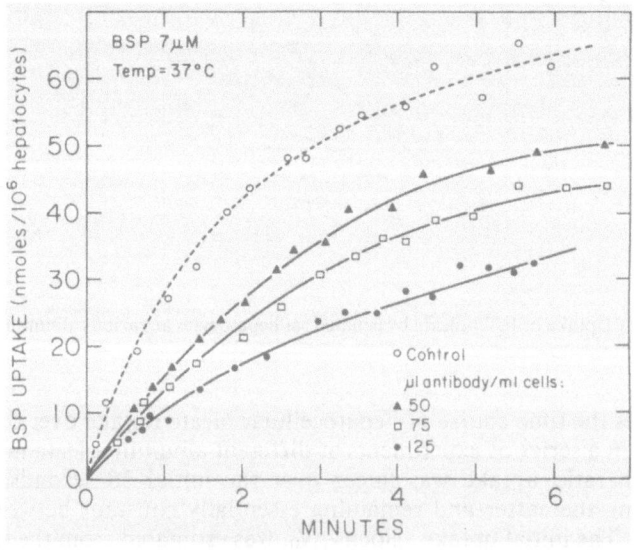

Figure 3.2 Influence of an antibody to the liver plasma membrane BSP/bilirubin binding protein on [35S]-BSP uptake by isolated rat hepatocytes

contrast, this antibody, raised against the liver plasma membrane fatty acid binding protein, had no effect on the hepatocellular uptake of either [^{14}C]-taurocholate, [^{35}S]-BSP, or [^{14}C]-cholic acid. Since anti LPM-FABP selectively inhibits the uptake of [^{14}C]-oleate by isolated hepatocytes, these studies indicate that the liver plasma membrane fatty acid binding protein must have a significant physiologic role in the hepatocellular uptake of free fatty acids.

Figure 3.2 illustrates the influence of an antibody to the liver plasma membrane BSP/bilirubin binding protein on hepatocellular uptake of [^{35}S]-BSP. Increasing concentrations of antibody, illustrated by the three lower curves, cause dose related inhibition of BSP uptake compared to the control

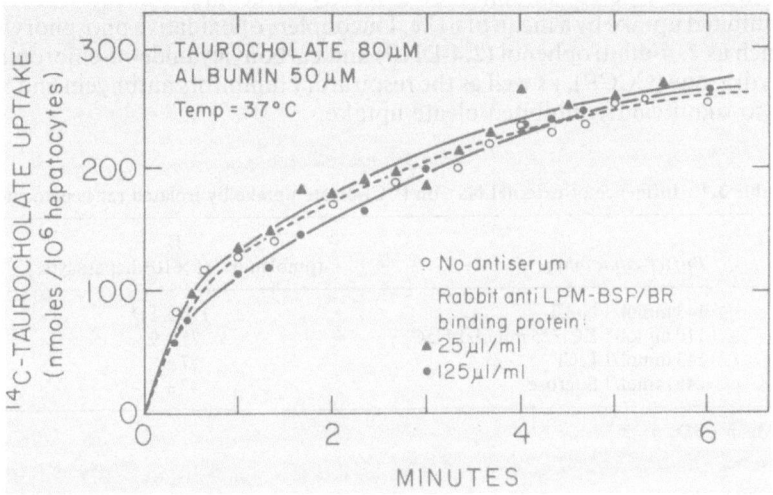

Figure 3.3 Influence of antibody to the liver plasma membrane BSP/bilirubin binding protein on [^{14}C]-taurocholate uptake by isolated rat hepatocytes

cells in the uppermost curve, which were again treated with an anti-rat fibronectin. In contrast to its effect on BSP uptake the anti LPM-BSP/bilirubin binding protein has no influence of the initial uptake of [^{14}C]-taurocholate by an analogous population of rat hepatocytes (Figure 3.3). These data, therefore, suggest an important role for the liver plasma membrane BSP/bilirubin binding protein in the hepatocellular uptake of this class of organic anions. In highly preliminary studies this role was also supported by uptake studies employing synthetic lecithin: cholesterol liposomes. BSP uptake was appreciably greater in liposomes to which the Triton X-100 extract of sinusoidal liver plasma membrane proteins had been incorporated, compared to its uptake in protein free liposomes or into liposomes containing red cell ghost membrane proteins.

Driving forces for free fatty acid and BSP uptake

Free fatty acids

We shall now turn our attention to studies of the driving forces mediating the hepatocellular uptake of free fatty acids. As shown in Table 3.2, hepatocellular uptake of [^{14}C]-oleate by isolated rat hepatocytes is significantly decreased when 143 mmol/l sodium chloride in the incubation medium is replaced by a solution containing 110 mmol/l potassium chloride and only 25 mmol/l sodium. Inhibition is even greater when sodium is totally replaced by lithium or by isosmotic replacement of inorganic salts by 246 mmol/l sucrose. Ouabain, which inhibits sodium–potassium ATPase, reduced the initial rate of oleate uptake by isolated hepatocytes by an average of 39%, suggesting that uptake might be linked to the activity of this enzyme. Phloretin, a potent inhibitor of a variety of cellular transport processes, inhibited uptake by a mean of 81%. Uncouplers of oxidative phosphorylation such as 2, 4-dinitrophenol (2,4-DNP) and carbonylcyanide-*m*-chlorophenyl-hydrazone (CCCP), as well as the respiratory inhibitors antimycin and KCN, also significantly inhibited oleate uptake.

Table 3.2 Influence of external Na$^+$ on [^{14}C]-oleate uptake by isolated rat hepatocytes

Buffer containing	V_0 (pmol min^{-1}/5 × 10^4 hepatocytes)
143 mmol/l NaCl	116 ± 11*
110 mmol/l KCl/25 mmol/l NaCl	75 ± 9
143 mmol/l LiCl	57 ± 8
246 mmol/l Sucrose	47 ± 7

*Mean ± SD, $n = 3$

Figure 3.4 illustrates the uptake of organic anions by isolated sinusoidal membrane vesicles in the presence of a buffer containing 10 mmol/l Tris-Hepes, pH 7.4, with 250 mmol/l sucrose, plus magnesium and calcium. These studies were conducted in duplicate in the presence or absence of 100 mmol/l sodium nitrate. As shown in the left hand panel, and as previously reported by others[28], uptake of [^{3}H]-taurocholate by sinusoidal membrane vesicles in the presence of sodium is significantly faster, with a greater maximal accumulation of anion, than occurs in the absence of sodium. The panel on the right illustrates the rapid uptake of tritiated oleate by analogous membrane vesicles in a sodium-containing medium. In confirmation of the data already presented with isolated hepatocytes, the uptake of [^{3}H]-oleate by sinosoidal membrane vesicles is significantly greater in the presence of external sodium than in the presence of external potassium (Figure 3.5). *In toto*, the data just presented support the concept that at least a component of the hepatocellular uptake of oleate is energy dependent, sodium linked and mediated by a specific liver plasma membrane fatty acid binding protein.

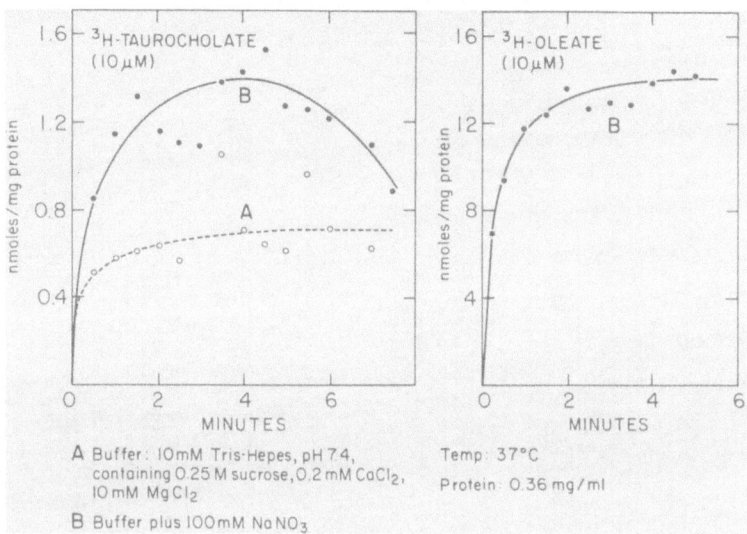

Figure 3.4 Uptake of [³H]-taurocholate (left) and [³H]-oleate (right) by rat liver sinusoidal plasma membrane vesicles

BSP

Numerous investigators, including ourselves, have attempted without success to define the driving forces for BSP uptake in the isolated perfused rat liver or in isolated hepatocytes. Figure 3.6 illustrates preliminary data on the effects of various inorganic ions on [³⁵S]-BSP uptake by rat liver sinusoidal

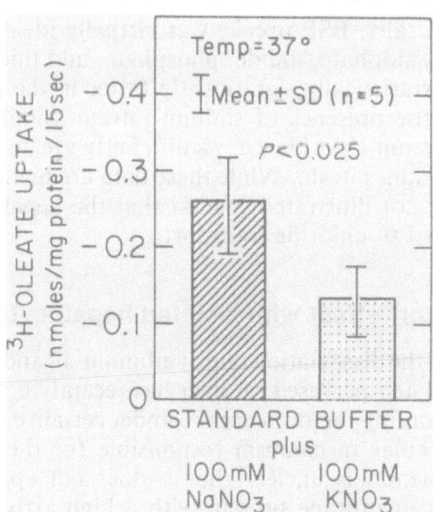

Figure 3.5 Influence of external sodium on [³H]-oleate uptake by isolated rat liver sinusoidal plasma membrane vesicles

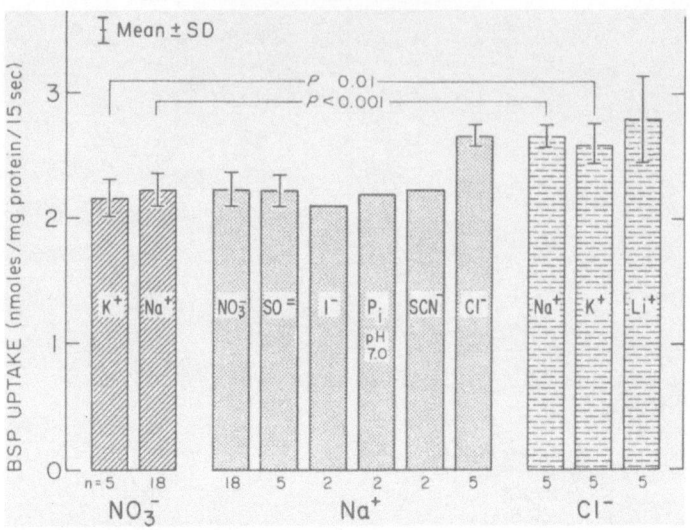

Figure 3.6 Effect of various inorganic ions on [^{35}S]-BSP uptake by rat liver sinusoidal plasma membrane vesicles. For a given cation, BSP uptake is significantly greater in the presence of chloride anion than in the presence of the other anions studied

membrane vesicles. As shown in the left hand pair of bars, when such vesicles were incubated in the presence of nitrate anion, substitution of potassium for sodium had no influence on the rate of BSP uptake. Correspondingly, when incubated in the presence of chloride anion, substitution of sodium by either potassium or lithium again had no significant influence on the rate of BSP uptake. When vesicles were incubated with [^{35}S]-BSP in the presence of a variety of sodium salts, BSP uptake was virtually identical in the presence of sodium nitrate, sulphate, iodide, phosphate, and thiocyanate. However, BSP uptake was statistically significantly faster in the presence of sodium chloride than in the presence of sodium nitrate. Similarly, uptake in the presence of potassium chloride was significantly greater than uptake in the presence of potassium nitrate. While these data are highly preliminary, they and other studies not illustrated suggest that the hepatocellular uptake of BSP may be linked to chloride transport.

'Albumin receptor' effect with isolated hepatocytes

The critical role of the dissociation rate of albumin–ligand complexes in ligand uptake by the isolated perfused rat liver has recently been emphasized, and shown to be the limiting factor in uptake under certain circumstances[13–16, 31]. The precise molecular mechanism responsible for the so-called 'albumin receptor' phenomenon is unclear, but it does not appear to result from the presence of a membrane protein with a high affinity for albumin, in the classical sense of the word 'receptor'[32]. It has been suggested that unstirred water layer effects within the space of Disse might play a role in the accelerated dissociation of albumin–ligand complexes near the hepato-cellular surface. In studies such as the one illustrated in Figure 3.7, the hepatocellular uptake of oleate appears to be limited more by an increasing albumin concentration than by the concentration of oleate *per se*. These data, which are virtually identical to those previously obtained with the isolated perfused rat liver[13], indicate that the albumin receptor phenomenon, what-ever it is, resides within the hepatocyte *per se* and is not dependent on anatomic features of the lobular architecture. Similar conclusions have also been drawn from studies of iopanoic acid uptake[33].

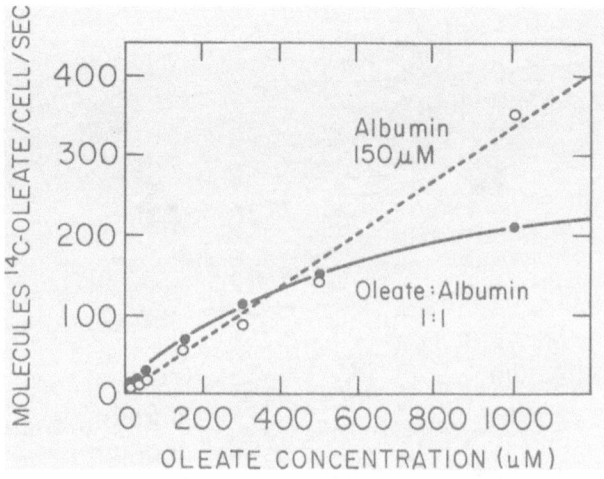

Figure 3.7 Influence of bovine serum albumin on uptake of [^{14}C]-oleate by isolated rat hepatocytes. In one study (O----O) a constant albumin concentration of 150 μmol/l was employed; in the other (●——●) various concentrations of [^{14}C]-oleate were incubated as a 1 : 1 complex with albumin

CONCLUSIONS

The hepatocellular uptake characteristics of such diverse classes of albumin bound organic anions as bile acids, free fatty acids and non-bile cholephils such as BSP and bilirubin have thus been shown to have numerous analogous features (Figure 3.8). All are transported in plasma tightly bound to albumin. For all three classes of albumin bound organic anions, some form of inter-action with the liver cell surface, presumably with the sinusoidal plasma membrane, accelerates the dissociation of ligand from albumin, making it more readily available to an intrinsic membrane binding protein which plays a critical role in the transport of the ligand into the cell. For each class of organic anion, a cytosolic binding protein is present in the cellular interior. Finally, for each anion class under discussion, some form of linkage with the transmembrane flux of an inorganic ion has been suggested by experimental

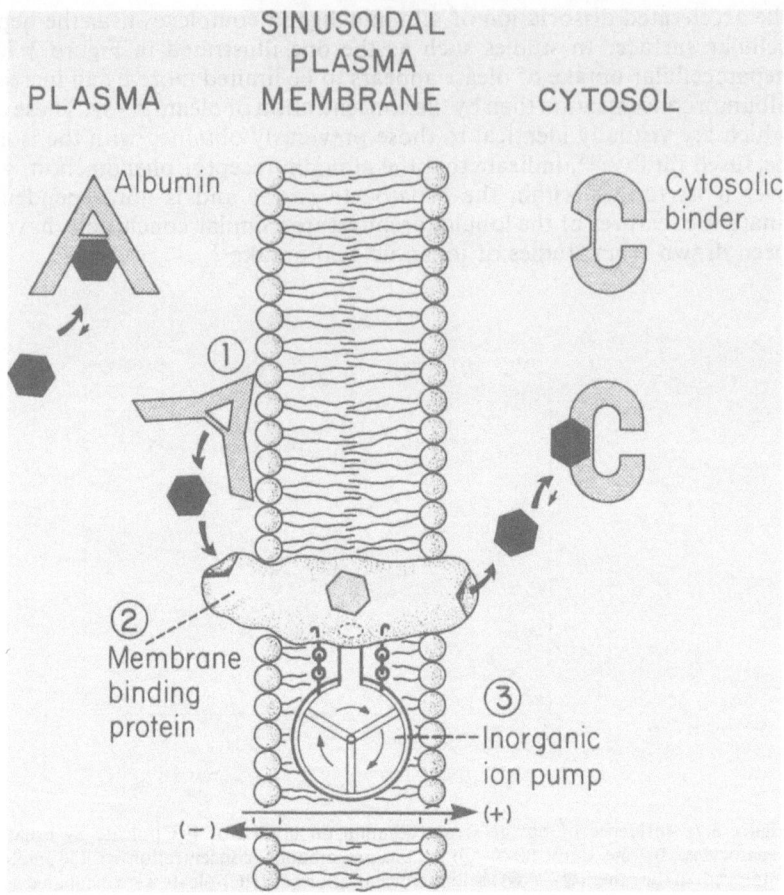

Figure 3.8 Scheme illustrating principal known features of the hepatocellular uptake mechanism for albumin-bound organic anions. Major areas of current interest include: (1) nature of the apparent surface-mediated dissociation of albumin : ligand complexes; (2) roles of the various liver plasma membrane organic anion binding proteins; and (3) nature of the relationship between organic anion transport and various membrane inorganic ion pumps

data, although the exact nature of the linkage between the pumping of inorganic ions and the transfer of organic anions remains to be established.

Research in the field of organic anion transport by the liver has moved progressively from intact man or animal to isolated organ, isolated liver cell, subcellular membrane fractions and purified proteins. A major direction of future work will certainly combine monoclonal antibody techniques with those of molecular biology to clone genes for the already identified membrane acceptor proteins. This step will open up new approaches to fundamental issues in membrane transport.

Acknowledgements

These studies were supported by Grants AM-26438 from the National Institute of Arthritis, Diabetes, Digestive and Kidney Disease (NIH), Bethesda, MD, USA, and Grant STR, 216/2-1/2 from the Deutsche Forschungsgemeinschaft, Bonn, West Germany, as well as generous gifts from the Jack Martin Fund and the Polly Annenberg Levee Charitable Trust. The authors are indebted to Sharon Bloomfield for the rapid and accurate preparation of the manuscript.

References

1. Heinz, E. (1978). *Mechanics and Energetics of Biological Transport*. (New York: Springer)
2. Reichen, J. and Paumgartner, G. (1975). Kinetics of taurocholate uptake by the perfused rat liver. *Gastroenterology*, **68**, 132-6
3. Scharschmidt, B. F. (1982). Bile formation and cholestasis. In Zakim, D. and Boyer, T. D. (eds.) *Hepatology*. pp. 297-335. (Philadelphia: W. B. Saunders)
4. Scharschmidt, B. F., Waggoner, J. G. and Berk, P. D. (1975). Hepatic organic anion uptake in the rat. *J. Clin. Invest.*, **56**, 1280-92
5. Stremmel, W., Tavoloni, N. and Berk, P. D. (1983). Uptake of bilirubin by the liver. *Semin. Liver Dis.*, **3**, 1-10
6. Wolkoff, A. W., Goresky, C. A., Sellin, J., Gatmaitan, Z. and Arias, I. M. (1979). Role of ligandin in transfer of bilirubin from plasma into liver. *Am. J. Physiol.*, **236**, E638-E648
7. Mahadevan, S. and Sauer, F. (1974). Effect of trypsin, phospholipases, and membrane-impermeable reagents on the uptake of palmitic acid by isolated rat liver cells. *Arch. Biochem. Biophys.*, **164**, 185-93
8. Berk, P. D., Stremmel, W., Okuda, H., Tavoloni, N., Kochwa, S., Potter, B., Nunes, R., Shepard, M. and Kiang, C.-L. (1985). Mechanisms of hepatic bilirubin uptake. In Brunner, H. and Thaler, H. (eds.) *Hepatology 1983: Festschrift for Hans Popper*. (New York: Raven)
9. Kramer, W., Buscher, H.-P., Gerok, K. and Kurz, G. (1979). Bile salt binding to serum components. Taurocholate incorporation into high-density lipoprotein revealed by photo-affinity labelling. *J. Biochem.*, **102**, 1-9
10. Baker, K. J. and Bradley, S. E. (1966). Binding of sulfobromophthalein (BSP) sodium by plasma albumin. Its role in hepatic BSP extraction. *J. Clin. Invest.*, **45**, 281-7
11. Jacobsen, J. (1969). Binding of bilirubin to human serum albumin - determination of the dissociation constants. *FEBS Lett.*, **5**, 112-14
12. Goodman, D. S. (1958). The interaction of human serum albumin with long-chain fatty acid anions. *J. Am. Chem. Soc.*, **80**, 3892-8
13. Weisiger, R., Gollan, J. and Ockner, R. (1981). Receptor for albumin on the liver cell surface may mediate uptake of fatty acids and other albumin-bound substances. *Science*, **211**, 1048-51
14. Ockner, R. K., Weisiger, R. A. and Gollan, J. L. (1983). Hepatic uptake of albumin-bound substances: albumin receptor concept. *Am. J. Physiol.*, **245**, G13-G18
15. Forker, E. L. and Luxon, B. A. (1981). Albumin helps mediate removal of taurocholate by rat liver. *J. Clin. Invest.*, **67**, 1517-22
16. Forker, E. L., Luxon, B. A., Snell, M. and Shurmantine, W. O. (1982). Effect of albumin binding on the hepatic transport of rose bengal: surface-mediated dissociation of limited capacity. *J. Pharmacol. Exp. Therapeut.*, **223**, 342-7
17. Kramer, W., Bickel, U., Buscher, H.-P., Gerok, W. and Kurz, G. (1982). Bile salt-binding polypeptides in plasma membranes of hepatocytes revealed by photoaffinity labeling. *Eur. J. Biochem.*, **129**, 13-24
18. Levy, D. and von Dippe, P. (1983). Reconstitution of the bile acid transport system derived from hepatocyte sinusoidal membranes. *Hepatology*, **3**, 837 (Abstr.)
19. Reichen, J. and Berk, P. D. (1979). Isolation of an organic anion binding protein from rat liver plasma membrane fractions by affinity chromatography. *Biochem. Biophys. Res. Commun.*, **91**, 484-9

20. Stremmel, W., Gerber, M. A., Glezerov, V., Thung, S. N., Kochwa, S. and Berk, P. D. (1983). Physicochemical and immunohistological studies of a sulfobromophthalein- and bilirubin-binding protein from rat liver plasma membranes. *J. Clin. Invest.*, **71**, 1796–805

21. Wolkoff, A. W. and Chung, C. T. (1980). Identification, purification and partial characterization of an organic anion binding protein from rat liver cell plasma membranes. *J. Clin. Invest.*, **65**, 1152–61

22. Stremmel, W., Strohmeyer, G., Borchard, F., Kochwa, S. and Berk, P. D. (1983). Isolation and partial characterization of a fatty acid binding protein from rat liver plasma membranes. *Hepatology*, **3**, 823 (Abstr.)

23. Levi, A. J., Gatmaitan, Z. and Arias, I. M. (1969). Two hepatic cytoplasmic protein fractions, Y and Z, and their possible role in the hepatic uptake of bilirubin, sulfobromophthalein and other anions. *J. Clin. Invest.*, **48**, 2156–67

24. Ockner, R. K., Manning, J. A., Poppenhausen, R. B. and Ho, W. K. L. (1972). A binding protein for fatty acids in cytosol of intestinal mucosa, liver, myocardium and other tissues. *Science*, **177**, 56–8

25. Sugiyama, Y., Yamada, T. and Kaplowitz, N. (1983). Newly identified bile acid binding proteins in rat liver cytosol: purification and comparison with glutathione-S-transferases. *J. Biol. Chem.*, **258**, 3602–7

26. De Grella, R. F. and Light, R. J. (1980). Uptake and metabolism of fatty acids by dispersed adult rat heart myocytes. *J. Biol. Chem.*, **255**, 9731–8 and 9739–49

27. Berry, M. N. and Friend, D. S. (1969). High yield preparation of isolated rat liver parenchymal cells: a biochemical and fine structural study. *J. Cell Biol.*, **43**, 506–20

28. Inoue, M., Kinne, R., Tran, T. and Arias, I. M. (1982). Taurocholate transport by rat liver sinusoidal membrane vesicles: Evidence of sodium co-transport. *Hepatology*, **2**, 572–9

29. Gerritsen, W. J., Verkley, A. J., Zwall, R. F. A. and Van Deenen, L. L. M. (1978). Freeze-fracture appearance and disposition of band 3 protein from the human erythrocyte membrane in lipid vesicles. *Eur. J. Biochem.*, **85**, 255–61

30. Reichen, J., Blitzer, B. L. and Berk, P. D. (1981). Binding of unconjugated and conjugated sulfobromophthalein to rat liver plasma membrane fractions *in vitro*. *Biochim. Biophys. Acta*, **640**, 298–312

31. Weisiger, R. A. (1983). Organic anion uptake limited by the rate of dissociation from albumin: predictions of a new general formulation for the "classical" uptake model. *Hepatology*, **3**, 869 (Abstr.)

32. Stremmel, W., Potter, B. J. and Berk, P. D. (1983). Studies of albumin binding to rat liver plasma membranes: Implication for the albumin receptor hypothesis. *Biochim. Biophys. Acta*, **756**, 20–7

33. Barnhart, J. L., Witt, B. L. and Hardison, W. G. (1983). Uptake of iopanoic acid by isolated rat hepatocytes in primary culture. *Am. J. Physiol.*, **244**, G630–G636

4
Biochemical pathways of transforming cholesterol

P. BACK

Cholesterol is virtually insoluble in water. Cholesterol is absorbed to a considerable extent from food sources and, in addition, is synthesized predominantly in the liver. The question, what happens to cholesterol, how is it excreted, is fundamental to our understanding of cholesterol homeostasis, and is intimately linked to problems related to pathological conditions of accumulation of cholesterol, such as hypercholesterolaemia, cholestasis, atherosclerosis and cholesterol gallstone disease.

In the plasma cholesterol is transported by lipoproteins, in the bile as a complex with phospholipids and bile acids. In the faeces water-insoluble neutral sterols are found in great amounts, but none of these mechanisms actually dissolve cholesterol.

We do not yet understand how cholesterol is transported throughout the cells; sterol carrier proteins mediating the transfer of molecules bound to membrane structures such as endoplasmic reticulum and mitochondria, are found in the cytosol[1-6].

This brief review, therefore, deals with the biochemical pathways encountered in man, which transform the molecule to a state of water-solubility. Obviously they have a long evolutionary history, and they are by no means fully explored.

The conventional view depicts the molecule as quite sheltered in the membrane. The single alcoholic group is positioned close to the positively charged end-group of choline of the phospholipid.

According to Danielsson and Sjövall[7] the first step in transforming cholesterol in the liver is the cytochrome P_{450}-mediated 7α-hydroxylation. This is a microsomally bound reaction requiring phospholipid in reconstituted systems which, however, need a cytosolic protein[8]. The formation of the reactive oxygen species during oxidation is not clear. It therefore seems permitted to recall Boyd's hypothesis[9] of 7α-hydroxylation, which postulates a fatty acid hydroperoxide in the reaction. This mechanism seems to be of interest[10] in view of the peroxidase function of cytochrome P_{450}.

There is also a mitochondrial 26-hydroxylation which, however, eventually leads to monohydroxy bile acids that remain lipophilic compounds, a true cul de sac pathway.

Other primary hydroxylations at the molecule are found in the adrenals, which will not be dealt with further, and in the animal kingdom, where 25-hydroxylation and 15-hydroxylation are pathways of high biological significance.

Esterification of cholesterol, on the other hand, renders the molecule more lipophilic. The acyl-CoA-cholesterolacyltransferase is stimulated by 25-hydroxycholesterol[11]. It is tempting to speculate that cholesterylesters are increasingly formed as soon as the first transforming reactions leading to the bile acids are impaired[12], such as in Wolman's disease. But the occurrence of 7α-hydroxycholesterylesters and 5,6-epoxycholesterylesters in this disease may equally well be explained by a deficiency of the next step in the transformation of the sterol nucleus, namely dehydrogenation of the 3β-hydroxy-group and isomerization of the Δ^5-configuration to a Δ^4-configuration.

The following 12α-hydroxylation is the branching point for synthesis of cholic and chenodeoxycholic acids. This reaction also takes place in the microsomal fraction. It requires coplanar steroidal substrates and is influenced by the thyroidal state. Hyper- and hypocholesterolaemias in dysfunction states of the thyroid gland may find their explanation, if the different solubilities required for intestinal reabsorption of the respective bacterial catabolites of the primary bile acids are considered. The reduction of the Δ^4-bond to 5β-H-compounds takes place in the cytosol. It seems, as if the microsomal 5α-reductase is inhibited in vivo[13], or that substrate does not normally reach the enzyme due to subcellular compartmentation. Studies performed by Cronholm[14] and Vlahcevic et al.[15], who labelled different NADPH-pools, support this contention. The 3α-steroid-dehydrogenase is again cytosolic.

In man the cholestane-diols and -triols formed are hydroxylated in position C_{26} by mitochondria. The 26-hydroxylation of cholesterol mentioned above may represent a minor pathway, possibly restricted to mitochondrial cholesterol, since the end product 3β-hydroxy-5-cholenoic acid as sulphate can be found only in trace amounts in bile of normal adults[16], and seems to originate from a different cholesterol pool, which is not labelled by exogenously administered labelled cholesterol[17]. However, this latter pathway seems to play a major role in the prenatal state[18] and under the conditions of cholestasis[17, 19].

The lack of mitochondrial 26-hydroxylase is the primary defect in cerebrotendinous xanthomatosis, a rare inherited disease[20]. It is compensated for by multiple microsomal side chain hydroxylations. These patients excrete large amounts of cholestane-tetrols and -pentols, in the urine, all of which are coupled to glucuronic acid[21] at C_3. Thus, side chain hydroxylations alone seemingly do not render the steroids water-soluble, but anionic groups at either part of the molecule at C_3 or at the side chain are required, as can be found elsewhere in nature[22].

Cytosolic enzymes catalyse the subsequent oxidations at C_{26} with formation of coprostanoic acids. These accumulate in Zellweger's syndrome because the subsequent step of 24-hydroxylation cannot be performed in these patients, who lack microbodies in the liver[23]. The peroxisomes have been shown to conduct β-oxidation of 24-hydroxylated coprostanoyl-CoA[24], similar to peroxisomal β-oxidation of fatty acids[25].

Conjugation with glycine or taurine are the final steps in the formation of the bile salts. The problem of making cholesterol soluble may seem to be solved at this stage of affairs. However, a considerable lipophilicity remains with the molecules ultimately formed, and is the reason for their efficient enterohepatic circulation and poor excretability with the urine.

In cholestatic liver disease the detergent-like properties may be harmful for the hepatocyte[26]. In addition, impaired 7α-hydroxylation in cholestatic liver disease[27] may result in increased formation of monohydroxy bile acids by the mitochondrial pathway of cholesterol catabolism[28], which itself may worsen the pathological condition.

There is, however, sulphation and glucuronidation at C_3 of bile acids in cholestasis. These typical phase-II-reactions yield quite soluble substances, which can be found preferentially in the urine of patients. However, their renal clearance is low[29], and these mechanisms remain inefficient in resolving a cholestatic condition.

Truly hydrophilic compounds eventually result from additional hydroxylation of the steroid nucleus. Atypical hydroxylations of steroids are common events in the prenatal phase, and it was a surprise to find these under the pathological conditions in cholestasis[30]. Tetrahydroxy bile acids are formed from cholic acid and trihydroxy compounds from chenodeoxycholic acid and deoxycholic acid. The hydroxylations occur mainly in the 1β- and 6α- and

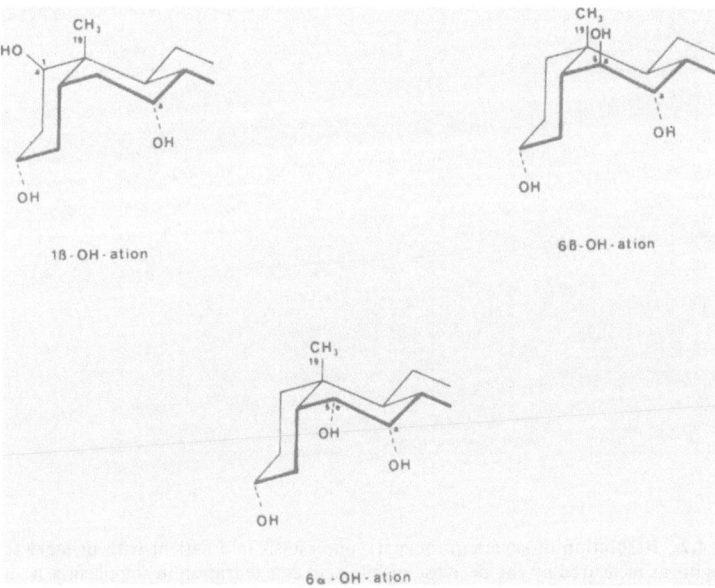

Figure 4.1 Atypical hydroxylations in cholestasis

6β-position. Since these hydroxylations are inducible by phenobarbital[31, 32] their microsomal site as well as the involvement of cytochrome P_{450} seems most likely. Particularly interesting is the attack on the lipophilic backbone of the steroid nucleus, most convincing in 1β- and 6β-hydroxylations, but also by the introduction of an equatorial hydroxyl group in the 6α-position. NMR studies[33] reveal considerable shielding effects on the C_{19} angular methyl protons due to the β-position of the hydroxy groups (Figure 4.1).

In the light of recent studies by Roda *et al.*[34], the introduction of an equatorial hydroxy group at C_6 may also alter the critical micellar concentrations of those compounds and possibly their hydrophilicity.

The biological concept of rendering the original cholesterol molecule water-soluble by virtue of converting it to atypically nucleus-hydroxylated bile acids has led to a recent therapeutic success in intrahepatic cholestasis. By stimulation of atypical hydroxylations with phenobarbital, severe intrahepatic cholestatic conditions can be treated effectively, as long as the inducing dose of the drug is high enough and is administered long enough. An example is given in Figure 4.2, where resolution of an extreme intrahepatic cholestasis resulted within several weeks.

The excretion of the new bile acid 1β, 3α, 7α, 12α-tetrahydroxy-5β-cholanoic acid into urine was high in phenobarbital treated patients, so that its isolation was possible as the methyl ester, and I am pleased to present those crystals, as Figure 4.3, on your 60th birthday to you, Dr Falk.

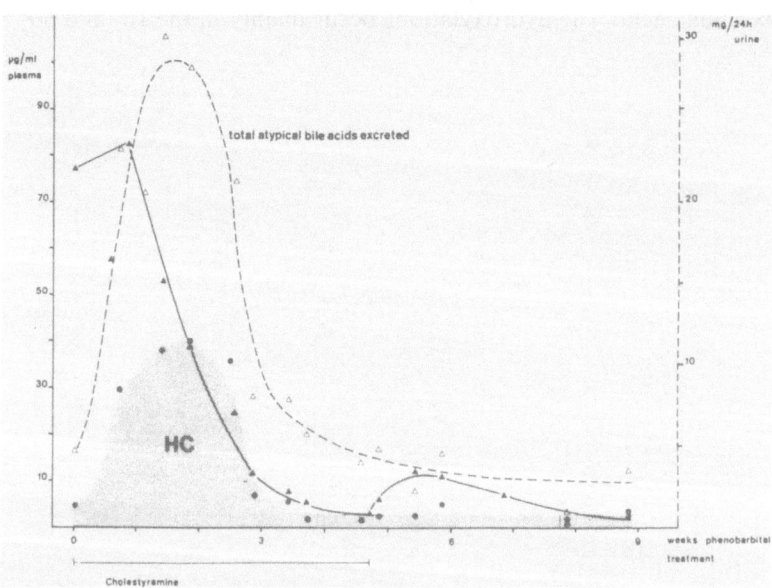

Figure 4.2 Resolution of severe intrahepatic cholestasis in a patient with primary sclerosing cholangitis as measured by the decrease of bile acid concentration in the plasma ▲——▲ and urinary excretion of atypically hydroxylated bile acids △------△ under induction therapy with phenobarbital. HC = hyocholic acid

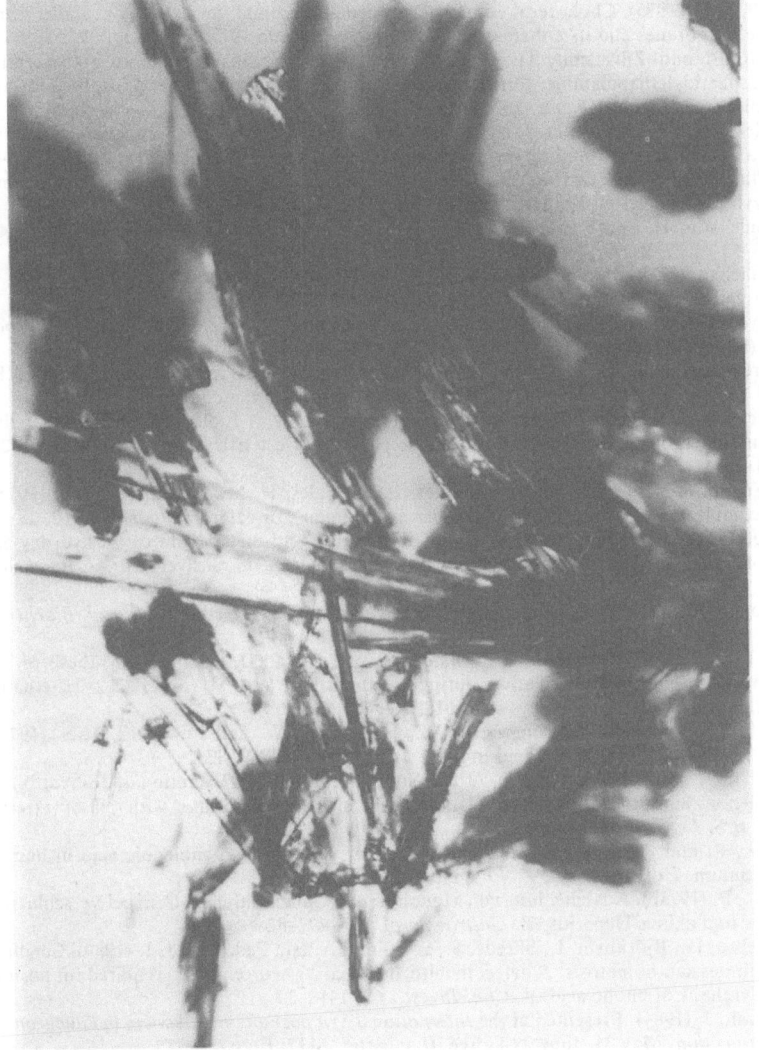

Figure 4.3 Methyl-1β,3α,7α,12α-tetrahydroxy-5β-cholanoate isolated from urine of a patient treated with phenobarbital because of recurrent intrahepatic cholestasis

References

1. Reyes, H., Levi, A. J., Gatmaitan, Z. and Arias, I. M. (1971). Studies of Y and Z, two hepatic cytoplasmic organic anion-binding proteins: Effect of drugs, chemicals, hormones, and cholestasis. *J. Clin. Invest.*, **50**, 2242-52
2. Ritter, M. C. and Dempsey, M. E. (1973). Squalene and sterol carrier protein: Structural properties, lipid binding, and function in cholesterol biosynthesis. *Proc. Nat. Acad. Sci. (USA)*, **70**, 265-9
3. Bell, F. P. (1975). Cholesterol exchange between microsomal, mitochondrial and erythrocyte membranes and its enhancement by cytosol. *Biochim. Biophys. Acta*, **398**, 18-27
4. Bloj, B. and Zilversmit, D. B. (1977). Rat liver proteins capable of transforming phosphatidylethanolamine. Purification and transfer activity for other phospholipids and cholesterol. *J. Biol. Chem.*, **252**, 1613-19
5. Erickson, S. K., Meyer, D. J. and Gould, R. G. (1978). Purification and characterization of a new cholesterol-binding protein from rat liver cytosol. *J. Biol. Chem.*, **253**, 1817-26
6. Billheimer, J. T. and Gaylor, J. L. (1980). Cytosolic modulators of activities of microsomal enzymes of cholesterol biosynthesis. *J. Biol. Chem.*, **255**, 8128-35
7. Danielsson, H. and Sjövall, J. (1975). Bile acid metabolism. *Ann. Rev. Biochem.*, **44**, 233-53
8. Danielsson, H., Kalles, I. and Wikvall, K. (1984). Regulation of hydroxylations in biosynthesis of bile acids. *J. Biol. Chem.*, **259**, 4258-62
9. Boyd, G. S. (1962). Effect of linoleate and estrogen on cholesterol metabolism. *Fed. Proc.*, **21** (Suppl. 11), 86-92
10. Orrenius, S. and Sies, H. (1982). Compartmentation of detoxication reactions. In Sies, H. (ed.) *Metabolic Compartmentation*. pp. 485-520. (London: Academic Press)
11. Erickson, S. K. (1984). Report on the American Society of Biological Chemists Satellite Conference on regulation of intracellular cholesterol esterification. *J. Lipid Res.*, **25**, 411-15
12. Assmann, G., Fredrickson, D. S., Sloan, H. R., Fales, H. M. and Highet, R. J. (1975). Accumulation of oxygenated steryl esters in Wolman's disease. *J. Lipid Res.*, **16**, 28-38
13. Björkhem, I. and Einarsson, K. (1970). Formation and metabolism of 7α-hydroxy-5α-cholestan-3-one and $7\alpha,12\alpha$-dihydroxy-5α-cholestan-3-one in rat liver. *Eur. J. Biochem.*, **13**, 174-9
14. Cronholm, T. (1972). Steroid metabolism in rats given [1-^{2}H$_2$] ethanol. *Eur. J. Biochem.*, **27**, 10-22
15. Vlahcevic, Z. R., Cronholm, T., Curstedt, T. and Sjövall, J. (1980). Biosynthesis of 5α- and 5β-cholanoic acid derivatives during metabolism of [1,1-^{2}H]- and [2,2,2-^{2}H]-ethanol in the rat. *Biochim. Biophys. Acta*, **618**, 369-77
16. Matern, S., Sjövall, J., Pomare, E. W., Heaton, K. W. and Low-Beer, T. S. (1975). Metabolism of deoxycholic acid in man. *Med. Biol.*, **53**, 107-13
17. Makino, I., Sjövall, J., Norman, A. and Strandvik, B. (1971). Excretion of 3β-hydroxy-5-cholenoic and 3α-hydroxy-5α-cholanoic acids in urine of infants with biliary atresia. *F.E.B.S. Lett.*, **15**, 161-4
18. Back, P. and Ross, K. (1973). Identification of 3β-hydroxy-5-cholenoic acid in human meconium. *Hoppe-Seyler's Z. Physiol. Chem.*, **354**, 83-9
19. Back, P. (1973b). Ausscheidung von Monohydroxy-Gallensäuren im Urin bei Verschlussikterus und akuter Hepatitis. *Z. Gastroenterol.*, **11**, 477-82
20. Oftebro, H., Björkhem, I., Skrede, S., Schreiner, A. and Pedersen, J. I. (1980). Cerebrotendinous xanthomatosis. A defect in mitochondrial 26-hydroxylation required for normal biosynthesis of cholic acid. *J. Clin. Invest.*, **65**, 1418-30
21. Sjövall, J. (1984). Presented at the *International Symposium on Advances in Glucuronide Conjugation*, May 31-June 2. Titisee. (Lancaster: MTP Press)
22. Haslewood, G. A. D. (1978). *The Biological Importance of Bile Acids*. (Amsterdam, New York, Oxford: North-Holland)
23. Hanson, R. F., Szczeponik-van Leuwen, P. A., Williams, G. C., Grabowski, G. and Sharp, H. L. (1979). Defects of bile acid synthesis in Zellweger's syndrome. *Science*, **203**, 1107-8
24. Pedersen, J. I. and Gustafsson, J. (1980). Conversion of 3α-, 7α-, 12α-trihydroxy-5β-cholestanoic acid into cholic acid by rat liver peroxisomes. *F.E.B.S. Lett.*, **121**, 345-8

25. Lazarow, P. B. (1982). Compartmentation of β-oxidation of fatty acids in peroxisomes. In Sies, H. (ed.) *Metabolic Compartmentation*. pp. 317–29. (London: Academic Press)
26. Greim, H. (1976). Bile acids in hepatobiliary diseases. In Nair, P. P. and Kritchevsky, D. (eds.) *The Bile Acids*. Vol. 3, pp. 53–80. (New York, London: Plenum Press)
27. Salen, G., Nicolau, G., Shefer, S. and Mosbach, E. H. (1975). Hepatic cholesterol metabolism in patients with gall-stones. *Gastroenterology*, **69**, 676–84
28. Back, P. (1973a). Die primäre Synthese von Mono-Hydroxy-Gallensäuren bei extrahepatischer Gallengangsatresie. *Klin. Wochenschr.*, **51**, 926–32
29. Back, P. and Gerok, W. (1977). Differences in renal excretion between glyco-, tauroconjugates, sulfoconjugates and glucuronoconjugates of bile acids in cholestasis. In Paumgartner, G. and Stiehl, A. (eds.) *Bile Acid Metabolism in Health and Disease*. pp. 93–100. (Lancaster: MTP Press)
30. Almé, B., Bremmelgaard, A., Sjövall, J. and Thomassen, P. (1977). Analysis of metabolic profiles of bile acids in urine using a lipophilic anion exchanger and computerized gas-liquid chromatography-mass spectrometry. *J. Lipid Res.*, **18**, 339–62
31. Back, P. and Gerok, W. (1978). Zum Effekt des Phenobarbitals bei intrahepatischer Cholestase. Stimulierung der Gallensäuren-6α-Hydroxylierung. *Inn. Med.*, **5**, 329–36
32. Back, P. (1982). Phenobarbital-induced alterations of bile acid metabolism in cases of intrahepatic cholestasis. *Klin. Wochenschr.*, **60**, 541–9
33. Back, P., Fritz, H. and Populoh, C. (1984). The isolation of tetrahydroxy bile acids as methyl esters from human urine and their characterization by ^{1}H- and ^{13}C-nuclear magnetic resonance spectroscopy. *Hoppe-Seyler's Z. Physiol. Chem.*, **365**, 479–84
34. Roda, A., Hofmann, A. F. and Mysels, K. J. (1983). The influence of bile salt structure on self-association in aqueous solutions. *J. Biol. Chem.*, **258**, 6362–70

5
Bile acid metabolism in hepatobiliary diseases

A. STIEHL

ENTEROHEPATIC CIRCULATION OF BILE ACIDS

Bile acids are formed in the liver from cholesterol, and before their excretion into bile they are conjugated at their carboxyl groups with the amino acids glycine or taurine. Monohydroxy bile acids in addition are in part sulphated at their hydroxyl group[1].

After their excretion in bile and intestine the bile acids are deconjugated and dehydroxylated by the intestinal flora. Most of the bile acids are re-absorbed by diffusion in the jejunum or by active transport in the ileum and return via the portal blood to the liver. Only 10% of the bile acid pool is excreted by the faeces per day.

URINARY AND BILIARY EXCRETION OF BILE ACIDS

In patients with hepatobiliary diseases the biliary excretion of bile acids may be diminished (Figure 5.1)[2-4], increased concentrations of bile acids appear in the peripheral blood and are excreted by the urine[5,6]. In patients with biliary obstruction urinary excretion becomes the main route of bile acid excretion[7,8].

In patients with hepatobiliary diseases many bile acids can be detected in urine which are not present in healthy man[9-11]. These bile acids include 3β-hydroxy-5-cholenoic acid, hyodeoxycholic acid, hyocholic acid, tetra-hydroxy bile acids and many others. The appearance of these atypical bile acids (Figure 5.2) is the result of abnormal hydroxylation reactions in the liver[11].

Another alteration of bile acid metabolism in hepatobiliary diseases represents the sulphation and glucuronidation of bile acids at their hydroxyl groups [5,6,12-19]. While in healthy man only monohydroxy bile acids are sulphated in greater amounts, patients with hepatobiliary diseases also

61

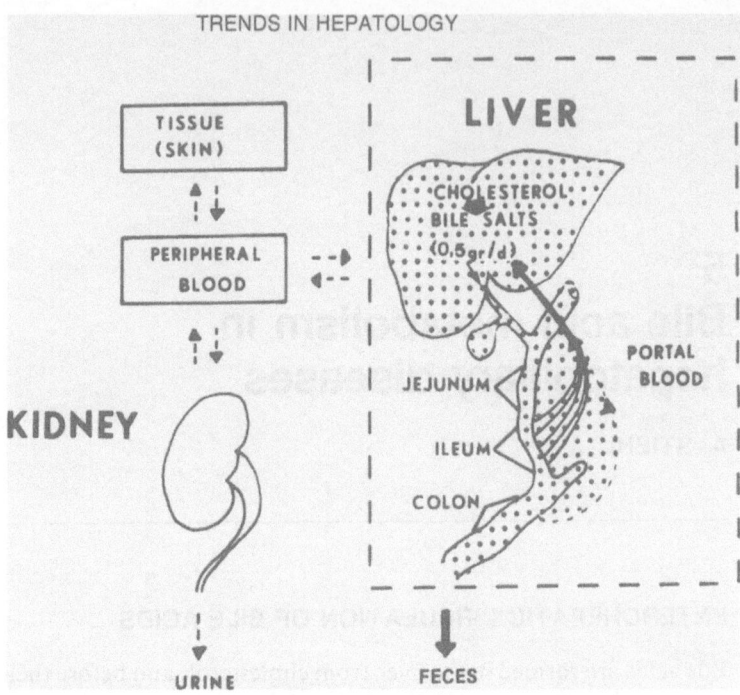

Figure 5.1 Enterohepatic circulation of bile acids in patients with hepatobiliary diseases. Plasma concentrations of bile acids increase and lead to increased urinary excretion of bile acids

sulphate and glucuronide di- and trihydroxy bile acids. More than 70% of the bile acids excreted in urine are sulphated or glucuronidated. Sulphation of bile acids decreases with the number of hydroxyl groups[10, 18]. The position of the hydroxyl group is of importance for the glucuronidation, with 6α-hydroxyl groups being a preferred substrate[20-22]. Tetrahydroxy bile acids are excreted in urine only in the non-sulphated, non-glucuronidated form. The majority of bile acid sulphates and bile acid glucuronides is in addition conjugated with taurine or glycine.

In the bile of patients with hepatobiliary diseases the proportion of sulphates and glucuronides is much smaller than in urine. Studies on the quantitative excretion of these molecules in bile of patients with cirrhosis of the liver indicate, however, that the biliary excretion of bile acid sulphates is 10 times greater and the biliary excretion of bile acid glucuronides is 20 times greater than in urine. It can be expected, however, that in the more severe forms of cholestasis the urinary excretion of sulphated and glucuronidated bile acids will become more important.

TURNOVER OF BILE ACIDS IN HEPATOBILIARY DISEASE

Data on the kinetics of bile acids are available for the non-sulphated, non-glucuronidated and for the sulphated bile acids but not for the glucuronides. In patients with cirrhosis of the liver, pool sizes and synthesis rates of cholic

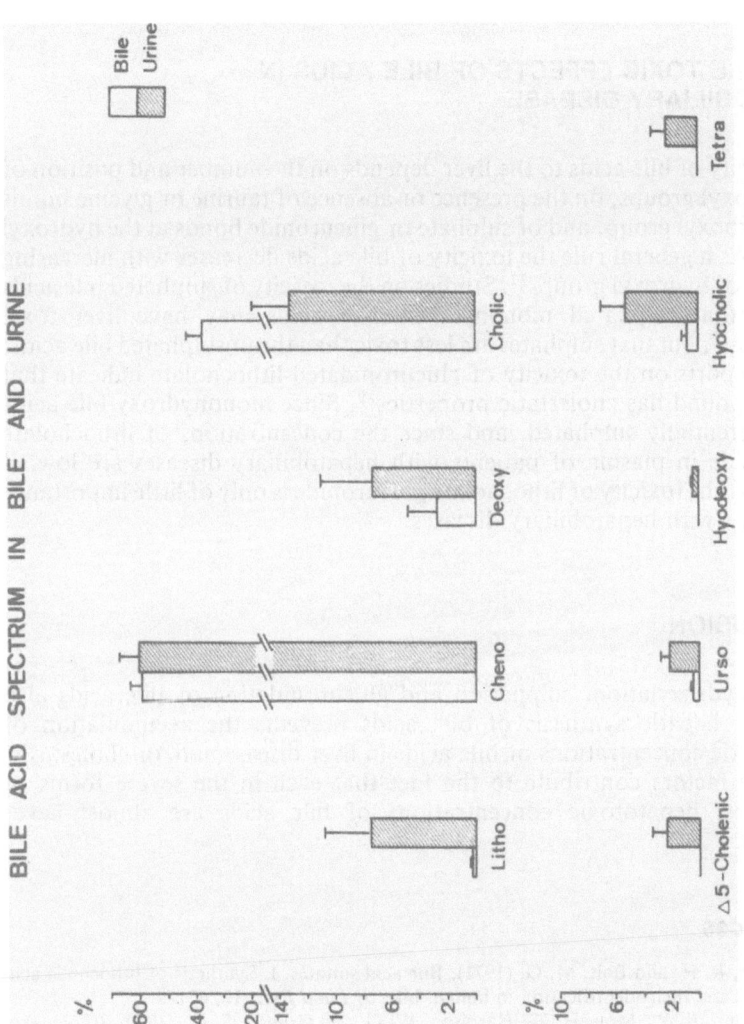

Figure. 5.2 Bile acid spectrum in bile and urine of patients with alcoholic cirrhosis of the liver. Litho = lithocholic acid; cheno = chenodeoxycholic acid; deoxy = deoxycholic acid; cholic = cholic acid; 5-cholenic = 3β-hydroxy-5-cholenoic acid; urso = ursodeoxycholic acid; hyodeoxy = hyodeoxycholic acid; hyocholic = hyocholic acid; tetra = tetrahydroxy bile acids. It is apparent that the 6α-hydroxylated bile acids (hyodeoxycholic acid and hyocholic acid) and the tetrahydroxylated bile acids appear preferentially or exclusively in urine

acid and of chenodeoxycholic acid are diminished[25, 26]. The metabolic half-life of sulphated bile acids is shorter than that of non-sulphated bile acids[23]. Chenodeoxycholate is sulphated to a much greater extent than cholate[23]. Greater clearance rates in the kidneys[13] and decreased absorption in the intestine[24] are the two factors which are responsible for the more rapid turnover of sulphated bile acids in comparison to the non-sulphated bile acids[23]. Thus sulphation contributes to a more rapid elimination of bile acids in hepatobiliary diseases.

POSSIBLE TOXIC EFFECTS OF BILE ACIDS IN HEPATOBILIARY DISEASE

The toxicity of bile acids to the liver depends on the number and position of the hydroxyl groups, on the presence or absence of taurine or glycine bonds at the carboxyl group, and of sulphate or glucuronide bonds at the hydroxyl groups. As a general rule the toxicity of bile acids decreases with increasing numbers of hydroxyl groups[27]. Studies on the toxicity of sulphated bile acids indicate that sulphated monohydroxy bile acids may have liver toxic properties[28], but that sulphates are less toxic than the unsulphated bile acids. Recent reports on the toxicity of glucuronidated lithocholate indicate that this compound has cholestatic properties[29]. Since monohydroxy bile acids are preferentially sulphated, and since the concentrations of lithocholate glucuronide in plasma of patients with hepatobiliary diseases are low, it seems that the toxicity of lithocholate glucuronide is only of little importance in patients with hepatobiliary diseases.

CONCLUSION

Besides hydroxylation, sulphation and glucuronidation of bile acids also decreased hepatic synthesis of bile acids prevents the accumulation of hepatotoxic concentrations of bile acids in liver disease and/or cholestasis. All these factors contribute to the fact that even in the severe forms of cholestasis, hepatotoxic concentrations of bile acids are almost never observed.

References

1. Palmer, R. H. and Bolt, M. G. (1971). Bile acid sulfates. I. Synthesis of lithocholic acid sulfates and their identification in human bile. *J. Lipid Res.*, **12**, 671-9
2. Bergmann, K. V., Mok, H. Y., Hardison, W. G. and Grundy, S. M. (1979). Cholesterol and bile acid metabolism in moderately advanced, stable cirrhosis of the liver. *Gastroenterology*, **77**, 1183-92
3. Schwartz, C. C., Almond, H. R., Vlahcevic, Z. R. and Swell, L. (1979). Bile acid metabolism in cirrhosis. V. Determination of biliary lipid secretion rates in patients with advanced cirrhosis. *Gastroenterology*, **77**, 1177-82

BILE ACID METABOLISM IN HEPATOBILIARY DISEASES

4. Raedsch, R., Stiehl, A., Gundert-Remy, U., Walker, S., Sieg, A., Czygan, P. and Kommerell, B. (1982). Hepatic secretion of bilirubin and biliary lipids in patients with alcoholic cirrhosis of the liver. *Digestion*, **26**, 80-8
5. Stiehl, A. (1972). Bile acid sulphates in intra- and extrahepatic cholestasis. In Back, P. and Gerok, E. (eds.) *Bile Acids in Human Diseases*. pp. 73-7. (Stuttgart: Schattauer)
6. Stiehl, A. (1974). Bile salt sulphates in cholestasis. *Eur. J. Clin. Invest.*, **4**, 59-63
7. Summerfield, J. A., Cullen, J., Barnes, S. and Billing, B. H. (1977). Evidence for renal control of urinary excretion of bile acids and bile acid sulfates in the cholestatic syndrome. *Clin. Sci.*, **52**, 51-65
8. Dooley, J. S., Bartholomew, C., Summerfield, J. A. and Billing, B. H. (1984). The biliary excretion of sulphated and non-sulphated bile acids and bilirubin in patients with external bile drainage. *Clin. Sci.*, **67**, 61-8
9. Summerfield, J. A., Billing, B. H. and Shackleton, C. H. L. (1976). Identification of bile acids in the serum and urine in cholestasis. Evidence for 6-alpha-hydroxylation of bile acids in man. *Biochem. J.*, **154**, 507-16
10. Alme, B., Bremmelgaard, A., Sjövall, J. and Thomassen, P. (1977). Analysis of metabolic profiles of bile acids in urine using a lipophilic anion exchanger and computerized gas liquid chromatography mass spectrometry. *J. Lipid Res.*, **18**, 339-61
11. Bremmelgaard, A. and Sjövall, J. (1980). Hydroxylation of cholic, chenodeoxycholic, and deoxycholic acids in patients with intrahepatic cholestasis. *J. Lipid Res.*, **21**, 1072-81
12. Makino, I., Shinozaki, K., Nakagawa, S. and Mashimo, H. (1975). Measurement of sulfated and nonsulfated bile acids in urine, serum, and bile of patients with hepatobiliary diseases. *Gastroenterology*, **68**, 545-53
13. Stiehl, A., Earnest, D. and Admirand, W. H. (1975). Sulfation and renal excretion of bile salts in patients with cirrhosis of the liver. *Gastroenterology*, **68**, 534-44
14. Back, P., Spaczynski, K. and Gerok, W. (1974). Bile acid glucuronides in urine. *Hoppe-Seyler's Z. Physiol. Chem.*, **335**, 749-52
15. Fröhling, W. and Stiehl, A. (1974). Identification and quantitative analysis of bile acid glucuronides in cholestasis. In Matern, S., Hackenschmidt, J., Back, P. and Gerok, W. (eds.) *Advances in Bile Acid Research*. pp. 153-6. (Stuttgart: Schattauer)
16. Back, P. (1976). Isolation and identification of a chenodeoxycholic acid glucuronide from human plasma in intrahepatic cholestasis. *Hoppe-Seyler's Z. Physiol. Chem.*, **357**, 213-17
17. Fröhling, W. and Stiehl, A. (1976). Bile acid glucuronides: identification and quantitative analysis in the urine of patients with cholestasis. *Eur. J. Clin. Invest.*, **6**, 67-74
18. Stiehl, A., Becker, M., Czygan, P., Fröhling, W., Kommerell, B., Rotthauwe, H. W. and Senn, M. (1980). Bile acids and their sulfated and glucuronidated derivatives in bile, plasma, and urine of children with intrahepatic cholestasis: effects of phenobarbital treatment. *Eur. J. Clin. Invest.*, **10**, 307-16
19. Stiehl, A., Raedsch, R., Rudolph, G., Czygan, P. and Walker, S. (1982). Analysis of bile acid glucuronides in urine: group separation on a lipophilic anion exchanger. *Clin. Chim. Acta*, **123**, 275-85
20. Alme, B., Norden, A. and Sjövall, J. (1970). Glucuronides of unconjugated 6-hydroxylated bile acids in urine of a patient with malabsorption. *Clin. Chim. Acta*, **86**, 251-9
21. Alme, B. and Sjövall, J. (1980). Analysis of bile acid glucuronides in urine. Identification of a 3 alpha, 6 alpha, 12 alpha-trihydroxy-5 beta-cholanoic acid. *J. Steroid Biochem.*, **13**, 907-16
22. Sacquet, E., Parquet, M., Riottot, M., Raizman, M., Jarrige, A., Huguet, C. and Infante, R. (1983). Intestinal absorption, excretion, and biotransformation of hyodeoxycholic acid in man. *J. Lipid Res.*, **24**, 604-13
23. Stiehl, A., Ast, E., Czygan, P., Fröhling, W., Raedsch, R. and Kommerell, B. (1978). Pool size, synthesis, and turnover of sulfated and nonsulfated cholic acid and chenodeoxycholic acid in patients with cirrhosis of the liver. *Gastroenterology*, **74**, 572-7
24. Cowen, A. E., Korman, M. G., Hofmann, A. F. and Cass, O. W. (1975). Metabolism of lithocholate in healthy man. II. Enterohepatic circulation. *Gastroenterology*, **69**, 67-76
25. Vlahcevic, Z. R., Juttijudata, P., Bell, C. C. et al. (1972). Bile acid metabolism in patients with cirrhosis. II. Cholic and chenodeoxycholic acid metabolism. *Gastroenterology*, **62**, 1174-81
26. Einarsson, K., Hellström, K. and Scjersten, T. (1975). The formation of bile acids in patients with portal cirrhosis. *Scand. J. Gastroenterol.*, **10**β, 311-14

27. Greim, H., Trülzsch, D., Czygan, P. *et al.* (1972). Mechanism of cholestasis. 6. Bile acids in human livers with or without biliary obstruction. *Gastroenterology*, **63**, 846-50
28. Yousef, I. M., Tuchweber, B., Vonk, R. J., Masse, M., Audet, M. and Roy, C. C. (1981). Lithocholate cholestasis: sulfated glycolithocholate induced intrahepatic cholestasis in rats. *Gastroenterology*, **80**, 233-41
29. Oelberg, D. G., Chari, M. V., Little, J. M., Adcock, E. W. and Lester, R. (1984). Lithocholate glucuronide is a cholestatic agent. *J. Clin. Invest.*, **73**, 1507-14

6
Effect of female sex hormones on bile acids

F. KERN Jr. AND G. T. EVERSON

The pathogenesis of cholesterol gallstones in women, especially during the childbearing years, and in association with the administration of female sex hormones, is a major interest of our research group. Studies in several laboratories, including ours, have revealed an increase in biliary cholesterol saturation and secretion in pregnant women and in those exposed to birth control pills. The physiological and biochemical mechanisms responsible for this relative increase in cholesterol in the bile are not understood. A list of possible mechanisms, probably an incomplete one, is shown in Table 6.1. We are currently studying several of them.

Increased cholesterol secretion due to altered secretory coupling of biliary lipids, secondary to an increase in the ratio of biliary cholic (CA) to chenodeoxycholic acid (CDCA) is one of the areas of special interest. The purpose of this paper is to briefly review the relevant data, to assess their possible importance and to present preliminary results of current studies.

Bennion and colleagues reported that in prepubertal and immediately post pubertal American Indian boys and girls, there was no sex difference in bile acid composition[1], but in a separate study of Indian and Caucasian adults,

Table 6.1 Possible mechanisms of female sex hormone-induced increase in biliary cholesterol

(1)	Increased cholesterol absorption
(2)	Increased cholesterol synthesis
(3)	Increased hepatic uptake of LP cholesterol
	(a) Exogenous – chylomicrons and VLDL
	(b) Endogenous – VLDL, LDL, HDL
(4)	Decreased hepatic cholesterol esterification
(5)	Differential effects of different bile acids on secretory coupling

VLDL = very low density lipoprotein
LDL = low density lipoprotein
HDL = high density lipoprotein

the same group reported that the total bile acid pool and the CDCA pool was smaller in women than in men[2]. This was not related to body weight, but it was associated with more saturated bile in the women.

We studied a large group of pregnant women and found that as pregnancy progressed the CA in bile increased and the CDCA decreased[3]. This led to an increase in the CA to CDCA ratio from unity in the non-pregnant state and in the first trimester of pregnancy, to a ratio of 2 : 1 in the third trimester. In the only other published study of bile acid composition in pregnant women, Laatikainen and colleagues in Finland found a similar change in all four subjects they studied[4]. In addition, in pregnant women with intrahepatic cholestasis of pregnancy, a group known to be at very high risk for developing cholesterol gallstones, the bile acid pool was 90% CA.

Since there is a wide difference in bile acid metabolism in different animal species, studies in many experimental animals may not be relevant to this problem, but observations in at least two animal species, the baboon and the hamster, are to some extent similar to those in man. In both species, the bile acid composition resembles that in man. In the pregnant baboon, Morrissey et al. reported a 50% decrease in CDCA synthesis rate and pool size, while CA synthesis and pool size did not change[5]. Kuroki et al. found that in female Syrian hamsters the CDCA pool was significantly smaller, and the CA to CDCA ratio was larger than in males[6]. Further, the hepatic and 12α-hydroxylase activity was proportionally increased in females.

Bennion et al. reported a decrease in percentage of chenodeoxycholic acid and an increase in cholic acid in the bile of women during treatment with oral contraceptive steroids containing a mixture of a synthetic oestrogen and progestin[7, 8]. In our study of women using such contraceptive steroids there were similar, but slight and not statistically significant, changes[9]. Thus, evidence suggests that exposure to a mixture of female sex steroid hormones leads to an increase in the biliary CA to CDCA ratio. Heuman et al. reported that ethinyl oestradiol alone had a similar effect in postmenopausal women[10], but Anderson et al. failed to find an effect of this agent on bile acid composition in male subjects[11].

We are currently studying the effects of Premarin on bile acid kinetics and on other aspects of hepatobiliary physiology in postmenopausal women. Thus far we have completed bile acid kinetic studies on eight women, age 28–47. In all of them, menopause had been surgically induced. Each had been given Premarin as replacement therapy for a period of 6 months to as long as 17 years.

Premarin is a complex mixture of nine conjugated oestrogens, about 50% oestrone sulphate, manufactured from pregnant mares' urine[12]. Despite its shortcomings as an ideal study drug and the fact that it has only fairly weak oestrogenic activity, we elected to use it in our study because it is taken by more than 80% of women who receive postmenopausal oestrogenic replacement in the United States. We studied our subjects during Premarin administration and after cessation of therapy for at least 6 weeks.

We estimated bile acid kinetics using [^{13}C]-24-cholic and [^{13}C]-24-chenodeoxycholic acids. We measured isotope ratios by gas chromatography/mass spectroscopy daily for 3–6 days and calculated the usual kinetic parameters by the Lindstedt technique. We measured bile acid isotope ratios in serum, not duodenal, bile acids, employing the techniques of sample preparation and analysis developed and validated in our laboratory[13]. Figure 6.1 shows the type of data obtained in this study.

The results thus far suggest the possibility that Premarin causes a decrease in CDCA pool and in per cent CDCA, but they are not statistically significant. It may be that progestin, not oestrogen, is responsible for this effect.

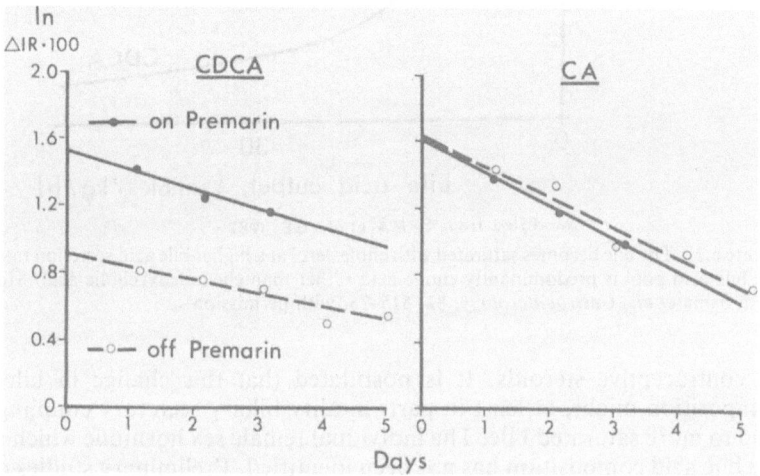

Figure 6.1 This shows the decay of [^{13}C]-24-chenodeoxycholic acid (CDCA) on the left and the decay of [^{13}C]-24-cholic acid (CA) on the right, on and off Premarin therapy, in a 32 year old woman who had undergone a bilateral oophorectomy 6 months before study

It is well established that chronic feeding of CDCA, increasing the proportion of this bile acid in the bile, decreases biliary cholesterol secretion and saturation. Feeding CA has no such effects. In addition, Lindblad et al.[14] and Sama et al.[15] acutely altered bile acid composition in man, and found that different bile acids had different effects on the secretion of biliary lipids. When they increased the percentage of CA in the bile, the bile became saturated with cholesterol at a higher rate of bile acid secretion than after a similar increase in the proportion of CDCA (Figure 6.2). It seems possible that an increased ratio of CA to CDCA circulating through the liver alters the secretory coupling of biliary lipids so that the bile is more lithogenic.

In summary, pregnancy and oral contraceptive steroid use, conditions known to increase the risk of cholesterol gallstones, are associated with more saturated bile due to increased cholesterol secretion. A number of possible mechanisms which might explain the phenomenon are being investigated. In this presentation we have focussed on the change in bile acid composition, namely, a decrease in chenodeoxycholic acid relative to cholic acid, which occurs in the 2nd and 3rd trimesters of pregnancy and during administration

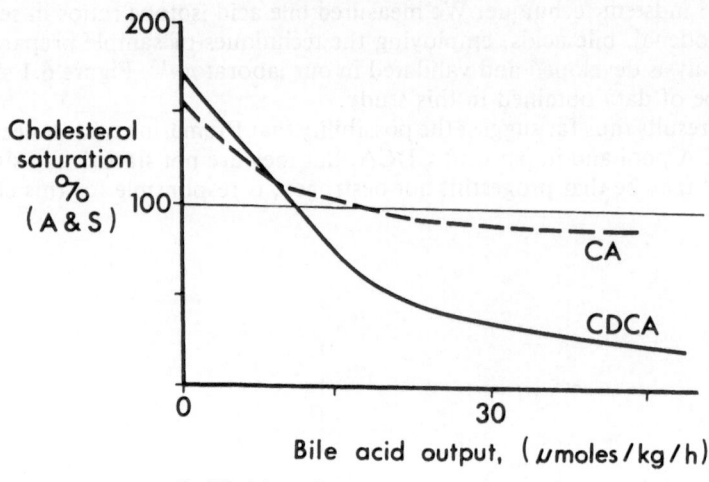

Modified from SAMA et al. GE 1982

Figure 6.2 The bile becomes saturated with cholesterol at a higher bile acid secretion rate when the bile acid pool is predominantly cholic acid rather than chenodeoxycholic acid. Modified from Sama *et al.*, *Gastroenterology*, **82**, 515-25, with permission

of contraceptive steroids. It is postulated that this change in bile acid composition might, at least in part, modify biliary secretory coupling and lead to more saturated bile. The individual female sex hormone which alters the bile acid composition has not been identified. Preliminary studies of the effect of Premarin in postmenopausal women are inconclusive to date.

Acknowledgements

This work was supported by grants from the US Public Health Service, National Institutes of Health, Research Grants AM 19605 and AM 31765. Dr Everson was supported in part by a National Institutes of Health Clinical Investigator Award AM 01156 and in part as a Teaching and Research Scholar of the American College of Physicians. The authors also acknowledge the support of the Kern Research Foundation.

References

1. Bennion, L. J., Knowler, W. C., Mott, D. M., Spagnola, A. M. and Bennett, P. H. (1979). Development of lithogenic bile during puberty in Pima Indians. *N. Engl. J. Med.*, **300**, 873-6
2. Bennion, L. J., Drobny, E., Knowler, W. C., Ginsberg, R. L., Garnick, M. B., Adler, R. D. and Duane, W. C. (1978). Sex differences in the size of bile acid pools. *Metabolism*, **27**, 961-9
3. Kern, F. Jr., Everson, G. T., DeMark, B., McKinley, C., Showalter, R., Erfling, W., Braverman, D. Z., Szczepanik-van Leeuwen, P. and Klein, P. D. (1981). Biliary lipids, bile acids, and gallbladder function in the human female. *J. Clin. Invest.*, **68**, 1229-42
4. Laatikainen, T., Lehtonen, P. and Hesso, A. (1978). Biliary bile acids in uncomplicated pregnancy and in cholestasis of pregnancy. *Clin. Chim. Acta*, **85**, 145-50

5. Morrissey, K., Panveliwalla, D., McSherry, C., Deitrick, J., Niemann, W. and Gupta, G. (1977). Effects of contraceptive steroids and pregnancy on bile composition and kinetics in the baboon. *J. Surg. Res.*, **22**, 598-604
6. Kuroki, S., Muramoto, S., Kuramoto, T. and Hoshita, T. (1983). Sex differences in gallbladder bile acid composition and hepatic steroid 12-hydroxylase activity in hamsters. *J. Lip. Res.*, **24**, 1543-9
7. Bennion, L. J., Ginsberg, R. L., Garnick, M. B. and Bennett, P. H. (1976). Effects of oral contraceptives on the gallbladder bile of normal women. *N. Engl. J. Med.*, **294**, 1189-92
8. Bennion, L. J., Mott, D. M. and Howard, B. V. (1980). Oral contraceptives raise the cholesterol saturation of bile by increasing biliary cholesterol secretion. *Metabolism*, **29**, 18-22
9. Kern, F. Jr., Everson, G. T., DeMark, B., McKinley, C., Showalter, R. and Braverman, D. Z. (1982). Biliary lipids, bile acids, and gallbladder function in the human female: effects of contraceptive steroids. *J. Lab. Clin. Med.*, **99**, 798-805
10. Heuman, R., Larsson-Cohn, U., Hammar, M. and Tiselius, H. G. (1979). Effects of postmenopausal ethinylestradiol treatment on gallbladder bile. *Maturitas*, **2**, 69-72
11. Anderson, A., James, O. F. W., Macdonald, H. S., Snowball, S. and Taylor, W. (1980). The effect of ethynyloestradiol on biliary lipid composition in young men. *Eur. J. Clin. Invest.*, **10**, 77-80
12. Johnson, R., Masserano, R., Haring, R., Kho, B. and Schilling, G. (1975). Quantitative GLC determination of conjugated estrogens in raw materials and finished dosage forms. *J. Pharmaceut. Sci.*, **64**, 1007-11
13. Everson, G. T., Hachey, D., Klein, P., Showalter, R., McKinley, C. and Kern, F. Jr. (1982). Simultaneous serum and biliary chenodeoxycholic (CDC) kinetics using [^{13}C]-CDC. *Gastroenterology*, **82**, 1051
14. Lindblad, L., Lundholm, K. and Schersten, T. (1977). Influence of cholic and chenodeoxycholic acid on biliary cholesterol secretion in man. *Eur. J. Clin. Invest.*, **7**, 383-8
15. Sama, C., LaRusso, N. F., Lopez Del Pino, V. and Thistle, J. L. (1982). Effects of acute bile acid administration on biliary lipid secretion in healthy volunteers. *Gastroenterology*, **82**, 515-25

7
The gallbladder after endoscopic papillotomy

M. CLASSEN, W. KURTZ AND F. HAGENMÜLLER

The extrahepatic part of the biliary system plays an important role in the storage of bile and its transport to the intestine. The gallbladder and the sphincter of Oddi regulate these functions both actively and passively. We have learned that the gallbladder fills when it is empty, and the closed sphincter of Oddi causes the pressure in the common bile duct to increase over the pressure within the gallbladder[1]. But after endoscopic papillotomy (EPT), we have observed patients with a wide open sphincter of Oddi and aerobilia whose gallbladder fills after intravenously administered contrast medium[2]. So, after EPT the gallbladder is not always a backwater for bile flow. Following EPT, potentially life threatening complications, for some patients, may originate here.

STUDY OF THE DIURNAL RHYTHM OF BILIARY LIPIDS AFTER EPT IN PATIENTS WITH AND WITHOUT GALLBLADDER

The investigations were carried out in 28 cholecystectomized patients and in seven patients with functioning gallbladder all of whom had cholecysto-lithiasis. In all patients an endoscopic papillotomy (EPT) had been carried

Table 7.1 Experimental design

Cholecystectomy ($n = 28$)
Functioning gallbladder ($n = 7$)
Endoscopic papillotomy
Nasobiliary drainage
Bile samples (2 ml) at 08.00, 12.00, 16.00, 20.00, 24.00, 04.00, 08.00 h
Cholesterol   : catalase method
Phospholipids   molybdate–vanadate reaction
Bile acids   : 3α-steroid dehydrogenase reaction
Saturation index: according to Carey

out for common bile duct stones, with the consecutive insertion of a nasobiliary drain. The investigations were performed at least one day after the
nasobiliary drain had been inserted; at the start of the investigation signs of
cholestasis had subsided. During the investigation the patients ate normal
hospital meals at 07.30, 11.45 and 17.30 h. 2 ml samples of bile were taken

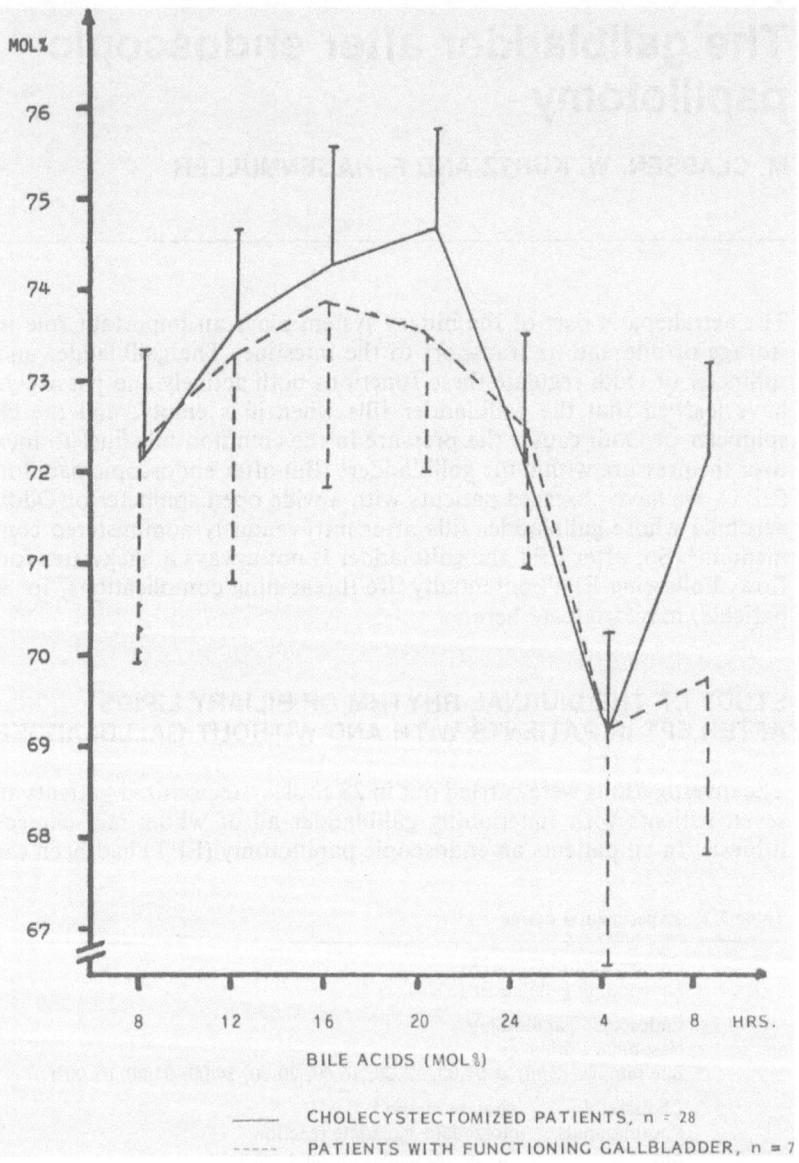

Figure 7.1

at 08.00, 12.00, 16.00, 20.00, 24.00 and 04.00 and 08.00 h the following day (Table 7.1).

In the functioning gallbladder, bile acid concentrations drop between 12.00 and 20.00 h and rise at night; after cholecystectomy the rhythm is always identical, but the diurnal changes always lag 4 h behind normal (Figure 7.1). This may be explained by the fact that in the functioning gallbladder bile acids are more rapidly available for secretion, while after cholecystectomy a greater part of the bile acid pool resides within the intestine, and may only be absorbed after reaching the terminal ileum. The possibility of other explanations, however, cannot be excluded.

So the gallbladder influences the diurnal rhythm of biliary bile acid concentrations but phospholipids (Figure 7.2) and cholesterol (Figure 7.3) are

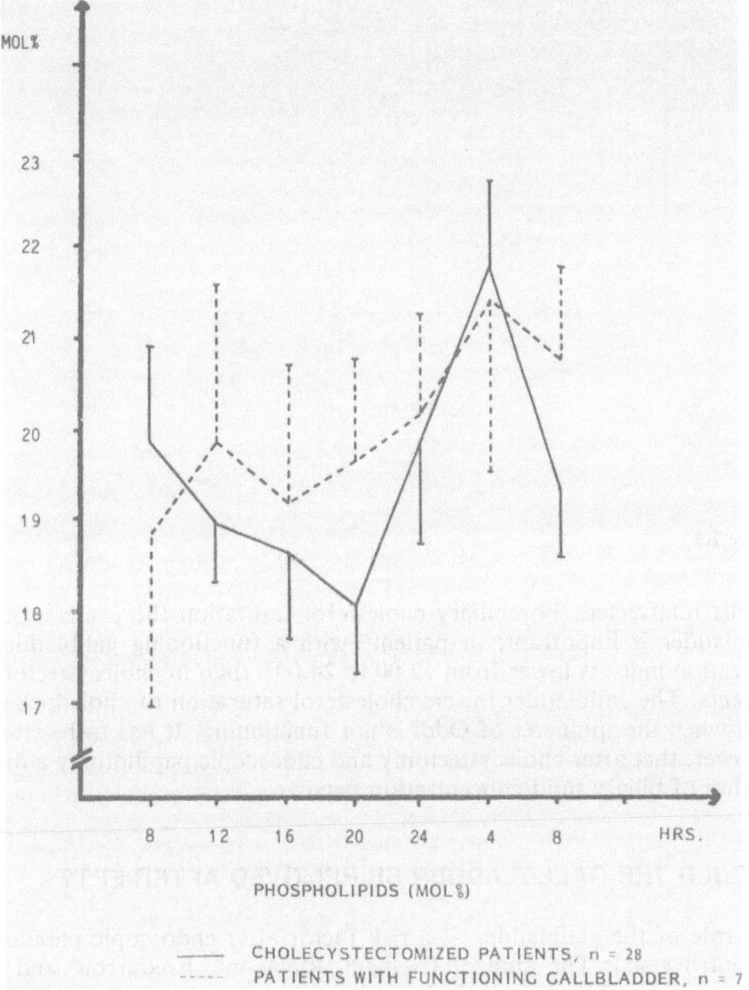

PHOSPHOLIPIDS (MOL%)

——— CHOLECYSTECTOMIZED PATIENTS, n = 28
- - - - PATIENTS WITH FUNCTIONING GALLBLADDER, n = 7

Figure 7.2

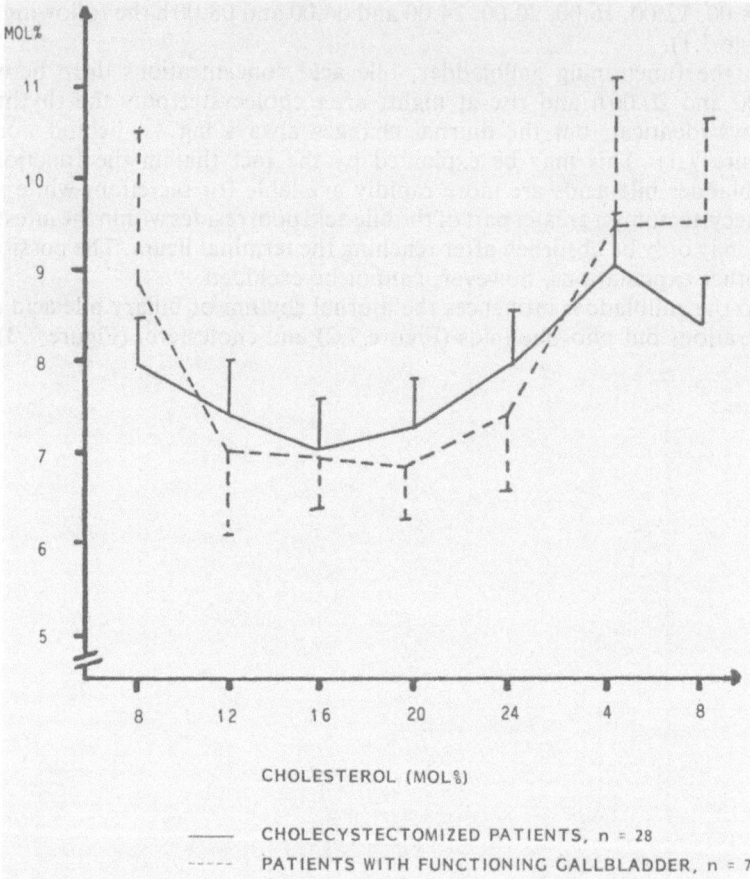

CHOLESTEROL (MOL%)

——— CHOLECYSTECTOMIZED PATIENTS, n = 28

------ PATIENTS WITH FUNCTIONING GALLBLADDER, n = 7

Figure 7.3

almost unaffected. For biliary cholesterol saturation the presence of the gallbladder is important: in patients with a functioning gallbladder the saturation index is lower from 12.00 to 24.00 h than in cholecystectomized patients. The gallbladder lowers cholesterol saturation of choledochal bile even when the sphincter of Oddi is not functioning. It has to be stressed, however, that after cholecystectomy and endoscopic papillotomy a diurnal rhythm of biliary lipid concentration persists.

SHOULD THE GALLBLADDER BE REMOVED AFTER EPT?

The role of the gallbladder as a risk factor after endoscopic papillotomy is controversial: The data of Cremer[6], Riemann[3], Escourrou[4] and from our group contain catamnestic data of patients up to 7 years after EPT, but only Hagenmüller[5] and Escourrou[4] compare patients with and without

Table 7.2 EPT in patients with gallbladder

Reference	n	% Total group	Observation period (months)	Average age (years)
Hagenmüller et al. (1979)[5]	68	38	12–60	
Cremer et al. (1981)[6]	486	61	4–75	74 (x)
Tulassay et al. (1983)	129	25	1–60	72 (x)
Riemann et al. (1984)[3]	184	?	16–84	75 (m)
Escourrou et al. (1984)[4]	130	57	6–66	79 (x)

gallbladder (Table 7.2). We found some very interesing points. The mean age of the patients was 75 years, exactly 10 years older than the patients who had undergone cholecystectomy before endoscopic papillotomy. So, these patients appear to belong to a particular group whose biliary problems appear only after stones are found in the gallbladder as well as in the common bile duct. Longterm biliary complications after papillotomy are found in 4–15% of the patients and are caused in up to 14% by the gallbladder (Table 7.3).

The results of Escourrou[4] and our group[5] show that patients without the gallbladder show significantly less longterm complications after EPT than patients with the gallbladder *in situ* (Tables 7.4 and 7.5). In over 50% of gallbladder carriers the complication originates within the gallbladder. In this patient group surgical intervention is necessary in most cases, while longterm biliary complications after cholecystectomy may, in most cases, be treated endoscopically. We have suggested elective cholecystectomy after

Table 7.3 Rate of late biliary complications in patients with gallbladder

Reference	Total (%)	Due to gallbladder (%)	Patient without gallbladder (%)
Hagenmüller et al.[5]	15	10–13	6
Cremer et al.[6]	4	4	?
Tulassay et al.	14	14	?
Riemann et al.[3]	7	1	?
Escourrou et al.[4]	12	7	5

Table 7.4 EPT in patients without gallbladder: late complications (n = 205*)

Cholangitis	4
Recurrent stone in DC	3
Restenosis of PV	2
Restenosis of PV in Ca	2
Restenosis of MPD orifice in acute pancreatitis	1
	12/205 (5.9%)

*From Hagenmüller et al.[5] and Escourrou et al.[4]

Table 7.5   EPT in patients with gallbladder: late complications ($n = 198^*$)

Cholecystitis	14
Cholangitis	5
Recurrent stone in DC	2
Restenosis of PV	2
Gallstone ileus	1
Liver abscess	1
Gallbladder Ca	1
	26/198 (13.1%)

*From Hagenmüller et al.[5] and Escourrou et al.[4]

endoscopic therapy for bile duct problems if the surgical risk is not elevated, but this has not been accepted by all authors. Riemann et al.[3] found 7% longterm complications in gallbladder carriers and only 1% of these complications was caused by the gallbladder *in situ*. A comparison with cholecystectomized patients, however, is lacking. As an argument against elective cholecystectomy after EPT the low lethality of complications after EPT is cited. It amounts to only 1% if data from the studies of Escourrou and Riemann and of our study are put together (Table 7.6). 16% of the total

Table 7.6   EPT in patients with gallbladder: fatalities

Reference	Total group (n)	Fatalities Biliary (%)	Fatalities Non-biliary cause (%)
Escourrou et al.[4]	226	0	28 (12)
Hagenmüller et al.[5]	68	1 (1.5)	14 (21)
Riemann et al.[3]	206	4 (2.0)	38 (18)
	500	5 (1)	80 (16)

group of 500 patients have died from non-biliary causes during the surveillance period. The low lethality from longterm complications after EPT in elderly patients with a short life expectancy span appears to justify the careful attitude towards cholecystectomy. According to the literature a simple cholecystectomy in patients over 80 years old has a lethality of 12%. In a total of 96 patients not a single fatality occurred in patients undergoing cholecystectomy after EPT (Table 7.7). This result confirms our attitude of advocating elective cholecystectomy after EPT in patients with a tolerable surgical risk.

The only available data concerning the role of the gallbladder after endoscopic papillotomy are all retrospective, some of the studies have resulted from questionnaires and only show a trend. The methodological structure of these data and the importance of the results show the urgent need for a prospective investigation. This study will shortly be started by the International Biliary Study Group.

Table 7.7   Elective cholecystectomy after EPT

Reference	Total group (n)	Elective CE n (%)	Fatalities
Cotton et al.	44	9 (20)	0
Cremer et al.[6]	496	20 (4)	0
Hagenmüller et al.[5]	68	5 (7)	0
Riemann et al.[3]	184	24 (13)	0
Tulassay et al.	74	38 (51)	0
Total	866	96 (11)	0

References

1. Hess, W. (1961). *Die Erkrankungen der Gallenwege und des Pankreas.* (Stuttgart: Thieme)
2. Paumgartner, G. and Sauerbruch, T. (1973). Secretion, composition and flow of bile. In *Clinics in Gastroenterology. Biliary Tract Disorders.* (London, Philadelphia, Toronto: W. B. Saunders)
3. Riemann, J. F., Gierth, K., Lux, G. and Altendorf, A. (1984). Die belassene Steingallenblase – ein Risikofaktor nach endoskopischer Papillotomie? *Z. Gastroenterol.*, **22**, 188–93
4. Escourrou, J., Cordoba, J. A., Lazorthas, F., Frexinos, J. and Ribet, A. (1984). Early and late complications after endoscopic sphincterotomy for biliary lithiasis with and without the gallbladder *in situ*. *Gut*, **25**, 598–602
5. Hagenmüller, F., Wurbs, D. and Classen, M. (1979). Long-term complications after endoscopic papillotomy (EPT) in patients with gallbladder *in situ*. *Endoscopy*, **4**, 283–4 (Abstract)
6. Cremer, M., Toussaint, J., Dunham, F. and Jeanmart, J. (1981). Endoscopic sphincterotomy (E.S.) with gallbladder *in situ*. *Gastroint. Endosc.*, **27**, 141 (Abstract)

8
Primary biliary cirrhosis: the present position

S. SHERLOCK AND O. EPSTEIN

Primary biliary cirrhosis is a disease with progressive granulomatous destruction of small intrahepatic bile ducts. It is of unknown aetiology. The disease is associated with a profound immunological disturbance and this has been related to bile duct destruction (Table 8.1). The final event seems to be an attack by cytotoxic lymphocytes on biliary epithelium. The antigen might be the individual's own human leukocyte antigens (HLA-ABC glycoproteins) which are present in high concentration on biliary epithelium. It is unclear why the reaction should be to normal rather than foreign proteins. Perhaps the patient's own lymphoid system is at fault so that self and self antigens are not recognized. This could be due to failure of schooling by cytotoxic T-cells in the thymus. These cells are regulated by suppressor cells which have been shown to be diminished both in number and function in primary biliary cirrhosis[1]. Alternatively, and perhaps more likely, the HLA proteins may have become foreign due to an extrinsic environmental factor. The identification of such a factor is an ongoing challenge to all those investigating primary biliary cirrhosis.

In many respects, primary biliary cirrhosis is analogous to the graft-versus-host syndrome as seen, for instance, after bone marrow transplant and where the immune system has become sensitized to foreign HLA proteins[2]. Structural changes in the bile ducts are similar. Other ducts with a high concentration of HLA antigens on their epithelium, such as the lachrymal and

Table 8.1 Immunological changes in primary biliary cirrhosis

Depressed skin energy
Granuloma formation
Circulating immune complexes
Complement activation
Reduction regulator suppressor cells

pancreatic[3], are involved. The condition can be viewed as a dry gland syndrome[2]. Ultrastructural changes in the bile ducts are similar.

The granulomas might be related to immune complexes, and indeed complement has been identified within them. However, they consist predominantly of cytotoxic T-cells, monocytes and macrophages, which suggest cell-mediated tissue injury. Patients with many granulomas are usually seen early in the disease where bile duct destruction is not prominent and the prognosis better. Such patients have normal or only slightly decreased concentrations of suppressor cells in the peripheral blood. This might be related to the rarity of diffuse bile duct destruction and the good prognosis[4].

Copper is retained in the liver, but in a non-hepatotoxic form[5].

EPIDEMIOLOGY AND GENETICS

The disease has been reported from all parts of the world. Asians, Caucasians, Jews, Negroes and Orientals are affected. There is family clustering and the prevalence of circulating mitochondrial antibodies is increased in relatives of patients. There is no excess of any particular ABO blood group, HLA antigen, or rhesus negativity[6].

PRESENTATION

The patient is usually female, only 10% being male. Presentation is usually between 40 and 60 years old. The usual onset is as pruritus. Jaundice may appear at the same time or later. The patient is usually pigmented. The liver is variably enlarged. The spleen is often palpable.

The asymptomatic patient

The widespread use of automated biochemical screening has resulted in an increasing number of patients being diagnosed when asymptomatic[7]. Similarly, the diagnosis may be made in patients under investigation for a condition known to be associated with primary biliary cirrhosis such as thyroid or collagen disease or in the course of family surveys. Such patients tend to be younger and abnormal physical signs may be absent. Mitochondrial antibody is always positive. Serum alkaline phosphatase and bilirubin may be normal or only minimally increased. Serum cholesterol and transaminases can also be normal.

ASSOCIATED DISEASES

Non-hepatic disorders are found in about two thirds especially the collagenoses, and autoimmune thyroiditis is also frequent. Primary biliary cirrhosis may be associated with scleroderma and with the whole CREST syndrome. Such patients usually have a nuclear centromere antibody[8]. A Sicca complex of dry eyes and mouth with or without the arthritis completing the Sjogren syndrome is found in about 75% of patients[2]. Associated skin lesions include immune complex capillaritis and lichen planus which is also a feature of graft-versus-host disease[9]. Primary biliary cirrhosis and jejunal villous atrophy, resembling coeliac disease, have been reported[10]. Other complications include IgM-associated membranous glomerulonephritis and renal tubular acidosis[11]. Bacteriuria develops in 35% and may be asymptomatic[12]. It is unexplained, but it has been postulated that urinary organisms might be invoked in the pathogenesis of primary biliary cirrhosis. Finger clubbing is common and occasionally, hypertrophic osteoarthropathy[13]. Gallstones, usually of the pigment type are present in a third.

INVESTIGATIONS

Biochemical tests

At the time of diagnosis, serum bilirubin values are rarely very high at the onset, usually less than 2 mg per 100 ml in asymptomatic patients. Serum alkaline phosphatase (gamma glutamyl transpeptidase) is raised. The total serum cholesterol is increased but not constantly. The serum albumin level is usually normal at presentation and the total serum globulin only moderately increased. Serum immunoglobulin M (IgM) is usually raised, and this estimation has been suggested for diagnosis. However, increases are not constant and this method is not reliable for diagnosis although an increase may add some diagnostic weight.

Serum mitochondrial (M) test

Circulating antibodies against mitochondria are found in virtually 100% patients with primary biliary cirrhosis, provided undiluted serum samples are used in a standard immunofluorescence test. They probably play no role in pathogenesis. Mitochondrial antibodies are not confined to primary biliary cirrhosis, being detected in 30% of patients with chronic active hepatitis (HBsAg negative) and 3% with connective tissue diseases. They are absent in patients with mechanical obstruction to the bile ducts including primary sclerosing cholangitis.

The antigen(s) concerned is a component of the mitochondrial inner membrane. These antigens are heterogenous, the ATPase associated is termed M2 and is said to be specific for primary biliary cirrhosis. A positive immunoassay for M2 may be specific for primary biliary cirrhosis[14]. A further antigen found on the outer mitochondrial membrane and termed M4 is associated with chronic active hepatitis, granulomas and bile duct proliferation, and must be distinguished from that found with classical primary biliary cirrhosis.

Liver biopsy

The only hepatic lesion diagnostic of primary biliary cirrhosis is the injured septal or interlobular bile duct. The disease begins with damage to the epithelium of small bile ducts. Histometric examinations show that bile ducts less than 70 to 80 μm in diameter are destroyed and particularly in the early stages. Surrounding the damaged duct is a cellular reaction which includes lymphocytes, plasma cells, eosinophils and histiocytes. Granulomas commonly form. Bile ducts become destroyed and are replaced by aggregates of lymphoid cells, and bile ducts begin to proliferate. Hepatic arterial branches can be identified in the portal zones but without accompanying bile ducts. Fibrosis extends from the portal tracts and there is a variable degree of piecemeal necrosis. Substantial amounts of copper and copper-associated protein can be demonstrated histochemically. The fibrous septa gradually come to distort the architecture of the liver and regeneration nodules form. These are often irregular in distribution and cirrhosis may be seen in one part of a biopsy but not in another. The histological appearances have been divided into four stages:

Stage I: florid bile duct lesions
Stage II: ductular proliferation
Stage III: scarring (septal fibrosis and bridging)
Stage IV: cirrhosis[15].

Such staging is of limited value as the changes in the liver are focal and evolve at different speeds in different parts. Stages overlap. It is particularly difficult to separate stages II and III. The disease has a very variable course and advanced stage III lesions may be seen in the asymptomatic patient. Moreover, serial biopsies have shown that the same stage may persist.

COURSE AND PROGNOSIS

Earlier diagnosis in the asymptomatic patient makes the duration seem much longer, and these patients usually survive at least 10 years[16]. In those with symptomatic disease and jaundice the survival is about 7 years.

The course of asymptomatic patients is variable and unpredictable, and counselling the patient and her family is very difficult. Overall, the life expectancy of these patients does not differ from that of the general population[16, 17]. Only 6 of 36 asymptomatic patients studied over 6–11.4 years died from liver disease[16]. Serum bilirubin values are the best indicators of prognosis[18]. When values are consistently greater than 6 mg/dl, the patient is unlikely to survive more than 2 years (Figure 8.1)[19].

Other features at diagnosis predicting decreased survival include symptoms, advanced age, hepatosplenomegaly, ascites and hypoalbuminaemia[20] (less than 3 g/dl)[20]. Histologically, piecemeal necrosis, cholestasis, bridging fibrosis and cirrhosis correlate with the worst prognosis. On the other hand, granulomas seen on an initial biopsy predict a longer survival[4], perhaps because they indicate a less aggressive immune response. Auto-immune diseases such as thyroiditis, Sicca syndrome or Raynaud's phenomenon correlate with decreased survival[16].

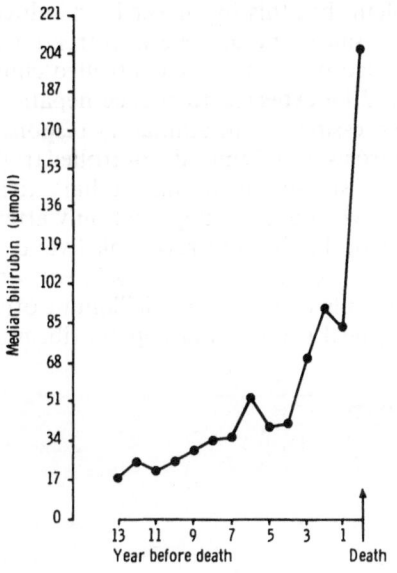

CONCLUSION

EXPECTED survival for any given bilirubin can be extrapolated from this nomogram

ie   Bilirubin (μmol/l)   Expected survival (years)

< 34	8-13
35-100	2-7
> 100	< 2

Figure 8.1   The evolution of liver failure in primary biliary cirrhosis. This nomogram is derived from the medians of pooled serum bilirubin results in patients followed serially from diagnosis to death. (Serum bilirubin 17 μmol/l equals 1 mg/dl)

TREATMENT

These regimens apply to all patients with cholestasis. They include the control of pruritus and the management of steatorrhoea. Fat soluble vitamins A, D and K must be given parenterally to all cholestatic patients. Vitamin E is given by mouth. Oral calcium supplements are indicated. The patient should be encouraged to sunbathe and an ultraviolet lamp may be useful in Northern climates. Medium chain triglycerides may be helpful. The patient is encouraged to lead as normal a life as possible, since the condition is compatible with a full domestic and professional life for many years.

Intractable pruritus and painful xantholmatous neuropathy can be treated by plasmapheresis. This is specialized and costly but may be considered in the exceptional patient. Corticosteroids might be expected to be beneficial, but accentuate the bone thinning of cholestasis. Indeed some of the most disastrous examples of skeletal crumbling that we have seen have been in patients with late stage primary biliary cirrhosis treated with prednisolone. Corticosteroids might be useful in the early, anicteric patient, where bone thinning is not a problem, but this has never been subjected to controlled trials. Azathioprine was said to be of benefit in treatment, but these good results were not confirmed in prospective controlled clinical trials[21, 22].

D-Penicillamine would be expected to reduce hepatic copper levels, act immunologically by depressing the inflammatory response and conceivably might reduce hepatic fibrosis. Randomized, controlled trials have shown that D-penicillamine increases survival in primary biliary cirrhosis[23, 24] (Figure 8.2). Improvement in survival became apparent only after 18 months treatment. Those dying early probably had irreversible liver disease. In surviving patients, D-penicillamine treatment was associated with improved biochemical tests, and a fall in liver copper. Penicillamine often reduces hepatic inflammation and piecemeal necrosis but hepatic fibrosis progresses.

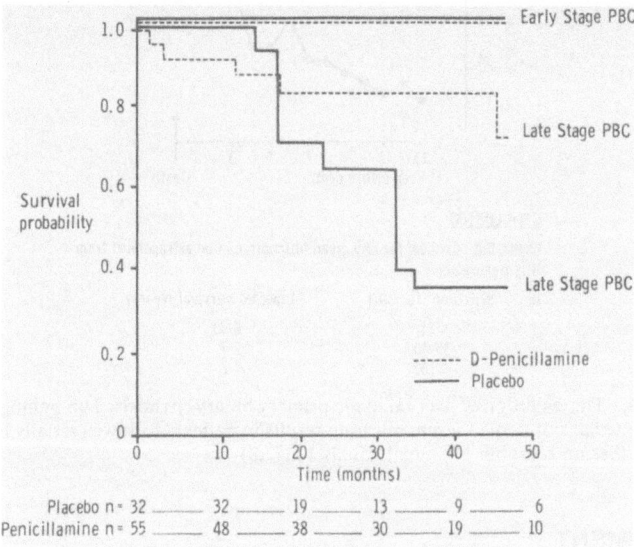

Figure 8.2 Survival probability in early and late histological stage primary biliary cirrhosis. Early PBC – stages I and II, late PBC – stages III and IV. From Epstein *et al.* (1981)[23]

Side effects of D-penicillamine unfortunately lead to non-compliance and withdrawal of therapy. The most frequent is dyspepsia with nausea and vomiting. Taste may be lost, but this returns whether or not the drug is discontinued. Serious reactions include skin rashes, proteinuria and blood dyscrasias, such as thrombocytopenia and neutropenia. These usually lead to permanent withdrawal of therapy. Various auto-immune syndromes, including myasthenia, polymyositis, systemic lupus and a Goodpasture-like picture are other complications[25].

Other trials have shown less satisfactory results with D-penicillamine recording a higher incidence of serious side effects[26]. Others have found no improvement in survival in those with fibrosis/cirrhosis on initial biopsy[24]. On small numbers, statistical analysis is difficult[19]. D-penicillamine is worth

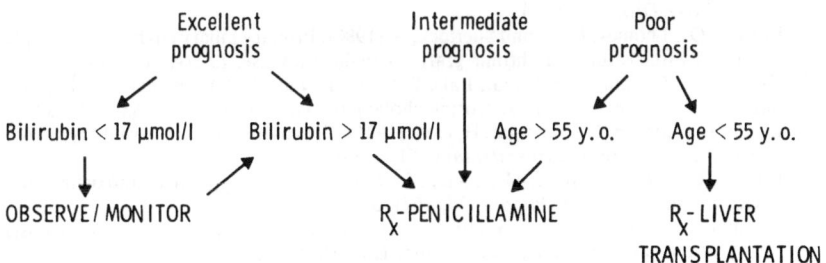

Figure 8.3 A rational approach to the treatment of PBC in 1984

a trial in those who are symptomatic with a rising serum bilirubin level, and who are unsuitable or have not reached the stage of consideration for liver transplantation (Figure 8.3). There is little else to offer. D-Penicillamine should not be given to the asymptomatic.

D-Penicillamine is commenced in a daily dose of 125 mg which is increased by 125 mg every 2 weeks until a maintenance dose of 500 mg daily is reached. Haemoglobin and white cell counts are measured, and proteinuria sought every week for the first 4 weeks, and then every month. The drug should be continued unless there is a serious complication or manifestations of the late stages of primary biliary cirrhosis such as haematemesis, ascites or precoma have developed.

Cyclosporin A has a marked effect on the suppressor-inducer T-lymphocytes in primary biliary cirrhosis[27]. However, the drug is nephrotoxic and difficult to justify for longterm use. Less toxic derivatives are awaited. Chlorambucil and colchicine are under trial, but preliminary results suggest that the improvement is not dramatic.

Haemorrhage from oesophageal varices may be early before a true nodular cirrhosis has developed. It is not surprising, therefore, that porta–caval shunting gives good results in these patients[28]. Hepatic encephalopathy is an unusual complication. These encouraging results apply particularly to good risk patients (Grade A and B), rather than those with poor hepatocellular function (Grade C). Gallstones should be left *in situ* unless causing severe symptoms or present in the common bile duct. Cholecystectomy is rarely indicated and is badly tolerated.

When the patient has developed chronic hepatocellular failure, particularly rapidly deepening jaundice and ascites, the outlook is extremely grave, survival being unlikely to exceed 1 year. In such patients hepatic transplantation must be considered[29]. Forty patients with primary biliary cirrhosis who were treated in Pittsburgh, had a 70% 1 year survival[30]. Twenty per cent needed a second transplant. Experience at the Royal Free Hospital is equally satisfactory. End-stage primary biliary cirrhosis is one of the best indications for liver transplantation. Recurrence of the disease in the transplanted liver has been reported[31], but this is difficult to distinguish from the graft-versus-host reaction of chronic rejection[32].

References

1. Thomas, H. C. (1982). Potential pathogenic mechanisms in primary biliary cirrhosis. *Semin. Liver Dis.*, **1**, 338-44
2. Epstein, O., Thomas, H. C. and Sherlock, S. (1980). Primary biliary cirrhosis is a dry gland syndrome with features of chronic graft-versus-host disease. *Lancet*, **1**, 1166-8
3. Epstein, O., Chapman, R. W. G., Lake-Bakaar, G. *et al.* (1982). The pancreas in primary biliary cirrhosis and primary sclerosing cholangitis. *Gastroenterology*, **83**, 1177-82
4. Lee, R. G., Epstein, O., Jauregui, H. *et al.* (1981). Granulomas in primary biliary cirrhosis: a prognostic feature. *Gastroenterology*, **81**, 983-6
5. Epstein, O., Arborgh, B. A. M., Sagiv, M. *et al.* (1981). Is copper hepatotoxic in primary biliary cirrhosis? *J. Clin. Pharm.*, **34**, 1071-5
6. Hamlyn, A. N. and Sherlock, S. (1974). The epidemiology of primary biliary cirrhosis: a survey of mortality in England and Wales. *Gut*, **15**, 473-9
7. Long, R. G., Scheuer, P. J. and Sherlock, S. (1977). Presentation and course of asymptomatic primary biliary cirrhosis. *Gastroenterology*, **72**, 1204-7
8. Makinen, D., Fritzer, M., Davis, P. and Sherlock, S. (1983). Anticentromere antibody in primary biliary cirrhosis. *Arthritis Rheum.*, **26**, 1914-16
9. Graham-Brown, R. A. C., Sarkany, I. and Sherlock, S. (1982). Lichen planus and primary biliary cirrhosis. *Br. J. Dermatol.*, **106**, 699-703
10. Iliffe, G. D. and Owen, D. A. (1979). An association between primary biliary cirrhosis and jejunal villous atrophy resembling celiac disease. *Dig. Dis. Sci.*, **24**, 802-6
11. Pares, A., Rimola, A., Bruguera, M. *et al.* (1981). Renal tubular acidosis in primary biliary cirrhosis. *Gastroenterology*, **80**, 681-6
12. Burroughs, A. K., Rosenstein, I. J., Epstein, O. *et al.* (1984). Bacteriuria and primary biliary cirrhosis. *Gut*, **25**, 133-7
13. Epstein, O., Dick, R. and Sherlock, S. (1981). Prospective study of periostitis and finger clubbing in primary biliary cirrhosis and other forms of chronic liver disease. *Gut*, **22**, 203-6
14. Berg, P. A., Klein, R., Lindenborn-Fotinos, J. *et al.* (1982). ATpase-associated antigen (M2): marker antigen for serological diagnosis of primary biliary cirrhosis. *Lancet*, **2**, 1423-5
15. Scheuer, P. J. (1980). Primary biliary cirrhosis. In *Liver Biopsy Interpretation. 3rd Ed.* pp. 47-56. (Baltimore: Williams and Wilkins)
16. Beswick, D. R., Klatskin, G. and Boyer, J. L. (1985). Asymptomatic primary biliary cirrhosis - long term follow-up and natural history. (In press)
17. James, O., Macklon, A. F. and Watson, A. J. (1981). Primary biliary cirrhosis - a revised clinical spectrum. *Lancet*, **1**, 1278-81
18. Shapiro, J. M., Smith, H. and Schaffner, F. (1979). Serum bilirubin; a prognostic factor in primary biliary cirrhosis. *Gut*, **20**, 137-46
19. Epstein, O., Cook, D. G., Jain, S. *et al.* (1984). D-Penicillamine in PBC - an untested (and unstable?) treatment. *Gut*. (In press)
20. Roll, J., Boyer, J. L., Barry, D. and Klatskin, G. (1983). The prognostic importance of clinical and histologic features in asymptomatic and symptomatic primary biliary cirrhosis. *N. Engl. J. Med.*, **308**, 1-7
21. Heathcote, J., Ross, A. and Sherlock, S. (1976). A prospective controlled trial of azathioprine in primary biliary cirrhosis. *Gastroenterology*, **70**, 656-60
22. Crowe, J., Christensen, E., Smith, M. *et al.* (1980). Azathioprine in primary biliary cirrhosis, a preliminary report of an international trial. *Gastroenterology*, **78**, 1005-10
23. Epstein, O., Jain, S., Lee, R. G. *et al.* (1981). D-Penicillamine improves survival in primary biliary cirrhosis. *Lancet*, **1**, 1275-7
24. Dickson, E. R., Wiesner, R. H., Baldus, W. P. *et al.* (1984). D-Penicillamine trial for primary biliary cirrhosis. *Gastroenterology*, **86**, 1062 A
25. Matloff, D. S. and Kaplan, M. M. (1980). D-Penicillamine-induced Goodpasture-like syndrome in primary biliary cirrhosis - Successful treatment with plasmapheresis and immuno-suppressives. *Gastroenterology*, **78**, 1046-9
26. Matloff, D. S., Alpert, E., Resnick, R. H. *et al.* (1982). A prospective trial of D-PCA in primary biliary cirrhosis. *N. Engl. J. Med.*, **306**, 319-26
27. Routhier, G., Epstein, O., Janossy, G. *et al.* (1980). Effects of cyclosporin A on suppressor and induced T-lymphocytes in primary biliary cirrhosis. *Lancet*, **2**, 1223-6

28. Spisni, R., Smith-Laing, G., Epstein, O. *et al.* (1981). Results of portal decompression in patients with primary biliary cirrhosis. *Gut*, **22**, 345–9
29. Sherlock, S. (1983). Hepatic transplantation: the state of play. *Lancet*, **2**, 778–9
30. Van Thiel, D. H. *et al.* (1984). The present results for liver transplantation. (In press)
31. Neuberger, J., Portmann, B., MacDougall, B. R. D. *et al.* (1982). Recurrence of primary biliary cirrhosis after liver transplantation. *N. Engl. J. Med.*, **306**, 1–4
32. Snover, D. C., Weisdorf, S. A., Ramsay, N. K. *et al.* (1984). Hepatic graft-versus-host disease: a study of the predictive value of liver biopsy in diagnosis. *Hepatology*, **4**, 123–30

28. Epstein, O., Dick, R. and Sherlock, S. (1981). Prospects for primary biliary cirrhosis. *Gut*, **22**, 84

29. Sherlock, S. (1959). *Diseases of the Liver and Biliary System*. 2nd ed.

30. Epstein, O. et al. (1981). D-penicillamine therapy in primary biliary cirrhosis: results of prolonged treatment. *Lancet*, **1**, 1275

31. Jain, S. et al. (1977). Controlled trial of D-penicillamine in primary biliary cirrhosis. *Lancet*, **1**, 831

9
Synthetic hepatology

K. DECKER

To consider trends in hepatology and to risk a look into the future of science is a dangerous task. Futurology backed by dubious authority has been known to inhibit rather than to foster scientific progress. However, we meet here to pay homage to a colleague who very early recognized a trend among hepatologists from differing disciplines – the desire to meet every year and exchange knowledge and ideas – and who was extremely successful in firmly establishing this trend. Thus, it may be appropriate to look at recent developments and to try to foresee future trends.

Hepatology as with every scientific endeavour began with analytical investigations. The measurements of arterio–venous differences, of hepatic clearance rates and, in particular, the studies of metabolites, enzymes and structural elements in cell extracts belong to the category of whole-organ analyses. With such a wealth of information available, kinetic measurements and studies on regulatory mechanisms were to follow. Finally, advances in methodology and new concepts of metabolism and its regulation allowed us to consider the spatial organization of cellular events, the importance of phases and phase transitions and the interactions of kinetic and topologic metabolic regulations.

The liver appeared to be particularly well suited for these kinds of biochemical and cell biological investigations as it is predominantly made up of *one* cell type, the hepatocyte. Quite often, 'liver metabolism' and 'hepatocyte metabolism' were used interchangeably. In recent years, however, it became increasingly evident that this approach was at best an approximation to reality, leaving many unsolved and paradoxical problems. The individual performances and functions of the different liver cells, the hepatocytes, endothelial, Kupffer and Ito cells (not to mention the specific cells of blood vessels and bile ductules) and their cooperation became targets for biochemical investigators. Metabolic zonation of the liver acinus, receptor and enzyme specificities and the interplay of signals and mediators of different liver cells will be used as examples to demonstrate the limits of whole organ studies, and to emphasize the importance of advances in the knowledge of the individual cell types for the understanding of liver functions.

The concept of *metabolic zonation* of the liver acinus has been initiated and considerably advanced by Jungermann's and Sasse's groups in Freiburg[1,2]. They proposed a metabolic (not a genetically determined) heterogeneity of the hepatocytes along the porto-venous distance. It is thought to result from gradients of oxygen, nutrients and hormones that develop as the fluid from the portal vein perfuses through the acinus. Metabolic zonation leads to different, sometimes even inverted metabolic processes in periportal and perivenous hepatocytes (Table 9.1). This concept allowed, for the first time, a consistent explanation of the apparently paradoxical fact that gluconeogenesis and glycolysis can be measured at the same time within the same liver. It is further supported by the elucidation of an intercellular hepatic glutamine cycle[3]. As metabolic zonation becomes an accepted fact it necessitates a reinterpretation of many data obtained with whole liver. In addition, one has to consider the possibility that not only physiological oscillations but also pathological deviations may be due to disturbances of the metabolic zonation of the liver acinus.

Table 9.1 Metabolic zonation of liver parenchyma. Predominant localization of major functions

Periportal zone	*Perivenous zone*
Glucose release	Glucose uptake
Glycogen degradation to glucose	Glycogen synthesis from glucose
Gluconeogenesis	Glycolysis
	Liponeogenesis
Oxidative energy metabolism	
Fatty acid oxidation	
Citrate cycle	
Respiratory chain	
	Biotransformation
Cholic acid excretion	
Bilirubin excretion	

From Jungermann and Katz[3a]

Gradients of hormones along the portal-venous distance cannot be explained by the binding and the relatively sluggish internalization by hepatocytes alone. An additional mechanism is proposed, that is derived from binding and degradation studies of peptide hormones with different liver cells[4]. The comparison of the rates of inactivation of insulin and glucagon by hepatocytes, Kupffer cells as well as by activated and non-activated alveolar macrophages (Table 9.2) reveals the enormous capability of Kupffer cells to inactivate these hormones, especially glucagon. Since the density of hormone receptors on Kupffer cells is not so different from that on hepatocytes[4] a faster turnover (membrane flow) in Kupffer cells appears to be responsible for this effect. Even considering the relative cell masses in the liver - Kupffer cells represent only 3% of the total mass - it is obvious that more than 50% of the glucagon removed by the liver is internalized by

Table 9.2 Degradative capacities at 37°C

Degradation of	Hepatocytes (pmol g^{-1} h^{-1})	Kupffer cells (pmol g^{-1} h^{-1})	Alveolar Mφ	
			non-activated (pmol g^{-1} h^{-1})	activated (pmol g^{-1} h^{-1})
Insulin (0.36 nmol/l)	3.65	152	0.03	0.15
Glucagon (10 nmol/l)	10.9	2440	—*	—*

*No binding observed

Kupffer cells. This effect of the Kupffer cells should contribute considerably to the glucagon gradient developing in the porto-venous distance and in the induction of a glycolytic–lipogenetic activity pattern in perivenous hepatocytes.

Differences in the *receptor outfit* of the various liver cells lead to various metabolic and functional specializations (Table 9.3). A telling example is to be found in the metabolism of low density lipoprotein (LDL) which is thought to be involved in certain forms of lipoproteinaemias and in the sclerotic process. Investigations by van Berkel's group[5] and others[6, 7] revealed that the vascular endothelial cells modify LDL, and that this modified LDL is taken up predominantly by the endothelial cells of the liver (Figure 9.1). These cells degrade the apoprotein of LDL. Free cholesterol liberated during this process is hardly metabolized by endothelial cells, but is exported to the hepatocytes for reutilization or bile salt synthesis.

Table 9.3 Receptor specificity of liver cells

Receptor or binding site for	Kupffer cells	Endothelial cells	Hepatocytes
Insulin	+	?	+
Glucagon	+	?	+
Lipoprotein lipase	−	+	+
Apolipoprotein B	+	−	(+)
Modified LDL (scavenger)	−	+	−
Galactose/GalNAc	+ (> 10 nm)	−	+ (< 10 nm)
Mannose/GlcNAc	+	+	−
F$_c$	+	+ (*in vitro*)	−
C$_3$b	+	−	−
Fibronectin	+	?	(−)
Yeast, bacteria	+	−	−

Lipid exchange between various liver cell types seems to be a frequently used mechanism. It has been shown[8] that retinol supplied to the liver is first taken up by hepatocytes, then transported to the Ito (fat storing) cells which are able to store large amounts of this vitamin. It must be assumed that retinol has to be carried back to the hepatocytes in order to become attached to the specific retinol-binding protein.

The individual liver cell types also show qualitative and quantitative differences in their *enzyme outfit*. This has been shown for lysosomal enzymes, especially for the protein-degrading activities; they are predominantly located in Kupffer cells but are also found in substantial concentrations in endothelial cells[9]. More interesting perhaps is the distribution of hexose-metabolizing activities within the liver: glucokinase appears to be exclusively located in hepatocytes, while the less specific hexokinase with its greater affinity for glucose is found predominantly in Kupffer cells[10]. Furthermore, the typical enzymes of the pentose phosphate pathway, glucose-6-phosphate

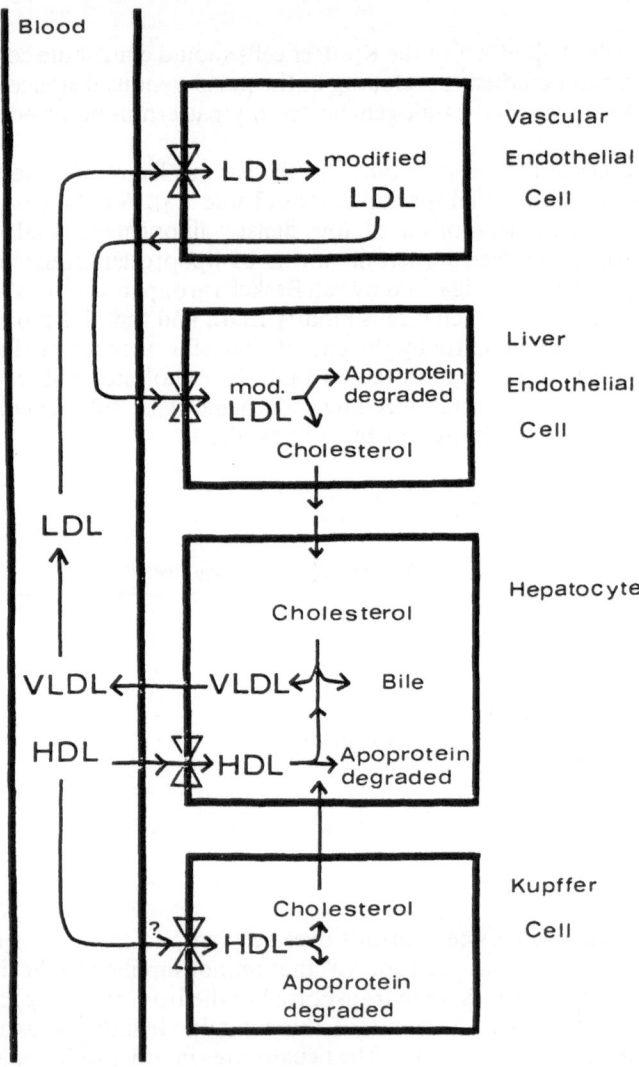

Figure 9.1 Scheme of LDL and HDL catabolism

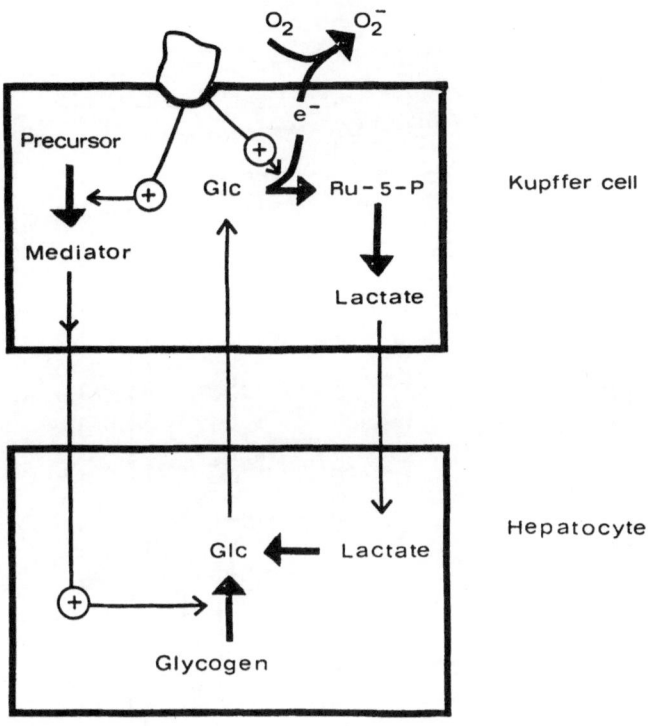

Figure 9.2 Metabolic cooperation of hepatocytes and Kupffer cells after external activation. Glc, glucose; Ru, ribulose

dehydrogenase and 6-phosphogluconate dehydrogenase, are almost exclusively localized in Kupffer cells. This surprising finding[11] has been corroborated by the elegant histochemical studies of Teutsch[12]. The distribution of the pentose phosphate pathway dehydrogenases is related to the mechanisms that furnish the reducing equivalents for lipid synthesis in hepatocytes. So far, the NADPH production in the pentose phosphate pathway has been seen as a major contributor. Obviously, that role has to be reconsidered. In Kupffer cells, however, this pathway is strongly involved in the generation of reactive oxygen species, in particular O_2^-, which are thought to play an important role in the inactivation of bacteria, viruses and oxygen-sensitive macromolecules. It has been shown[13] that contact with phagocytosable particles leads to an activation of the NADPH oxidase of Kupffer cells. The electrons necessary for the partial O_2 reduction are provided by a strongly enhanced flux of glucose to the pentose phosphate pathway[13]. The rather low mitochondrial capacity of Kupffer cells cannot cope with the increased pyruvate production; thus, mainly lactate is formed in the activated state. A metabolic cooperation can now develop between activated Kupffer cells and hepatocytes: while excess lactate is offered to the parenchymal cells for gluconeogenesis, the mediator-activated (*see* below) hepatocytes, on the

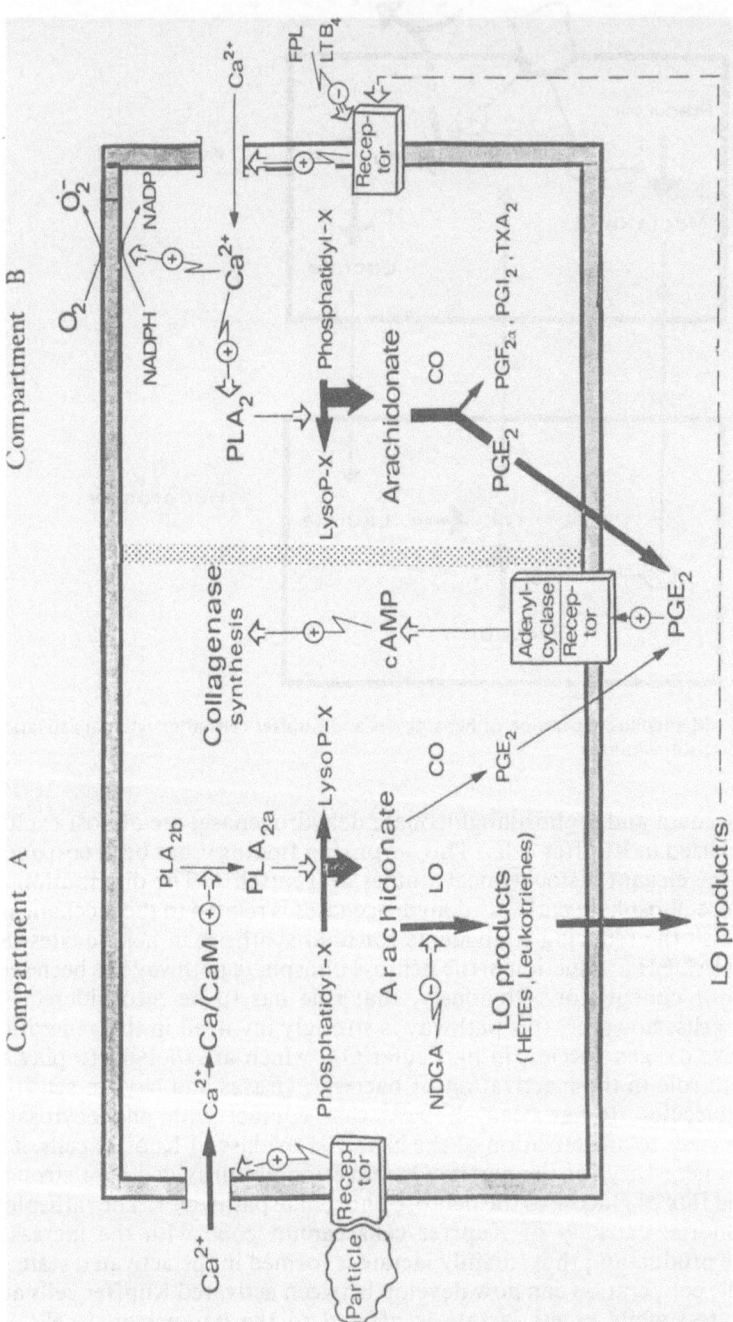

Figure 9.3 Tentative scheme of the phagocytic cascade. PGE₂ (B) > (A); CaM-dependent in A only; cyto-oxygenase (CO) mainly in B; lipoxygenase (LO) in A only; no exchange A ⇌ B

Table 9.4 Eicosanoids released by rat Kupffer cells

Cyclo-oxygenase products:
  prostaglandin E_2
  prostaglandin $F_{2\alpha}$
  prostacyclin (PGI_2, measured as $PGF_{1\alpha}$)
  thromboxane A_2 (measured as TXB_2)

Lipoxygenase products:
  5-hydroxyeicosatetraenoic acid
  leukotriene C_4 (D_4)

other hand, show an increased glucose production that may help Kupffer cells to meet their increased demand for glucose during phagocytosis (Figure 9.2).

Contact with phagocytosable material[14, 15] but also with substances such as endotoxins[16] or calcium ionophores leads to the synthesis and release of *signal molecules* from Kupffer cells. Immunocomplexes and zymosan particles elicit the production of mediators, mainly of the arachidonic acid family (Table 9.4), of which PGE_2 is quantitatively the most predominant. Their synthesis and release depends on a transiently increased influx of calcium ions[17]. It is suppressed by inhibitors of calmodulin-dependent reactions, of cyclo-oxygenase and of lipoxygenase, and is also blocked[15] by leukotriene B_4 (Figure 9.3).

Much less is known about the effects that these mediators have on the liver or on other organs than about their synthesis in Kupffer cells. There is evidence, of course, for interactions of activated Kupffer cells and hepatocytes. We have learned that PGE_2 is degraded very rapidly by hepatocytes but not by Kupffer cells. By maintaining physiological PGE_2 concentrations ($\leqslant 1\,\mu mol/l$) in primary cultures of rat hepatocytes, it was possible to show a 2-4 fold stimulation of adenylate cyclase and glycogenolysis, and to observe a pattern of protein phosphorylation that resembles the action of noradrenaline rather than that of glucagon. Similar effects on hepatocytes can be obtained with supernatants of activated Kupffer cells. It is assumed that in situations which lead to an activation of Kupffer cells, protection is offered to hepatocytes by providing a PGE_2-dependent stimulation of the energy metabolism. Conversely, an amplifier mechanism of liver cell damage (Figure 9.4) would be established through the above mentioned inhibition by LTB_4 of prostaglandin synthesis in Kupffer cells because data reported by Bissell and associates[18] suggest that increased amounts of LTB_4 are formed by damaged hepatocytes.

Kupffer and parenchymal cells also cooperate in the synthesis of acute phase proteins, e.g. α_2-macroglobulin, by primary cultures of hepatocytes[19]. Substances formed by Kupffer cells and released into the medium were able to stimulate, in the presence of permissive concentrations (1 nmol/l) of glucocorticoids α_2-macroglobulin synthesis, while neither the Kupffer cell product nor 1 nmol/l dexamethasone alone had any effect. It should be mentioned here that hepatocytes and Kupffer cells react inversely to glucocorticoids. For example, fibronectin (FN) synthesis is enhanced by dexamethasone in hepatocytes, but it is depressed in Kupffer cells[14] (Table 9.5).

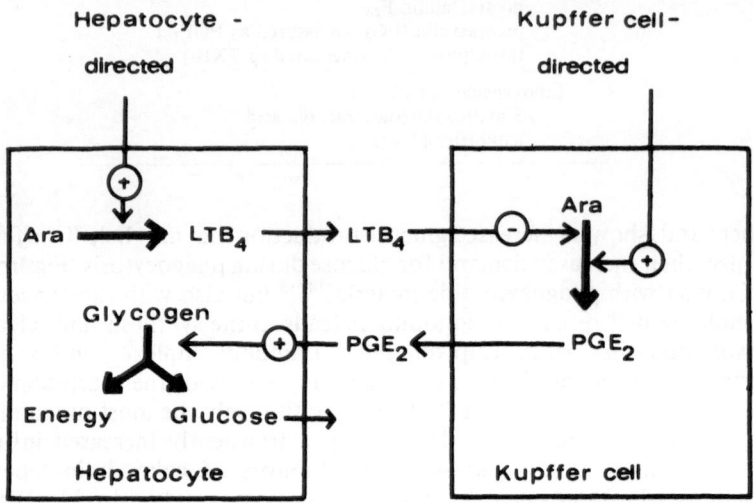

Figure 9.4. Possible mechanism of injury amplification in hepatocytes. Ara, arachidonic acid

Table 9.5 Relative rate of fibronectin synthesis

	Hepatocytes	Kupffer cells
In unstimulated cells	100	100
In presence of 1 μmol/l dexamethasone	190	50
After treatment with lipopolysaccharide (30 μg/ml, 24 h)	90	200

Rate of synthesis in hepatocytes 400, in Kupffer cells 4.4 μg FN d^{-1}g^{-1} liver wet wt

Hardly anybody will doubt that a better understanding of metabolism and function, physiology and pathology of the liver will depend on deeper insights into the performances of the individual liver cell types and in their cooperation. At the same time we must be fully aware that many traps and pitfalls are waiting on our way to amalgamate individual findings into a coordinated picture of the whole organ. The route we travelled from the intact liver to the cell extract in a *tour de force*, we will have to go back now by many small, well controlled steps passing over subcellular structures, isolated cells, the isolated organ until we reach the liver as it functions within the framework of the whole organism.

As we travel towards this final goal we may expect not only to gain new knowledge and insight but also new opportunities for action. The existence of different and specific receptors and binding sites should offer possibilities of making individual cell types targets for site-directed agents and, thereby, to modify their function or viability. Selective activation of Kupffer cells, e.g. with glucan, is being discussed as a therapeutic strategy for liver protection. Similar considerations may apply to endothelial cells and LDL metabolism. Beyond that, restitution or improvement of failing cell functions may be envisaged by the application of molecular engineering. Areas of liver regeneration or the mobile stages of Kupffer cell precursors are, in principle, targets for gene transfer techniques. When this will be accomplished is still a matter of conjecture, but is, nevertheless, an option that will enlarge our knowledge and spectrum of action.

References

1. Jungermann, K. and Sasse, D. (1978). Heterogeneity of liver parenchymal cells. *Trends Biochem. Sci.*, **3**, 198-202
2. Sasse, D., Katz, N. and Jungermann, K. (1975). Functional heterogeneity of rat liver parenchyma and of isolated hepatocytes. *FEBS Lett.*, **57**, 83-8
3. Häussinger, D., Gerok, W. and Sies, H. (1984). Hepatic role in pH regulation: role of the intercellular glutamine cycle. *Trends Biochem. Sci.*, **9**, 300-2
3a. Jungermann, K. and Katz, N. (1982). Functional hepatocellular heterogeneity. *Hepatology*, **2**, 385-95
4. Decker, K. and Kreusch, J. (1982). *9th International RES Congress*, Davos. See also Kreusch, J., Thesis, Medical Faculty, The University of Freiburg (FRG) 1979. Binding, uptake and degradation of peptide hormones by macrophages.
5. Nagelkerke, J. F., Barto, K. P. and van Berkel, T. J. C. (1983). *In vivo* and *in vitro* uptake and degradation of acetylated low density lipoprotein by rat liver endothelial, Kupffer and parenchymal cells. *J. Biol. Chem.*, **258**, 12221-7
6. Henriksen, T., Mahoney, E. M. and Steinberg, D. (1981). Enhanced macrophage degradation of low density lipoprotein previously incubated with cultured endothelial cells: recognition by receptors for acetylated low density lipoprotein. *Proc. Natl. Acad. Sci. USA*, **78**, 6499-503
7. Goldstein, J. L., Basu, S. K. and Brown, M. S. (1983). Receptor-mediated endocytosis of low-density lipoprotein in cultured cells. *Meth. Enzymol.*, **98**, 241-60
8. Blomhoff, R., Holte, K., Naess, L. and Berg, T. (1984). Newly administered |³H|retinol is transferred from hepatocytes to stellate cells in liver for storage. *Exp. Cell Res.*, **150**, 186-93
9. Blouin, A., Bolender, R. P. and Weibel, E. R. (1977). Distribution of organelles and membranes between hepatocytes and non hepatocytes in the rat liver parenchyma. A stereological study. *J. Cell. Biol.*, **72**, 441-55
10. Dileepan, K. N., Wagle, S. R., Hofmann, F. and Decker, K. (1979). Distribution profile of glucokinase and hexokinase in parenchymal and sinusoidal cells of rat liver during development. *Life Sci.*, **24**, 89-96
11. Knook, D. L., Sleyster, E. C. and Teutsch, H. F. (1980). High activity of glucose-6-phosphate dehydrogenase in Kupffer cells isolated from rat liver. *Histochemistry*, **69**, 211-16
12. Teutsch, H. F. (1981). Chemomorphology of liver parenchyma. Qualitative histochemical distribution patterns and quantitative sinusoidal profiles of G-6-Pase, G-6-PDH and malic enzyme activity and of glycogen content. *Progr. Histochem. Cytochem.*, **14**, 1-92
13. Bhatnagar, R., Schirmer, R., Ernst, M. and Decker, K. (1981). Superoxide release by zymosan-stimulated rat Kupffer cells *in vitro*. *Eur. J. Biochem.*, **119**, 171-5
14. Rieder, H., Birmelin, M. and Decker, K. (1982). Synthesis and functions of fibronectin in rat liver cells *in vitro*. In Knook, D. L. and Wisse, E. (eds.) *Sinusoidal Liver Cells*. pp. 193-200. (Amsterdam, New York, Oxford: Elsevier Biomedical Press)
15. Birmelin, M. and Decker, K. (1984). Synthesis of prostanoids and cyclic nucleotides by phagocytosing rat Kupffer cells. *Eur. J. Biochem.*, **142**, 219-25

16. Bhatnagar, R., Schade, U., Rietschel, Th.E. and Decker, K. (1982). Involvement of prostaglandin E and cyclic adenosin $3',5'$-monophosphate in lipopolysaccharide-stimulated collagenase release by rat Kupffer cells. *Eur. J. Biochem.*, **125**, 125–30

17. Birmelin, M. and Decker, K. (1983). Ca^{2+} flux as an initial event in phagocytosis by rat Kupffer cells. *Eur. J. Biochem.*, **131**, 539–43

18. Perez, H. D., Roll, F. J., Bissell, D. M., Shak, S. and Goldstein, I. M. (1984). Production of chemotactic activity for polymorphonuclear leukocytes by cultured rat hepatocytes exposed to ethanol. *J. Clin. Invest.*, **74**, 1350–57

19. Bauer, J., Birmelin, M., Northoff, G.-H., Northemann, W., Tran-Thi, T. A., Ueberberg, H., Decker, K. and Heinrich, P. (1984). Induction of rat α_2-macroglobulin *in vivo* and in hepatocyte primary cultures: synergistic action of glucocorticoids and a Kupffer cell-derived factor. *FEBS Lett.*, **177**, 89–94

10
Studies on the molecular basis of polymorphic drug oxidation (debrisoquine/sparteine-type) in man

U. A. MEYER, P. DAYER, J. GUT AND T. KRONBACH

In 1977, physicians at St Mary's Hospital Medical School in London made the serendipitous observation that a volunteer's hypotensive response to *debrisoquine*, a sympathicolytic antihypertensive drug, was markedly increased, and that this was due to the impaired benzylic 4-hydroxylation of debrisoquine[1]. At the same time a group of physicians in Bonn independently observed increased side effects associated with decreased oxidative metabolism of *sparteine*, an oxytocic and antiarrhythmic alkaloid[2]. Both reactions, the hydroxylation of debrisoquine[3] and the oxidation of sparteine to dehydrosparteine[4] (Figure 10.1) are catalysed by microsomal mono-oxygenases and appear to be under identical or linked monogenic control in most populations studied[3]. The commonly determined urinary metabolic ratio (MR) of debrisoquine to 4-hydroxydebrisoquine or of sparteine to dehydrosparteine separates subjects into extensive (EM) and poor metabolizers (PM) after standard doses of these compounds. Family studies indicate that PMs are homozygous for an autosomal recessive gene[4].

Since the discovery of the debrisoquine/sparteine-type polymorphism in 1977 considerable clinical information has accumulated from many different laboratories, indicating that poor metabolizer subjects represent 3–10% of the white populations in Europe and North America[3-6]. Most importantly, these subjects also have an impaired oxidation of to date near to 20 other drugs including phenformin, perhexiline, guanoxan, encainide, nortriptylin and the β-adrenergic receptor blocking drugs bufuralol and metoprolol[3, 5, 6]. Clinical studies have clearly demonstrated that PMs are in increased danger of suffering toxic side effects from several of these drugs when given the usual doses[3, 5-8]

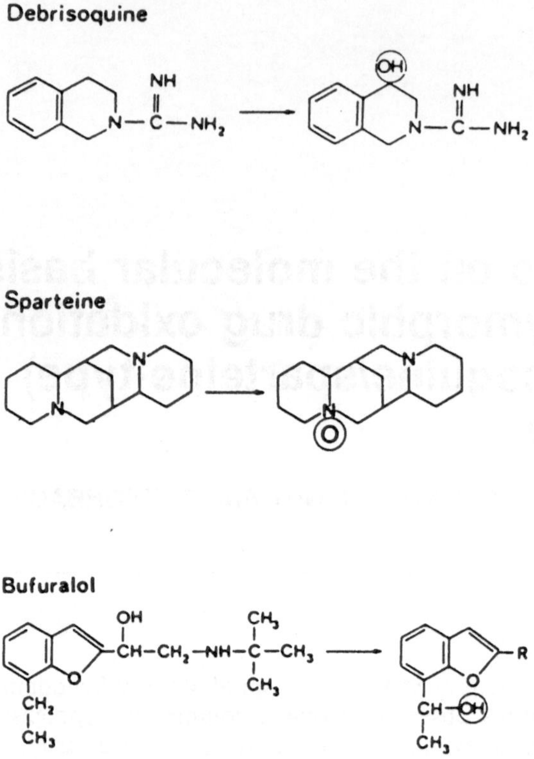

Debrisoquine

Sparteine

Bufuralol

Figure 10.1   Structures and major oxidative pathways of debrisoquine, sparteine and bufuralol

Because the reactions which are deficient in poor metabolizers are mediated by cytochrome P_{450}-type haemoprotein mono-oxygenases, we and others have tested the hypothesis that the polymorphic metabolism of debrisoquine and other drugs may be caused by a quantitative or functional deficiency of one (or more) cytochrome P_{450} isozyme(s)[9-12].

ESTABLISHMENT OF A BANK OF HUMAN LIVER TISSUE

In order to investigate this hypothesis we have established a bank of human liver tissue. This bank presently contains 18 human livers collected immediately after circulatory arrest from kidney transplant donors. Tissue from these livers was used to adapt and optimize fractionation procedures, storage conditions and enzyme assays. In addition, 70 wedge biopsies of 0.5–2 g wet-weight were obtained from the livers of patients which had been subjected to either diagnostic or therapeutic laparotomy. Many methods and techniques have been developed for the fractionation, storage and enzymatic characterization of human liver tissue and for the study of cytochrome P_{450}-dependent mono-oxygenase reactions[9].

IN VIVO–IN VITRO CORRELATION OF THE METABOLISM OF DEBRISOQUINE IN HUMAN LIVER MICROSOMES

In liver microsomes of two individuals identified as poor metabolizers by *in vivo* tests (urinary metabolic ratio), we found a markedly reduced hydroxylation rate of debrisoquine[9] confirming and extending previous studies by Davies *et al.*[11], who had observed a lack of 4-OH debrisoquine formation in the liver biopsy of one poor metabolizer. This indicates that the deficient metabolism of debrisoquine in poor metabolizers is caused by a deficiency of a mono-oxygenase reaction in the liver. Moreover, our data demonstrated that defective hydroxylation of debrisoquine is not related to a general impairment of microsomal oxidation reactions.

IN VIVO–IN VITRO CORRELATION OF THE METABOLISM OF BUFURALOL

Bufuralol is a β-adrenergic receptor blocking drug which is under clinical investigation (Figure 10.1). One of the major pathways of bufuralol metabolism is its oxidation to 1'-OH-bufuralol (or carbinol). This reaction is under the same or linked genetic control as the metabolism of debrisoquine[13]. We have developed a highly sensitive HPLC-assay for the measurement of carbinol formation in small liver samples and in reconstituted cytochrome P_{450}[10] (Kronbach *et al.*, in preparation). The metabolism of bufuralol to carbinol showed substrate selectivity, preferring the (+) isomer of bufuralol and exhibited saturation kinetics. The activity was competitively inhibited by other substrates sharing the same oxidation polymorphism *in vivo*. Moreover, the kinetics of the reaction were compatible with a one enzyme reaction, in contrast to the 4-hydroxylation of debrisoquine which shows a low K_m and high K_m component[12]. To rule out that the defect is related to a soluble modifier of enzyme activity, we mixed microsomes of a poor metabolizer with those of an extensive metabolizer. The rate of carbinol production of the mixture was equal to the sum of the two components[10]. This excludes a transferable inhibitor in the PM microsomes or a transferable factor in the EM microsomes able to correct the defect in the PM microsomes.

Our indirect studies in microsomes thus strongly support the concept that a genetically variant cytochrome P_{450} isozyme with high affinity for these substrates is defective in subjects of the poor metabolizer phenotype. They also support the conclusions drawn from cross-over population studies that the metabolism of drugs involved in this polymorphism is co-incidentally regulated by the same gene locus[3, 5, 6]. These investigations, however, do not answer the question as to the nature of the oxidation impairment at the molecular level in poor metabolizers.

MICHAELIS CONSTANT (K_m) AND STEREOSELECTIVITY OF BUFURALOL 1'-HYDROXYLATION IN MICROSOMES OF POOR METABOLIZERS

During the investigation of the kinetics of bufuralol-1'-hydroxylation in human liver microsomes we observed that in extensive metabolizers the oxidation of bufuralol to carbinol is stereoselective, preferring the (+) isomer, in agreement with *in vivo* studies[14]. However, in microsomes of two poor metabolizers, this stereoselectivity was virtually lost, suggesting that an isozyme stereoselective for (+) bufuralol is deficient[10, 14-16]. Moreover, the markedly decreased V_{max} for (+) bufuralol was associated with a 4–5-fold increase in the K_m[15]. This increase in K_m has to be confirmed with other substrates involved in this polymorphism.

PURIFICATION AND FUNCTIONAL CHARACTERIZATION OF P$_{450}$ BUF, A CYTOCHROME P$_{450}$ ISOZYME WITH HIGH ACTIVITY FOR BUFURALOL-1'-HYDROXYLATION

By using the specific enzymatic activity of bufuralol-1'-hydroxylation in a reconstituted system (i.e. P$_{450}$ reductase, NADPH, phospholipids) to optimize hydrophobic and ion-exchange chromatography, we have purified, to electrophoretic homogeneity, a cytochrome P$_{450}$ isozyme with high activity for bufuralol hydroxylation, named 'P$_{450}$ buf'[16]. The purified isozyme has an apparent molecular weight of 50 000 and shows a striking increase in stereoselectivity for the (+) isomer of bufuralol when compared to microsomes. A polyclonal non-inhibiting antibody against P$_{450}$ buf was raised in rabbits[17]. Monoclonal and polyclonal inhibiting antibodies are under development. The non-inhibiting polyclonal antibody recognized the same amount of immunoreactive material in the microsomes of poor and extensive metabolizers, but these data have to be interpreted with caution, as the isozyme specificity of this antibody is not precisely established.

CONCLUSIONS

We conclude that a quantitative or qualitative deficiency of a highly stereoselective cytochrome P$_{450}$ buf is likely to be the cause of this common genetic variation of drug oxidation. An isozyme-specific antibody will be required to test for the presence or absence of the corresponding isozyme in poor metabolizer liver. Whether the high K_m for bufuralol in microsomes of poor metabolizers is due to a structural variant of P$_{450}$ buf or reflects metabolism by other less specific microsomal isozyme(s) not affected by the genetic polymorphism is presently under investigation.

We are convinced that the elucidation of common genetic defects in drug oxidation deserves a major effort as numerous additional drugs may be involved, and because these polymorphisms may be prototypes for other defects of cytochrome P_{450} isozymes. Moreover, this form of interindividual variability may be mechanistically related to the extreme multiplicity and functional variability of cytochrome P_{450} isozymes[18].

Acknowledgment

This research was supported by grant 3.893.81 from the Swiss National Science Foundation, the Geigy-Jubiläums-Foundation and the Sandoz-Foundation for Therapeutic Research.

References

1. Mahgoub, A., Idle, J. R., Dring, G. L., Lancaster, R. and Smith, R. L. (1977). Polymorphic hydroxylation of debrisoquine in man. *Lancet*, **ii**, 584-6
2. Eichelbaum, M., Spannbrucker, N., Steincke, B. and Dengler, H. J. (1979). *N*-oxidation of sparteine in man: a new pharmacogenetic defect. *Eur. J. Clin. Pharmacol.*, **16**, 183-7
3. Eichelbaum, M. (1984). Polymorphic drug oxidation in humans. *Fed. Proc.*, **43**, 2298-302
4. Price-Evans, D. A. P., Mahgoub, A., Sloan, T. P., Idle, J. R. and Smith, R. L. (1980). A family and population study of the genetic polymorphism of debrisoquine oxidation in a white British population. *J. Med. Genet.*, **17**, 102-5
5. Kalow, W. (1982). The metabolism of xenobiotics in different populations. *Can. J. Physiol. Pharmacol.*, **60**, 1-12
6. Idle, J. R. and Smith, R. L. (1979). Polymorphisms of oxidation at carbon centers of drugs and their clinical significance. *Drug Metab. Rev.*, **9**, 301-17
7. Cooper, R. G. and Evans, D. A. P. (1984). Oxidation polymorphism has clinical relevance. *Lancet*, **ii**, 227
8. Idle, J. R., Oates, N. S., Shah, R. R. and Smith, R. L. (1983). Protecting poor metabolisers, a group at high risk of adverse drug reactions. *Lancet*, **i**, 1388
9. Meier, P. J., Müller, H. K., Dick, B. and Meyer, U.A. (1983). Hepatic monooxygenase activities in subjects with genetic defects in drug oxidation. *Gastroenterology*, **85**, 682-92
10. Minder, E., Meier, P. J., Müller, H. K. and Meyer, U. A. (1984). Bufuralol Metabolism in Human Liver - A sensitive probe for the debrisoquine-type polymorphism of drug oxidation. *Eur. J. Clin. Invest.*, **14**, 184-9
11. Davies, D. S., Kahn, G. C., Murray, S., Brodie, M. J. and Boobis, A. R. (1981). Evidence for an enzymatic defect in the 4-hydroxylation of debrisoquine by human liver. *Br. J. Clin. Pharmacol.*, **11**, 89-91
12. Boobis, A. R., Murray, S., Kahan, G. C., Robertz, G. M. and Davies, D. S. (1983). Substrate specificity of the form of cytochrome P_{450} catalyzing the 4-hydroxylation of debrisoquine in man. *Mol. Pharmacol.*, **23**, 474-81
13. Dayer, P., Balant, L., Courvoisier, F., Küpfer, A., Kubli, A. and Fabre, J. (1982). The genetic control of bufuralol metabolism in man. *Eur. J. Drug Metab. Pharmacokin.*, **7**, 73-7
14. Dayer, P., Leeman, T., Gut, J., Kronbach, T., Küpfer, A., Francis, R. and Meyer, U. A. (1985). Steric configuration and polymorphic oxidation of lipophilic beta-adrenoceptor blocking agents: *In vivo - in vitro* correlations. *Biochem. Pharmacol.*, **34**, 399-400
15. Dayer, P., Gasser, R., Gut, J., Kronbach, T., Robertz, G. M., Eichelbaum, M. and Meyer, U. A. (1984). Characterization of a common genetic defect of cytochrome P_{450} function (Debrisoquine-Sparteine type polymorphism) - Increased Michaelis constant (K_m) and loss of stereoselectivity of bufuralol 1'-hydroxylation in poor metabolizers. *Biochem. Biophys. Res. Comm.*, **125**, 374-80
16. Gut, J., Gasser, R., Dayer, P., Kronbach, T., Catin, T. and Meyer, U. A. (1984). Debrisoquine-type polymorphism of drug oxidation: Purification from human liver of a cytochrome P_{450} isozyme with high activity for bufuralol hydroxylation. *FEBS Lett.*, **173**, 287-90

17. Gasser, R., Gut, J., Marti, U., Catin, T. and Meyer, U. A. (1984). Debrisoquine-type polymorphism: Immunochemical studies on human cytochrome P_{450} (P_{450}) isozymes with different bufuralol hydroxylation activity. *Xenobiotica*, **14**, 101 (Suppl. No. 1)
18. Meyer, U. A. (1984). The clinical pharmacology of cytochrome P450. In Lemberger, L. and Reidenberg, M. M. (eds.) *Proceedings of the 2nd World Conference on Clinical Pharmacology and Therapeutics ASPET*. pp. 331–41. (Bethesda)

11
The role of tumour-promoting chemical in hepatocarcinogenesis

H. GREIM, E. DEML AND D. OESTERLE

INTRODUCTION

In animal experiments, clear evidence has been established for the existence of a two-stage mechanism in chemical carcinogenesis. This was first demonstrated in mouse skin epidermal carcinogenesis[1]. The existence of similar stages of initiation and promotion in other organs of epithelial origin, e.g. liver, urinary bladder and mamma, have been demonstrated[2].

A number of compounds have been identified as promoters of hepatocarcinogenesis. These chemicals include persistent halogenated hydrocarbons, e.g. DDT, polychlorinated and polybrominated biphenyls, alpha-HCH and phenobarbital (for review *see* Reference 3), which are either ubiquitous environmental contaminants or frequently used drugs. None of these compounds reveal any mutagenic effects in *in vitro* test systems. *In vivo*, tumours have been observed mostly in mice, and only after long term treatment. Therefore, these chemicals have been classified as promoters, which do not possess initiating activity.

The relevance of these findings for human carcinogenesis has yet to be established. For this purpose two questions should be answered. Firstly, is there any evidence that there is a threshold for the tumour promoting effect? This question is of special interest in respect to risk evaluation. Secondly, do epidemiologic data reveal a correlation between intake of known promoting chemicals and tumour incidence?

Unfortunately, only a few studies have been performed on the dose dependency of promoting effects which may indicate the existence of thresholds. Furthermore, the mechanisms of promotion are mostly unknown. Thus, the theoretical basis for assuming the existence of a threshold is still lacking. In spite of these limitations, this paper aims to give at least a preliminary answer to these open questions.

The promoting effect of phenobarbital on liver tumours and preneoplastic lesions has previously been studied in detail, and dose-dependent studies have been performed[4,5]. For polychlorinated biphenyls (PCBs), we studied the dose–dependency of the promoting effect. Epidemiologic data, which may be related to the intake of the putative promoter, exist for phenobarbital, and, more limited, for PCBs. The following considerations will, therefore, be restricted to these two compounds.

POLYCHLORINATED BIPHENYLS

Material and methods

The experiments have been performed based on the two-step model of experimental hepatocarcinogenesis, using the histochemical detection of preneoplastic hepatocellular foci[6]. As a representative of the tumour promoting agents we choose Clophen A 50, a mixture of polychlorinated biphenyls, which is comparable to Aroclor 1254 in the degree of chlorination, and diethylnitrosamine for initiation. Weanling female Sprague-Dawley rats received a single dose of 8 mg/kg b.wt. diethylnitrosamine. One week later, doses of 0.1–50 mg/kg b.wt. Clophen A 50 were applied by gavage three times a week for 11 weeks. Twelve weeks after the initiation the livers were screened histochemically for adenosine triphosphatase-deficient and γ-glutamyltranspeptidase-positive islands.

Results

The higher doses significantly increased the number and area of preneoplastic islands. No such effects were observed at doses of 1 mg/kg and lower (Figure 11.1). This suggests a no-effect level in the promoting activity of these chemicals.

Simultaneously the dose-dependent induction of a microsomal monooxygenase reaction, the aldrine epoxidase[7], and the increase in the content of cytochrome P-450 were measured. A positive correlation between enzyme induction as well as the increase in the amount of cytochrome P-450 and the promoting effect has been found. A no-effect on enzyme induction was observed with 1 mg/kg b.wt. Clophen A 50 applied three times a week (Figure 11.2).

The activity of these enzyme reactions can be readily determined in humans. Furthermore, in experimental animals and in man microsomal enzyme induction is associated with a proliferation of the hepatic smooth endoplasmic reticulum, which can be diagnosed by electron microscopic investigation of liver biopsies. Such a proliferation of the endoplasmic reticulum has been observed in the liver of a patient who had ingested significant amounts of PCBs in the Yusho accident[8].

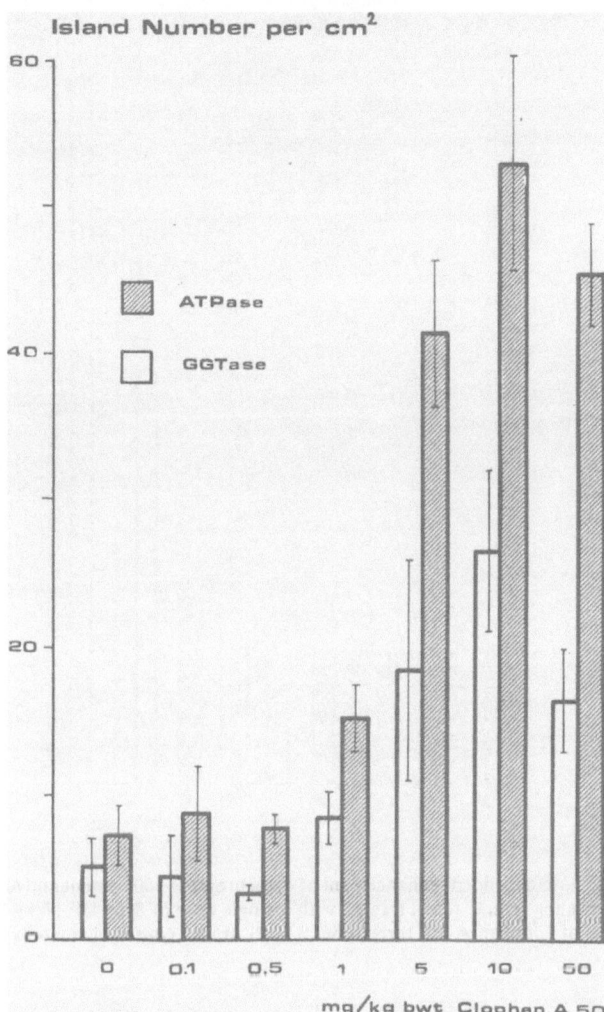

Figure 11.1 Dose-dependent enhancement in the number of adenosine triphosphatase deficient and γ-glutamyltranspeptidase positive islands in female Sprague-Dawley rats, treated with a single dose of 8 mg DE N/kg b.wt., and with various doses of Clophen A 50, three times a week for 11 consecutive weeks

Epidemiologic data

Considering these points, we have evaluated the possible role of poly-chlorinated biphenyls as promoters in human carcinogenesis.

From 1930 to 1970 PCBs were used in a wide variety of industrial applications. Since then their use has been voluntarily restricted to closed systems. This reduced the extent of human exposure by environmental pollution, industrial accidents and by migration from food packaging materials into

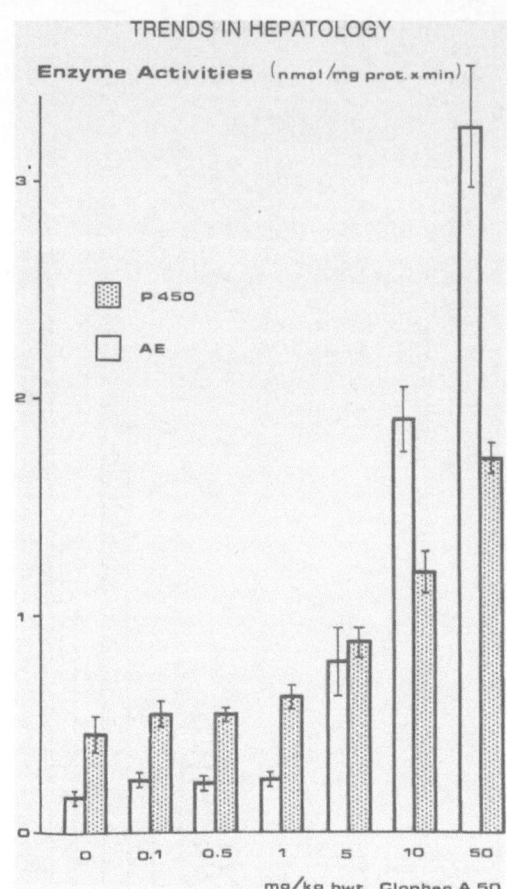

Figure 11.2 Dose-dependent enhancement of cytochrome P-450 content and aldrine epoxidase activity in weanling female rates, treated with a single dose of 8 mg DE N/kg b.wt., and with various doses of Clophen A 50, three times a week for 11 consecutive weeks

food[9]. The present intake by the general public is estimated to be[10] $5-10\,\mu g/$day $(0.07-0.14\,\mu g\,kg\,b.wt.^{-1}\,day^{-1})$. In a fish-eating population a 5-30 fold higher intake has been suggested, since fish still contains significant amounts[9]. Due to their lipophilicity, PCBs accumulate in adipose tissue. The majority of human adipose tissue contains 1-2 mg/kg PCBs with a range of 0.11-6.6 mg/kg in the Canadian population[11]. In spite of this relatively high exposure no adverse effects have been observed in the latter population.

In the Yusho food poisoning outbreak a commercial brand of rice oil was contaminated with polychlorinated biphenyls, dibenzofurans and quaterphenyls. The poisoning occurred in Western Japan in 1968, involving more than 1600 people[8].

The patients ingested, on average, 633 mg PCBs during a period of approximately 10 weeks. The clinical manifestation of the disease persisted for approximately 2 years with chloracne as the predominant symptom.

Other symptoms of the disease were pigmentation of the skin, visual disturbances, feeling of weakness, headaches and disturbances in liver function. The lowest dose producing overt effects was 500 mg total intake[12].

Epidemiologic data on the tumour incidence of this population or of other groups highly exposed to PCBs are incomplete. In the Yusho follow-up study at the end of 1977, 51 of the known patients had died and neoplasms accounted for 35.4% of the 31 classified deaths. This is a 21% higher mortality rate from neoplasms than the unexposed population of this region[13].

Although drug metabolism has not been studied in the Yusho patients, in one patient who had been subjected to liver biopsy a marked proliferation of the endoplasmic reticulum was found[8]. Together with the observation of an induced drug metabolism in workers who have been highly exposed to polychlorinated biphenyls[14] this suggests that Yusho patients have been exposed to amounts with a tumour promoting capacity. Further epidemiologic studies in this group of patients will be of great interest.

The general population is much less exposed, having a daily intake of 5–10 μg. Even the highly exposed fishermen who ingest approximately 0.5–4 μg/kg b.wt. daily do not reach the doses which have promoting effects in animal experiments (Table 11.1).

Thus, tumour promotion exerted by polychlorinated biphenyls in the general population is unlikely, although highly exposed people may be at a certain risk.

Table 11.1 Doses of polychlorinated biphenyls used in animal promotion experiments and intake by humans

Doses used in tumour promotion experiments	50–100 mg kg^{-1} week^{-1}
Dose without effect	3 × 0.5 mg kg^{-1} week^{-1} (~200 μg kg^{-1} day^{-1})
Estimated intake in Yusho patients within 10 weeks	600–700 mg (~160 μg kg^{-1} day^{-1})
Estimated daily intake in the general public in lake Michigan fishermen	0.07–0.14 μg kg^{-1} day^{-1} 0.5–4 μg kg^{-1} day^{-1}

PHENOBARBITAL

Results from experimental studies

For phenobarbital the dose-dependency of the promoting effect on preneoplastic islands in rat liver was studied by Kunz et al.[5]. They showed that daily oral application of 75 mg/kg b.wt. phenobarbital for 18 weeks enhanced the number of preneoplastic islands, whereas 7.5 and 0.75 mg/kg did not (Table 11.2). These data indicate that promotion by chemicals is dose-dependent and that a no-effect level can be considered.

No-effect levels in phenobarbital promotion have previously been observed. After feeding 0.02% 2-acetylaminofluorene (AAF) for 2 weeks, Peraino et al.[4] observed no increase in tumour incidence, and only a slight

Table 11.2 Dose-dependency in the promotion of preneoplastic islands in rat liver by oral phenobarbital

Initiation	18 weeks of daily phenobarbital treatment (mg/kg)	Preneoplastic areas (n/cm²) ATPase(–)	GT(+)
NNM	Water	288	780
NNM	0.75	270	657
NNM	7.5	285	720
NNM	75	612	1597
Water	75	10	10
Water	Water	10	10

(Data from Kunz et al.[5])

enhancement of tumour frequency by 0.002% phenobarbital in the diet, even after 84 subsequent weeks of treatment. The latter observation is of special significance, since most authors use short term experiments to study the tumour promoting effects of chemicals. The reliability of such short term experiments on no-effect concentrations could be questioned with the objection that the experiments have been conducted for an insufficient period of time.

Considering these points, the possible role of phenobarbital as a promoter of human carcinogenesis is evaluated.

Epidemiologic data

Phenobarbital is a long-acting central nervous system depressant. In antiepileptic therapy phenobarbital is given in daily doses of 50–200 mg, representing 0.7–3 mg/kg b.wt. Generally an increased hepatic microsomal enzyme activity is observed, resulting in a higher tolerance of the patients to other drugs which are metabolized by these enzymes (for review see reference 15).

Two epidemiological studies on 9136 epileptic patients treated with anticonvulsant drugs, including phenobarbital, were performed[16]. They revealed that in those patients treated for up to 10 years the incidence of cancer at all sites, except the liver, was the same or lower than that expected when compared with the incidence in the general population. In patients treated for more than 10 years, four cases of liver cancer were observed in males, whereas 1.1 were expected. However, when reconsidering these data, it turned out that three out of the four male patients with liver tumours had previously been treated with thorotrast[17] which is known to induce liver tumours in man[18].

The apparent negative findings in these studies are supported by dose-effect considerations. In promotion experiments, usually 0.05–0.1% phenobarbital in the drinking water or in the diet corresponding to approximately 40 mg kg b.wt.$^{-1}$ day^{-1} are given. According to Kunz et al.[5] a dose of 7.5 mg/kg phenobarbital is ineffective in rats. The therapeutic dose in epileptics of maximally 4 mg/kg is even lower (Table 11.3). This dose is given only for short periods of time since it produces intensive sleepiness.

Table 11.3 Doses of phenobarbital in promotion experiments and in medical use

Doses used in tumour promotion experiments	$20-80 \, mg \, kg^{-1} day^{-1}$
Dose without effect	$7.5 \, mg \, kg^{-1} day^{-1}$
Daily dose in epileptics	$100-300 \, mg$ ($\sim 0.7-4 \, mg/kg$)

Although not substantiated by the epidemiologic studies one has also to note that there is some indication of a reduced incidence of cancer at all sites in the patients treated for up to 10 years with phenobarbital. This would support the observations that phenobarbital reduces the liver tumour incidence in rats when it is given prior to aflatoxin[19].

Thus, this evaluation so far indicates that the continuous therapeutic use of relatively high doses of phenobarbital which results in an enhanced drug metabolism in these patients[15] may have no tumour promoting capability. This may be mostly related to the low therapeutic doses as compared to those required for tumour promotion in experimental animals.

TUMOUR PROMOTION IN OTHER ORGANS

Saccharin, when given as 5% (50 000 p.p.m.) in the diet, after an initiating treatment of FANFT, acted as a promotor[20]. In a different experiment using the urinary carcinogen dibutylnitrosamine, Nakanishi et al.[21] observed a dose-response effect in the tumour promoting capacity of saccharin in rats. No such effect was found at saccharin doses below 1% in the diet. Again, there is no epidemiologic evidence that saccharin increases the tumour incidence in humans[22].

For various experimental systems, e.g. mouse lung and rat mammary gland, the action of tumour promoters has been demonstrated[3], but no corresponding epidemiologic data exist.

POSSIBLE MECHANISMS OF TUMOUR PROMOTION AND THE EXISTENCE OF THRESHOLDS

As mentioned above, in experimental hepatocarcinogenesis there is clear evidence that promoters exist which may be distinguished from initiators and complete carcinogens. Furthermore, experimental data support the suggestion that the promoting effect is dose-dependent and, in contrast to initiators, is reversible and possesses a no-effect level.

Epidemiologic data from humans are in agreement with this hypothesis. No indication exists for enhanced tumour formation in people who are exposed to putative promoting agents over a long period. Taken together, experimental and epidemiologic data suggest that promotion is a reversible and thresholded process.

Table 11.4 Phenobarbital doses with no tumour-promoting effect in rats

Dose	Time of promotion (weeks)	Reference
20 ppm in diet	81	4
20 ppm in drinking water	24	25
7.5 mg/kg i.p. (daily)	18	5

The crucial task is now to establish a theoretical base for this hypothesis, which must include the mechanisms of promoting action. At present, the mechanisms of promotion are mostly unknown, and there is no unifying theory.

The main effect of tumour promoters, regardless of type, is the expansion of the initiated cell population within a target tissue[23]. One factor involved in the promotion process may be the enhancement of cell proliferation, as indicated by the promoting effect of regenerative growth after partial hepatectomy[24], or, correspondingly, inflammation and concomitant hyperplasia of the skin. The induction of cell proliferation may be of greater importance in liver, as a resting organ than in other tissues such as skin.

Another factor which may play a role is the inhibition of intercellular communication as demonstrated in liver cell culture[25]. This inhibitory effect may support the escape of preneoplastic cells from growth control.

Based on the effects of phorbolesters and teleocidin B on cell differentiation in the skin[26] another mechanism is suggested, which includes the completion of conversion of partially transformed cells into neoplastic cells. The possible mechanisms of skin tumour promotion have been discussed in detail[27] (for review *see* reference 23).

Williams[28] summarized a number of cellular effects that could facilitate the growth of neoplastic cells into tumours. The main points are the enhancement of expression of neoplastic phenotype, the stimulation of cell proliferation, mediated by cytotoxicity or by hormone-like effects, immunosuppression and cell membrane effects, e.g. the inhibition of intercellular communication. Promotion could, according to Williams[28], be a consequence of any of these actions alone or in combination.

In conclusion, the effects mentioned above are not contradictory to the suggestion of a possible threshold. Nevertheless, some recent observations indicate that promoting agents may cause irreversible, genotoxic effects: Montesano and Slaga[29] pointed out that skin promoters like TPA can produce DNA damage due to the formation of free radicals[30] and that some effects are irreversible[31]. This and the observation of chromosomal aberrations[32] caused the IARC[33] to express strong reservations to a hypothesis of a general differentiation of the effects of initiators and promoters in carcinogenesis.

According to some authors (e.g. Weinstein[34], Lijinsky[35]) the present distinction between 'initiating' and 'promoting' carcinogens which implicates a difference in the risk to humans is not justified, since a substantial theoretical base is still lacking. These considerations must not be neglected. Further work should focus on this subject.

References

1. Berenblum, I. and Shubik, P. (1947). A new, quantitative approach to the study of the stages of chemical carcinogenesis in the mouse's skin. *Br. J. Cancer*, **1**, 383-6
2. Pitot, H. C. (1983). Contributions of our understanding of the natural history of neoplastic development in lower animals to the cause and control of human cancer. *Cancer Surv.*, **2**, 519-37
3. Pitot, H. C. and Sirica, A. E. (1980). The stages of initiation and promotion in hepatocarcinogenesis. *Biochim. Biophys. Acta*, **605**, 191-215
4. Peraino, C., Staffeldt, E. F., Haugen, D. A., Lombard, L.S., Stevens, F. J. and Fry, R. J. M. (1980). Effects of varying the dietary concentration of phenobarbital on its enhancement of 2-acetylaminofluorene-induced hepatic tumorigenesis. *Cancer Res.*, **40**, 3268-73
5. Kunz, W., Schaüde, G., Schwarz, M. and Tennekes, H. (1982). Quantitative aspects of drug-mediated tumour promotion in liver and its toxicological implications. In Hecker, E., Fusenig, N. E., Kunz, W., Marks, F. and Thielmann, H. W. (eds.) *Cocarcinogenesis and Biological Effects of Tumor Promoters, Carcinogenesis*. Vol. 7, pp. 111-26. (New York: Raven Press)
6. Oesterle, D. and Deml, E. (1983). Promoting effect of polychlorinated biphenyls on development of enzyme-altered islands in livers of weanling and adult rats. *J. Cancer Res. Clin. Oncol.*, **105**, 141-7
7. Wolff, T., Deml, E. and Wanders, H. (1979). Aldrin epoxidation, a highly sensitive indicator specific for cytochrome P-450-dependent monooxygenase activities. *Drug Metab. Dispos.*, **7**, 301-5
8. Kuratsune, M. (1980). Yusho. In Kimbrough, R. D. (ed.) *Halogenated biphenyls, terphenyls, naphthalenes, dibenzodioxins and related products.* pp. 287-302. (Elsevier: North Holland Biomedical Press)
9. Cordle, F., Corneliussen, P., Jelinek, C., Hackley, B., Lehman, R. and Shapiro, R. (1978). Human exposure to polychlorinated biphenyls and polybrominated biphenyls. *Environ. Health Persp.*, **24**, 157-72
10. Humphrey, H. E. B., Price, H. A. and Budd, M. L. (1976). Evaluation of changes of the level of polychlorinated biphenyls (PCBs) in human tissue. *Final Report of FDA contract No. 223-73-2209*
11. Grant, D. L., Mes, J. and Frank, R. (1976). PCB residues in human adipose tissue and milk. In *Proceedings of National Conference on Polychlorinated biphenyls*, Chicago 1975. EPA-560/6-75-04. (Washington: US Environ. Protect. Agency)
12. Kuratsune, M., Masuda, Y. and Nagayama, J. (1976). Some of the recent findings concerning Yusho. In *Proceedings of a National Conference on Polychlorinated Biphenyls*, Chicago 1975. pp. 14-29. EPA-560/6-75-004. (Washington DC: Environmental Protection Agency)
13. Urabe, H., Koda, H. and Asahi, M. (1979). Present state of Yusho patients. *Ann. NY Acad. Sci.*, **320**, 273-6
14. Alvares, A. P., Fischbein, A., Anderson, K. E. and Kappas, A. (1977). Alterations in drug metabolism in workers exposed to polychlorinated biphenyls. *Clin. Pharmacol. Therap.*, **22**, 140-6
15. Greim, H. A. (1981). An overview of the phenomena of enzyme induction and inhibition: Their relevance to drug action and drug interactions. In Jenner, P. and Testa, B. (eds.) *Concepts in Drug Metabolism*. pp. 219-63. (New York: Dekker Inc.)
16. Clemmesen, J., Fuglsang-Frederiksen, V. and Plum, C. M. (1974). Are anticonvulsants oncogenic? *Lancet*, **i**, 705-7
17. Clemmesen, J. (1975). Phenobarbitone, liver tumours and thorotrast. *Lancet*, **i**, 37-8
18. Kiely, J. M., Titus, J. L. and Orvis, A. (1973). Thorotrast-induced hepatoma presenting as hyperparathyroidism. *Cancer*, **31**, 1312-14
19. McLean, A. E. M. and Marshall, A. (1971). Reduced carcinogenic effects of aflatoxin in rats given phenobarbitone. *Br. J. Exp. Pathol.*, **52**, 322-9
20. Cohen, S. M., Arai, M., Jacobs, J. B. and Friedell, G. H. (1979). Promoting effect of saccharin and DL-tryptophan in urinary bladder carcinogenesis. *Cancer Res.*, **39**, 1207-17
21. Nakanishi, K., Hagiwara, A., Shibata, M., Imaida, K., Tatematsu, M. and Ito, N. (1980). Dose response of saccharin in the induction of urinary bladder lesions in rats pretreated with N-butyl-N-(4-hydroxybutyl)nitrosamine. *J. Natl. Cancer Inst.*, **65**, 1005-10

22. Wynder, E. L. and Stellman, S. D. (1980). Bladder cancer and artificial sweeteners: A methodological issue. *Science*, **210**, 447-8
23. Slaga, T. J. (1983). Cellular and molecular mechanisms of tumour promotion. *Cancer Surv.*, **2**, 595-612
24. Scherer, E. and Emmelot, P. (1975). Foci of altered liver cells induced by a single dose of diethylnitrosamine and partial hepatectomy: Their contribution to hepatocarcinogenesis in the rat. *Eur. J. Cancer*, **11**, 145-54
25. Williams, G. M. (1981). Liver carcinogenesis: The role for some chemicals of an epigenetic mechanism of liver-tumour promotion involving modification of the cell membrane. *Food Cosmet. Toxicol.*, **19**, 577-83
26. Fujiki, H., Mori, M., Nakayasu, M., Terada, M. and Sugimura, T. (1979). A possibly naturally occuring tumor promoter teleocidin B from Streptomyces. *Biochem. Biophys. Res. Commun.*, **90**, 976
27. Weinstein, I. B., Horowitz, A. D., Mufson, R. A., Fisher, P. B., Ivanovic, V. and Greenebaum, E. (1982). Results and speculations related to recent studies on mechanisms of tumor promotion. In Hecker, E., Fusenig, N. E., Kunz, W., Marks, F. and Thielmann, H. W. (eds.) *Cocarcinogenesis and Biological Effects of Tumor Promoters, Carcinogenesis.* Vol. 7, pp. 599-613. (New York: Raven Press)
28. Williams, G. M. (1984). Modulation of chemical carcinogenesis by xenobiotics. *Fund. Appl. Toxicol.*, **4**, 325-44
29. Montesano, R. and Slaga, T. J. (1983). Initiation and promotion in carcinogenesis: An appraisal. *Cancer Surveys*, **2**, 613-21
30. Marx, J. C. (1983). Do tumour promoters affect DNA after all? *Science*, **219**, 158-9
31. Fürstenberger, G., Sorg, B. and Marks, F. (1983). Tumor promotion by phorbol esters in skin: Evidence for a memory effect. *Science*, **220**, 89-91
32. Birnboim, H. C. (1982). DNA strand breakage in human leukocytes exposed to a tumour promoter, phorbol myristate acetate. *Science*, **215**, 1247-9
33. IARC (1983). Approaches to classifying chemical carcinogens according to mechanism of action. *IARC Internal Technical Report No. 83/001*, Lyon, 1983
34. Weinstein, I. B. (1983). Carcinogen Policy at EPA. *Science*, **219**, 794-6
35. Lijinsky, W. (1983). Carcinogenic risk. *Science*, **221**, 810

12
Recent trends in studies of the pathogenesis of hepatic encephalopathy

E. A. JONES

Hepatic encephalopathy precipitated by hepatocellular failure has been extensively studied, but the neural mechanisms that mediate this syndrome remain unknown[1-3]. It is still uncertain whether hepatic encephalopathy is due to diminished hepatic synthesis of a substance necessary for normal brain function or diminished hepatic metabolism of a substance which can induce neural inhibition. Two observations tend to favour the second of these possibilities. One is the clinical observation that therapeutic manoeuvres which reduce the interaction between nitrogenous substances and the enteric bacterial flora are often followed by the amelioration of hepatic encephalopathy in patients with cirrhosis[1]. The other is the result of carefully conducted experiments in which normal and liverless rats were cross-circulated and the E.E.G. monitored; brain function of liverless rats improved more rapidly when their aortic blood was infused into the portal vein rather than the jugular vein of normal rats[4].

Until recently there have been three principal hypotheses of the pathogenesis of hepatic encephalopathy. These have implicated ammonia-induced neurotoxicity[1-3], the synergistic interactions between ammonia, mercaptans and fatty acids[2] and false-neurotransmitter-induced neural inhibition[5]. These hypotheses have been based largely on studies in which concentrations of neuroactive substances or their metabolites have been measured in plasma, CSF or brain. Studies of this type have not led to an understanding of the neural mechanisms responsible for hepatic encephalopathy[6]. If a positive correlation is found between the increased level of a substance and the stage of hepatic encephalopathy three explanations are possible: (1) the increased level of the substance may contribute to the encephalopathy; (2) production of the substance may occur secondary to encephalopathy, and (3) some entirely unrelated phenomenon precipitated by liver failure is responsible for the mediation of the encephalopathy. Furthermore, because of subcellular compartmentalization of substances within the brain[7] mean changes in the concentration of a neuroactive substance in whole brain may not be relevant to the pathogenesis of hepatic encephalopathy. For example, the concentrations of neurotransmitters in synaptic clefts may be important, but such concentrations may not be reflected in mean concentrations of neurotransmitters in whole brain.

An alternative approach is to consider which well characterized neurophysiologic mechanisms could conceivably mediate hepatic encephalopathy. Clearly, this syndrome is characterized by profound neural inhibition. The best characterized mechanism for inducing neural inhibition in the brain is the interaction between γ-amino butyric acid (GABA) and its receptors on postsynaptic neurons. This interaction promotes chloride ion conductance across the postsynaptic neural membrane and hence hyperpolarization of the membrane and an inhibitory post-synaptic potential[8, 9] (Figure 12.1). Accordingly, the question arises whether GABA could be implicated in the pathogenesis of hepatic encephalopathy.

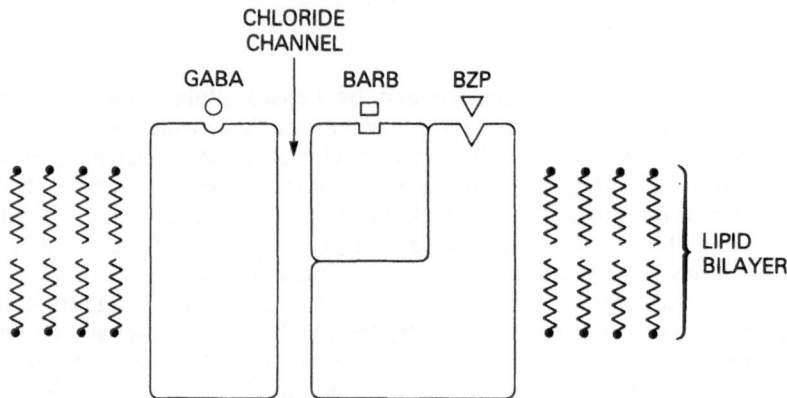

Figure 12.1 A simplified model of the GABA-receptor/ionophore complex embedded in a postsynaptic neural membrane. Binding of any of the depicted ligands: GABA, a barbiturate (BARB) or a benzodiazepine (BZP), to its specific binding site promotes chloride ion conductance through the membrane and hence hyperpolarization of the membrane and an inhibitory postsynaptic potential. (From reference 16)

SOME RELEVANT PROPERTIES OF GABA

GABA is the principal inhibitory neurotransmitter of the mammalian brain[8, 9]. It is a potent inhibitor of single neurons[10] and it can induce coma. Within 10 seconds of the instillation of less than 1 μmole of GABA into the hippocampus of conscious rabbits the animals *'became quiet; the spontaneous locomotor activity declined and the animals mostly lay on the cage floor'*[11]. These behavioural changes were associated with spreading delta wave E.E.G. activity[11] similar to that seen in hepatic coma[12].

It would be expected that a substance of importance in the pathogenesis of hepatic encephalopathy would be synthesized by gut bacteria[1]. GABA has this property. Not only is the concentration of GABA in portal venous plasma about twice that in aortic plasma of normal rabbits, but *Escherichia coli* and *Bacteroides fragilis*, isolated from human faeces, synthesize abundant quantities of GABA when cultured anaerobically[13].

In rabbits the liver contains more than 80% of the total body activity of GABA-transaminase, the enzyme responsible for the catabolism of GABA[14], and it seems likely that the liver plays a major role in the metabolism of gut-derived GABA[15]. Decreased hepatic metabolism of gut-derived GABA presumably contributes to the markedly increased concentrations of GABA that have been found in a (galactosamine-induced) rabbit model of acute liver failure before the onset of overt encephalopathy[15].

For gut-derived GABA to be implicated in the pathogenesis of hepatic encephalopathy, it has been postulated that GABA in plasma crosses the blood–brain barrier in liver failure[16]. Intravenously administered ^{14}C-labelled α-aminoisobutyric acid has been used as a marker to study non-specific changes in the permeability of the blood–brain barrier in a (galactosamine-induced) rabbit model of acute liver failure. The magnitude of transfer of the marker across the barrier can be assessed from colour-referenced auto-radiograms of the brain. In normal rabbits transfer is minimal. The onset of acute liver failure is associated with a selective increase in the permeability of the barrier in certain grey matter areas of the brain. This non-specific increase in permeability occurs before the onset of overt encephalopathy, and is compatible with GABA in plasma gaining access to the brain in liver failure[17].

STUDIES OF VISUAL EVOKED POTENTIALS

An attempt has been made to determine whether the pattern of neuronal activity in the brain in experimental hepatic encephalopathy is similar to or different from that in a variety of other experimentally-induced encephalopathies. The approach adopted was to record visual evoked potentials (VEPs). VEPs represent the summation of volleys of excitatory and inhibitory postsynaptic potentials in response to repeated flashes of light. They are derived from the E.E.G. by averaging signals that are time-locked to the visual stimulus using a computer of average transients[18] (Figure 12.2). The normal VEP in rabbits consists of a series of peaks that occur reproducibly between 15 and 1000 ms after the photic stimulus. These peaks are defined in terms of their orientation (positive or negative), their amplitude and their latency (time of occurrence after photic stimulation)[18] (Figure 12.3). Hepatic coma (induced by galactosamine) is associated with distinctive and reproducible changes in the VEP waveform[18] (Figure 12.3). Encephalopathy, in the absence of seizures, induced by infusing a solution of ammonium chloride, is associated with changes in the VEP waveform that do not resemble those associated with hepatic coma[19] (Figure 12.3). Furthermore, coma in the absence of seizures, induced by administering subcoma doses of ammonium chloride,

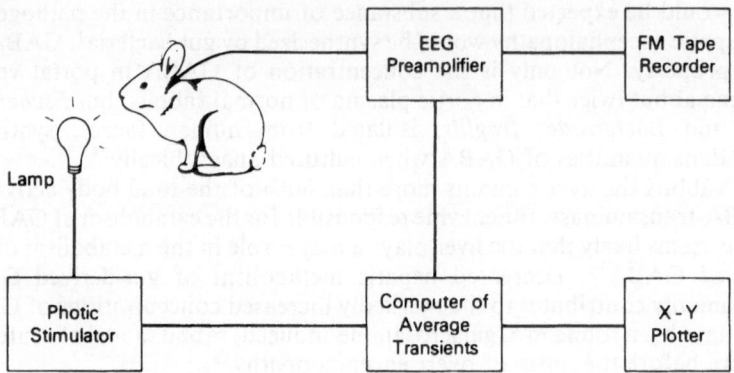

Figure 12.2 Diagram illustrating the method of recording visual evoked potentials (VEPs) in rabbits. The EEG preamplifier signal serves as the input to a signal averager (computer of average transients). The E.E.G. can be simultaneously recorded on FM tape. The photic stimulator is triggered by a circuit of the signal averager to allow analysis of E.E.G. activity time-locked to the visual stimulus. The X–Y plotter is used to record the VEP. (From reference 18)

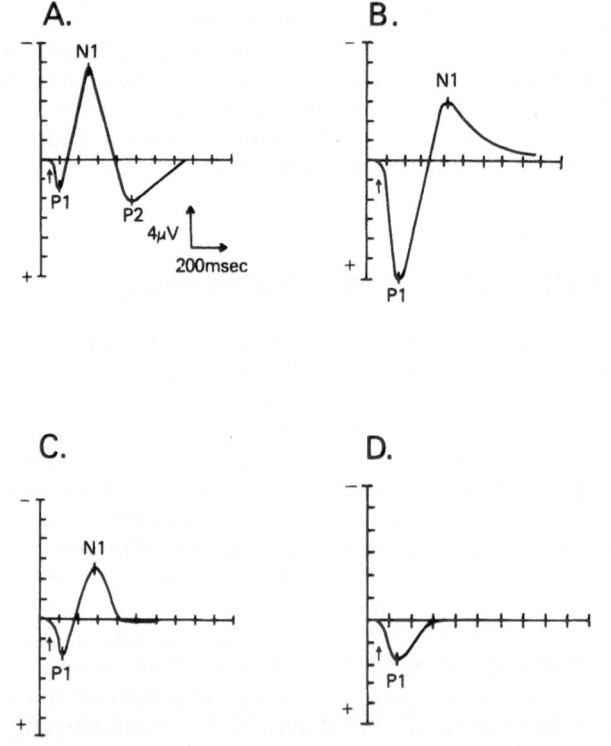

Figure 12.3 Visual evoked potentials in rabbits. A: Normal. B: Hepatic coma or coma induced by pentobarbital, diazepam or muscimol. C: Preseizure hyperammonaemic encephalopathy. D: Preseizure coma induced by the simultaneous administration of subcoma doses of ammonium chloride, dimethyldisulphide and octanoic acid. (From references 18 and 19)

dimethyldisulphide (a mercaptan precursor) and octanoic acid, is also associated with changes in the VEP waveform that do not resemble those associated with hepatic coma[19] (Figure 12.3). It should be emphasized that these findings in rabbits are at variance with the results of an analogous study in rats[20], possibly due, at least in part, to different routes of administration of ammonium chloride, different doses of the three toxins administered and the different species studied.

The GABA receptor complex has sites on its surface for the binding of not only GABA but also barbiturates and benzodiazepines. The specific binding of a barbiturate or a benzodiazepine to its binding site on this complex promotes GABA-mediated neural inhibition[8, 21–23] (Figure 12.1). Coma, induced by administering the barbiturate, pentobarbital, the benzodiazepine, diazepam or the potent GABA agonist, muscimol, is associated with changes in the VEP waveform that are identical to those observed in hepatic coma[18] (Figure 12.3). One explanation for these findings is that the pattern of post-synaptic neuronal activity in hepatic coma is similar to that associated with activation of the GABA inhibitory neurotransmitter system.

STUDIES OF NEUROTRANSMITTER RECEPTORS

To study the status of neurotransmitter receptors in the brain in hepatic encephalopathy the classical experimental approach applied in most ligand-receptor binding studies has been adopted. Data on the binding of a neuro-transmitter to neural membranes isolated from the brain are obtained at equilibrium and corrected for non-specific binding. Such data have been subjected to Scatchard analysis using the LIGAND computer program[24].

Data on the binding of GABA to neural membranes isolated from rabbit brain are consistent with the existence of two classes of binding site for this ligand, each with a characteristic (high or low) affinity[25]. Hepatic coma (induced by galactosamine) is associated, with no change in the affinities of these receptors but with increases in the densities of both the high and low affinity receptors[25] (Figure 12.4). Similar findings have been reported in rats[26]. Hyperammonaemia in the absence of liver failure in rabbits is associated with no changes in the affinities or densities of GABA receptors[27]. Corresponding data for the binding of glutamate, the principal excitatory neurotransmitter of the brain, indicate the presence of a single class of receptors. Hepatic coma is associated with no change in the affinity but with a decrease in the density of glutamate receptors. In contrast, hyperammonaemia in the absence of liver failure is associated with an increase in both the affinity and density of glutamate receptors[28] (Figure 12.5). Analogous studies of seven other neurotransmitter receptors have been conducted. The binding data are compatible with two classes of binding site for glycine, and single classes of binding site for aspartate, kainic acid, dopamine and muscarinic acetylcholine receptors. Hepatic coma is associated with an increase in the density of glycine receptors, a decrease in the density of aspartate and kainic acid receptors and no change in the density of μ-opiate, δ-opiate, dopamine and muscarinic acetylcholine receptors[29]. Thus, in hepatic coma there is an increase in the density of receptors for inhibitory amino acid neurotransmitters (GABA,

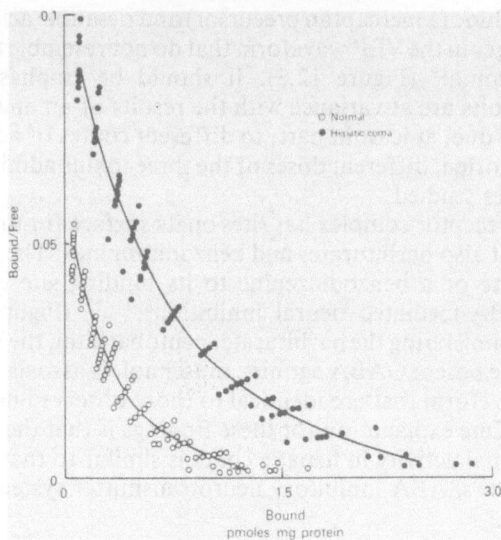

Figure 12.4 Scatchard plots of the specific binding of GABA to synaptic membranes isolated from the brains of normal control rabbits and rabbits with hepatic coma induced by galactosamine. (From reference 25.) The corresponding Scatchard plot for rabbits with preseizure hyperammonaemic encephalopathy in the absence of liver failure is superimposable on that of controls

glycine), a decrease in the density of receptors for excitatory amino acid neurotransmitters (glutamate, aspartate, kainic acid) and no change in the density of receptors for non-amino acid neurotransmitters (μ-opiate, δ-opiate, dopamine, acetylcholine).

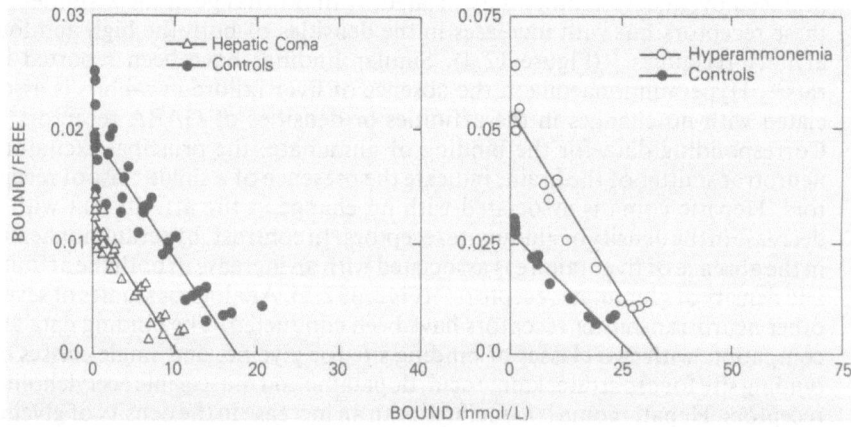

Figure 12.5 Scatchard plots of the specific binding of glutamate to synaptic membranes isolated from the brains of normal control rabbits, rabbits with hepatic coma induced by galactosamine and rabbits with preseizure hyperammonaemic encephalopathy in the absence of liver failure. (From reference 28)

124

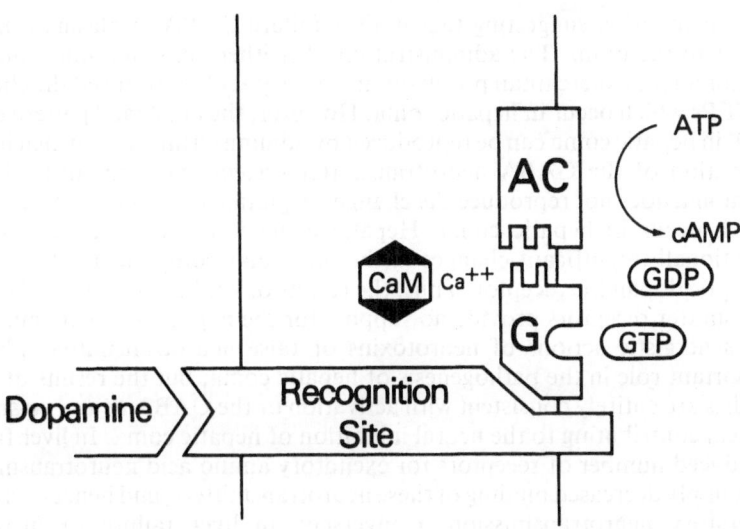

Figure 12.6 A model of the postsynaptic dopamine receptor. CaM, calmodulin; G, G coupling protein (regulatory subunit); AC, adenylate cyclase; GTP, guanosine triphosphate; GDP, guanosine diphosphate; ATP, adenosine triphosphate; cAMP, cyclic adenosine monophosphate

The function of dopamine receptors in the corpus striatum can be studied by assaying cyclic AMP production catalysed by dopamine-sensitive adenylate cyclase[30]. Binding of dopamine to its receptors mediates activation of adenylate cyclase via the G coupling protein (regulatory subunit) and calmodulin (Figure 12.6). The dopamine concentration–adenylate cyclase stimulation response relationship does not shift in rabbits with hepatic coma (induced by galactosamine) relative to the corresponding response relationship in normal rabbits[31]. Furthermore, the adenylate cyclase responses to stimulating the G coupling protein with sodium fluoride and to a specific dopamine receptor agonist in hepatic coma were similar to corresponding control responses[31] indicating, respectively, that hepatic coma is not associated with any changes in the stimulatory or inhibitory regulatory subunits of adenylate cyclase. These negative findings make it unlikely that impaired dopaminergic neurotransmission plays an important role in the mediation of hepatic coma, and consequently are at variance with a component of the false neurotransmitter hypothesis of the pathogenesis of hepatic encephalopathy.

SUMMARY, CONCLUSIONS AND SPECULATIONS

GABA, the principal inhibitory neurotransmitter of the mammalian brain, posseses properties that would be expected of a substance of importance in the pathogenesis of hepatic encephalopathy. It can cause coma and it is synthesized by gut bacteria. In acute liver failure a non-specific increase in the permeability of the blood–brain barrier occurs before the onset of overt encephalopathy, suggesting that in liver failure GABA in plasma can gain access to the brain. The administration of neither ammonia nor a mixture of ammonia, a mercaptan precursor and a fatty acid reproduced the changes in VEPs which occur in hepatic coma. However, the abnormal pattern of the VEP in hepatic coma can be reproduced by administering drugs which induce activation of the GABA neurotransmitter system. The administration of ammonia does not reproduce the changes in glutamate and GABA receptors which occur in hepatic coma. Hepatic coma is not associated with any functionally significant changes in the molecular components of the post-synaptic dopamine receptor. Thus, the results of studies of VEPs and neurotransmitter receptors provide no support for the hypotheses that ammonia, the synergistic actions of neurotoxins or false neurotransmitters play an important role in the pathogenesis of hepatic coma; but the results of these studies are entirely consistent with activation of the GABA neurotransmitter system contributing to the neural inhibition of hepatic coma. In liver failure a reduced number of receptors for excitatory amino acid neurotransmitters may imply decreased binding of these neurotransmitters, and hence decreased excitatory neurotransmission. Conversely, in liver failure an increased number of receptors for inhibitory amino acid neurotransmitters, including GABA, may imply increased binding of these neurotransmitters and hence increased inhibitory neurotransmission. Such changes in neurotransmission may constitute the neuropathophysiologic basis of the syndrome of hepatic encephalopathy.

References

1. Conn, H. O. and Lieberthal, M. M. (1978). *The Hepatic Coma Syndromes and Lactulose.* (Baltimore: Williams and Wilkins)
2. Zieve, L. (1982). Hepatic encephalopathy. In Schiff, L. and Schiff, E. R. (eds.) *Diseases of the Liver.* 5th Edn., pp. 433–59. (Philadelphia: Lippincott)
3. Duffy, T. E. and Plum, F. (1982). Hepatic encephalopathy. In Arias, I. M., Popper, H., Schacter, D. and Shafritz, D. A. *The Liver: Biology and Pathobiology.* pp. 693–715. (New York: Raven Press)
4. Roche-Sicot, J., Sicot, C., Peignous, M., Bourdiau, D., Degos, F., Degos, J.-D., Prandi, D., Rueff, R. and Benhamou, J.-P. (1974). Acute hepatic encephalopathy in the rat. The effect of cross circulation. *Clin. Sci. Molec. Med.*, **47**, 609–15
5. James, J. H., Jeppson, B., Ziparo, V., Fischer, J. E. (1979). Hyperammonemia, plasma amino acid imbalance and blood brain amino acid transport: a unified theory of portal systemic encephalopathy. *Lancet*, **i**, 86–7
6. Zieve, L. (1981). The mechanism of hepatic coma. *Hepatology*, **1**, 360–5
7. Balazs, R. and Cremer, J. E. (1972). *Metabolic Compartmentalization in the Brain.* (New York: John Wiley and Sons)
8. Costa, E., Di Chiara, G., Gessa, G. L. (eds.) (1981). GABA and benzodiazepine receptors. *Advances in Biochemical Psychopharmacology.* Volume 26. (New York: Raven Press)
9. Roberts, E. (1984). The γ-aminobutyric acid (GABA) system and hepatic encephalopathy. *Hepatology*, **4**, 342–5
10. Krnjevic, K. and Phillis, J. W. (1963). Iontophoretic studies of neurones in the mammalian cerebral cortex. *J. Physiol.*, **165**, 274–304
11. Smialowski, A. (1978). The effects of intra-hippocampal administration of γ-aminobutyric acid (GABA). In Fonnum, F. (ed.) *Amino Acids as Chemical Transmitters.* pp. 1977–80. (New York: Plenum Press)

12. Blitzer, B. L., Waggoner, J. G., Jones, E. A. *et al.* (1978). A model of fulminant hepatic failure in the rabbit. *Gastroenterology*, **74**, 664–71
13. Schafer, D. F., Fowler, J. M., Jones, E. A. (1981). Colonic bacteria: A source of γ-aminobutyric acid in blood. *Proc. Soc. Exp. Biol. Med.*, **167**, 301–3
14. Ferenci, P., Schafer, D. F., Shrager, R. and Jones, E. A. (1981). Metabolism of the inhibitory neurotransmitter γ-aminobutyric acid in a rabbit model of acute hepatic failure. *Hepatology*, **1**, 509 (Abstr.)
15. Ferenci, P., Covell, D., Schafer, D. F. *et al.* (1983). Metabolism of the inhibitory neurotransmitter γ-aminobutyric acid in a rabbit model of fulminant hepatic failure. *Hepatology*, **3**, 507–12
16. Schafer, D. F. and Jones, E. A. (1982). Hepatic encephalopathy and the γ-aminobutyric acid neurotransmitter system. *Lancet*, **1**, 18–20
17. Horowitz, M. E., Schafer, D. F., Molnar, P. *et al.* (1983). Increased blood–brain transfer in a rabbit model of acute liver failure. *Gastroenterology*, **84**, 1003–11
18. Schafer, D. F., Pappas, S. C., Brody, L. E. *et al.* (1984). Visual evoked potentials in a rabbit model of hepatic encephalopathy. I. Sequential changes and comparisons with drug-induced comas. *Gastroenterology*, **86**, 540–5
19. Pappas, S. C., Ferenci, P., Schafer, D. F. and Jones, E. A. (1984). Visual evoked potentials in a rabbit model of hepatic encephalopathy. II. Comparison of hyperammonemic encephalopathy, post-ictal coma, and coma induced by synergistic neurotoxins. *Gastroenterology*, **86**, 546–51
20. Zeneroli, M. L., Ventura, E., Baraldi, M. *et al.* (1982). Visual evoked potentials in encephalopathy induced by galactosamine, ammonia, dimethyldisulfide and octanoic acid. *Hepatology*, **2**, 532–8
21. Tallman, J. F., Paul, S. M., Skolnick, P. *et al.* (1980). Receptors for the age of anxiety: Pharmacology of benzodiazepines. *Science*, **207**, 274–81
22. Skolnick, P., Moncada, V., Barker, J. L. *et al.* (1981). Phenobarbital: dual actions to increase brain benzodiazepine receptor affinity. *Science*, **211**, 1448–50
23. Paul, S. M., Marangos, P. J. and Skolnick, P. (1981). The benzodiazepine-GABA-chloride ionophore receptor complex: common site of minor tranquilizer action. *Biol. Psychol.*, **16**, 213–29
24. Munson, P. J. and Rodbard, D. (1980). LIGAND: A versatile computerized approach for characterization of ligand-binding systems. *Anal. Biochem.*, **107**, 220–39
25. Schafer, D. F., Fowler, J. M., Munson, P. J. *et al.* (1983). Gamma-aminobutyric acid and benzodiazepine receptors in an animal model of fulminant hepatic failure. *J. Lab. Clin. Med.*, **102**, 870–80
26. Baraldi, M. and Zeneroli, M. L. (1982). Experimental hepatic encephalopathy: changes in the binding of γ-aminobutyric acid. *Science*, **216**, 427–9
27. Ferenci, P., Pappas, S. C. and Jones, E. A. (1982). Does hyperammonemia reproduce the changes in neurotransmitter receptors associated with hepatic encephalopathy? *Hepatology*, **2**, 726 (Abstr.)
28. Ferenci, P., Pappas, S. C., Munson, P. J. and Jones, E. A. (1984). Changes in glutamate receptors on synaptic membranes associated with hepatic encephalopathy or hyperammonemia in the rabbit. *Hepatology*, **4**, 25–9
29. Ferenci, P., Pappas, S. C., Munson, P. J., Henson, R. and Jones, E. A. (1984). Changes in the status of neurotransmitter receptors in a rabbit model of hepatic encephalopathy. *Hepatology*, **4**, 186–91
30. Memo, M., Lovenberg, W. and Hanbauer, I. (1982). Agonist-induced subsensitivity of adenylate cyclase coupled with a dopamine receptor in slices from rat corpus striatum. *Proc. Natl. Acad. Sci. USA*, **79**, 4456–60
31. Ferenci, P., Hanbauer, I. and Jones, E. A. (1983). Lack of evidence for impaired dopaminergic neurotransmission in experimental hepatic coma. *Hepatology*, **3**, 849 (Abstr.)

13
Urea synthesis and its enzymatic regulation

K. P. MAIER

Ammonia plays a central role in nitrogen metabolism. It is both a product of protein and nucleic acid catabolism and a precursor of non-essential amino acids and other nitrogenous substances.

The schematic representation of ammonia metabolism (Figure 13.1) demonstrates the:

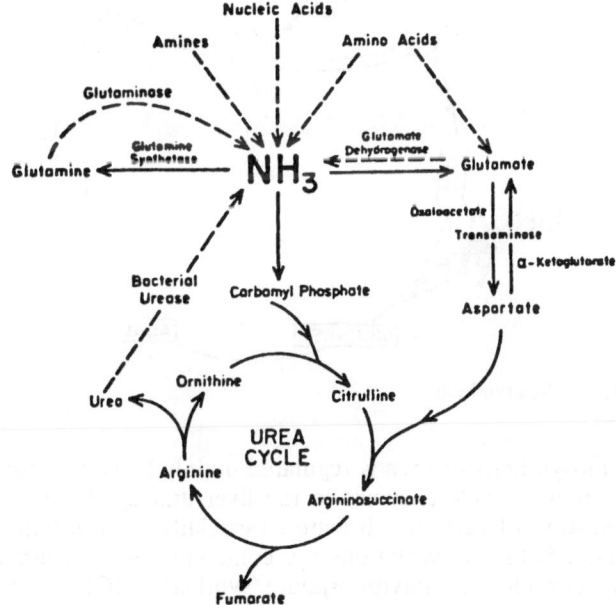

Figure 13.1 Ammonia metabolism

(1) Conversion of urea to ammonia in the gut – quantitatively the most important source of hepatic ammonia,

(2) Release of nitrogen from amino acids and the deamination of glutamate,

(3) Synthesis of glutamine – a storage and transport form of ammonia, and

(4) Urea cycle, which operates to dispose of surplus nitrogen.

In this enzymatically catalysed cycle urea is formed from ammonia. Ornithine, citrulline, argininosuccinate and arginine serve as carrier compounds.

Urea biosynthesis is an exclusive liver function, located in the periportal zone of the liver lobule. Subcellularly, urea formation is associated both with the cytoplasmic and the mitochondrial space (Figure 13.2).

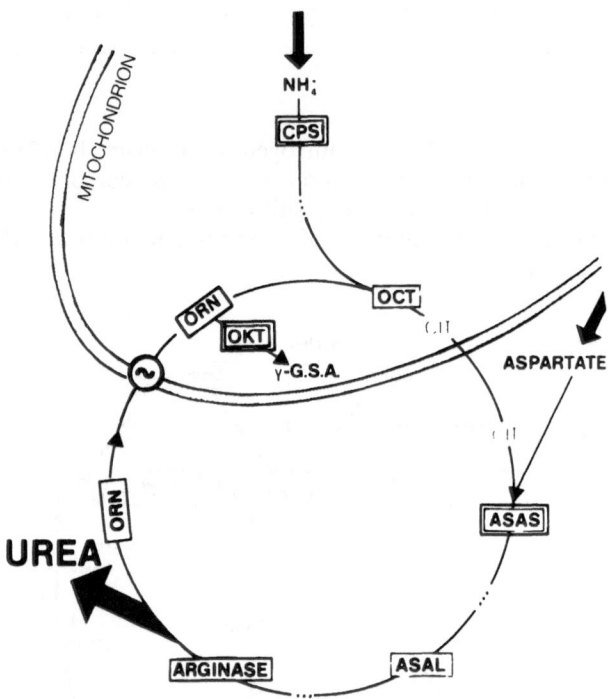

Figure 13.2 Urea synthesis

The biosynthesis of urea is regulated mainly by two factors: the concentration of urea cycle enzymes in the liver and by the intramitochondrial concentration of certain substrates, especially of ornithine and N-acetylglutamate. Substrate variations are controlled by the mitochondrial rate-limiting enzyme carbamylphosphate synthetase (CPS)[1]. An immediate, intermediate and longterm adaptation of urea synthesis according to the varying metabolic needs of the organism can be differentiated.

SUBSTRATE ACTIVATION OF MITOCHONDRIAL ENZYMES

Ornithine (ORN) is transported continuously into the mitochondria by an active transport system in order to maintain urea synthesis (Figure 13.3). The metabolite is first degraded by the action of OKT to form γ-glutamyl-semialdehyde, then by its reaction in the urea cycle to form citrulline.

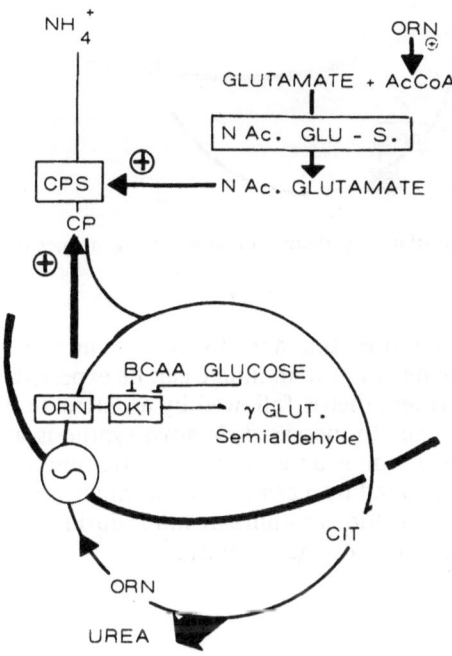

Figure 13.3 Regulation of urea synthesis – role of ornithine (ORN)

ORN stimulates CPS, which is markedly inhibited in the absence of ORN. Thus, increased mitochondrial concentrations of ORN 'open' one of the entrance ports to the ammonia detoxifying cycle. For instance, this may occur when ingesting a high protein diet, where intramitochondrial concentrations of this intermediate of the cycle increase markedly.

N-Ac-Glu serves as a positive allosteric effector of CPS[2] (Figure 13.4). It is formed in the mitochondria by the action of N-Ac-Glu-synthetase. This enzyme is only slightly induced by a high protein diet, but up to six-fold by the addition of arginine[3]. Arginine, derived from dietary protein, is thought to be the main source of N-Ac-Glu and of ORN. In the liver of rats subjected to dietary changes the concentrations of ORN and N-Ac-Glu were found to increase prior to activity changes in urea-cycle enzymes[4]. N-Ac-Glu has a

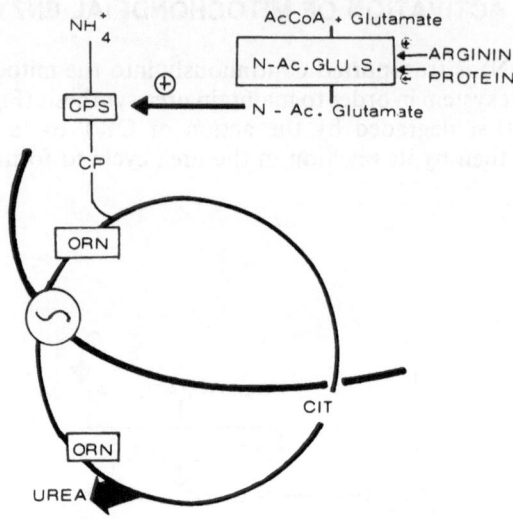

Figure 13.4   Regulation of urea synthesis – role of *N*-acetyl glutamate synthesis (NAc.GLU.-S.)

half-life of only 25 minutes, thus a relatively rapid increase in urea formation in response to a change in protein intake can be expected. Long term application of a high protein diet is followed by an increase in the rate limiting enzymes, probably due to increased *de novo* synthesis within 5–8 days. In summary, urea formation is an exclusive hepatic function with a very high capacity, tightly regulated by a cascade of enzymatically controlled steps to hold ammonia concentrations within safe limits during the varying metabolic and hormonal conditions of the organism.

PATHOPHYSIOLOGICAL CONDITIONS IN CHRONIC LIVER DISEASE

In cirrhotic patients several findings suggest impairment of the capacity for urea synthesis. Normally, an increased protein load is followed by high increase in urea excretion. Following a high protein load, patients with cirrhosis excrete only slightly more urea, than controls, but for a longer period of time[5]. This and other studies suggest that, at least in cirrhosis, the metabolic capacity of urea biosynthesis is limited. *In vitro* studies confirmed a marked reduction in urea formation in slices of liver biopsies from cirrhotic patients as compared to controls[6].

This reduction in urea formation can be attributed to: (1) reduced enzymatic machinery in the cirrhotic liver, (2) blood shunting around the liver, and (3) a combination of both.

As far as the enzymatic machinery is concerned it has been shown that in liver biopsies, as well as in the whole liver, the concentration of urea cycle enzymes is markedly reduced. However, their physicochemical properties remained unchanged[7]. We were able to demonstrate that this reduction in enzyme activity occurs in the precirrhotic stage, in patients suffering from severe alcoholic hepatitis or chronic active hepatitis[8, 9]. In the latter group of patients, histologically characterized by a marked inflammation of the periportal region, the rate-limiting enzymes of the urea cycle, CPS and argininosuccinate synthetase (ASAS), are markedly reduced as compared to healthy controls ingesting the same amount of protein.

The same holds true for patients with persistent periportal infiltration despite steroid treatment; in fact, a reduction in the degree of periportal infiltration is followed by enhanced enzyme activity, indistinguishable from normal controls[8] (Figure 13.5).

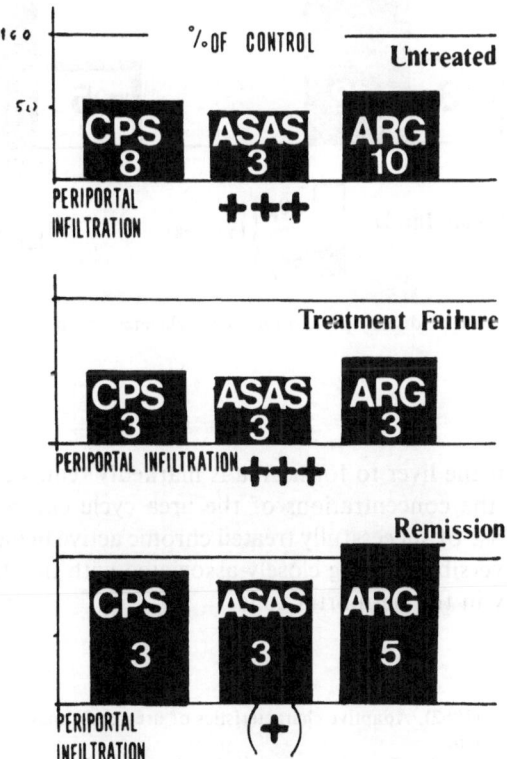

Figure 13.5 Urea cycle enzymes in chronic active hepatitis

As previously mentioned, urea cycle enzyme activity in patients with cirrhosis is less than half that of controls. Preliminary data, however, show that a stepwise increase in protein intake is followed by a marked increase in the activities of the rate-limiting enzymes of urea synthesis[10] (Figure 13.6). Moreover, the physicochemical properties of urea cycle enzymes from cirrhotic and normal liver are identical. At the moment, it is still a matter of speculation whether the regulation of urea synthesis in chronic liver disease is the same as in healthy people.

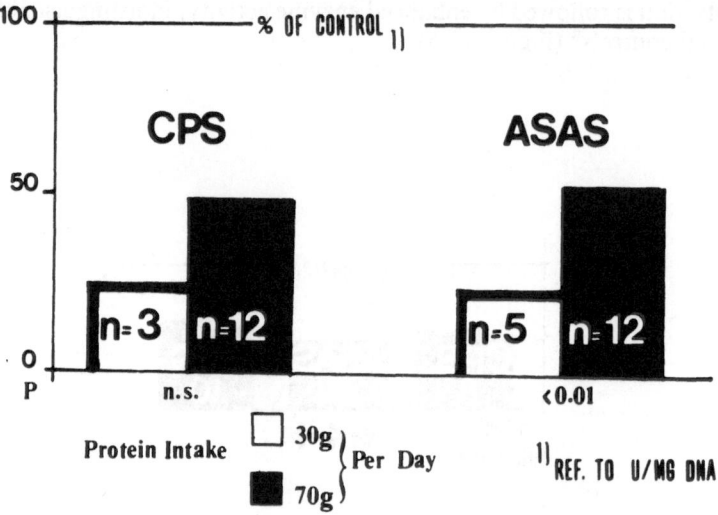

Figure 13.6 Influence of dietary protein on urea cycle enzymes in cirrhosis

SUMMARY

The capacity of the liver to form urea is markedly reduced in chronic liver disease as are the concentrations of the urea cycle enzymes in the whole organ. In the case of successfully treated chronic active hepatitis this process seems to be reversible – being closely associated with the degree of inflammatory activity in the periportal zone.

References

1. Schimke, R. T. (1962). Adaptive characteristics of urea cycle enzymes in the rat. *J. Biol. Chem.*, **237**, 459–68
2. Saheki, T., Katsunuma, T. and Sase, M. (1977). Regulation of urea synthesis in rat liver, changes of ornithine and acetylglutamate concentration in the livers of rats subjected to dietary transitions. *J. Biochem.*, **82**, 551–6

3. Shigesada, K., Aoyagi, K. and Tatibana, M. (1978). Role of acetylglutamate in ureotelism: variations in acetylglutamate level and its possible significance in control of urea synthesis in mammalian liver. *Eur. J. Biochem.*, **85**, 385-91

4. Saheki, T., Hosoya, M., Fujinami, S. and Katsunuma, T. (1982). Regulation of urea synthesis: changes in the concentration of ornithine in the liver corresponding to changes in urea synthesis. In Lowenthal, A., Mori, A. and Marescau, B. (eds.) *Urea Cycle Diseases*. p. 255. (New York, London: Plenum Press)

5. Rudmann, D., Difulco, T. J., Glambos, J. T. *et al.* (1973). Maximal rates of urea synthesis in normal and cirrhotic subjects. *J. Clin. Invest.*, **52**, 2241-9

6. Maier, K. P., Talke, H. and Gerok, W. (1977). Harnstoffzyklusenzyme und Harnstoffsynthese bei chronischen Lebererkrankungen. In *Aminosäuren, Ammoniak und hepatische Encephalopathie*, Vol. III, p. 33. *Internationales Ammoniak-Symposium*, May, Wien. (Stuttgart, New York: G. Fischer Verlag)

7. Summer, B. and Manning, R. T. (1965). Crystallization of arginase from normal and cirrhotic human liver. *Nature*, **207**, 79-80

8. Maier, K. P., Talke, H., Heimsoeth, H. and Gerok, W. (1978). Influence of steroids on urea-cycle enzymes in chronic human liver disease. *Klin. Wschr.*, **56**, 291-5

9. Maier, K. P., Volks, B. and Gerok, W. (1974). Urea-cycle enzymes in normal liver and in patients with alcoholic hepatitis. *Eur. J. Clin. Invest.*, **4**, 25-7

10. Maier, K. P., Wichmann, B. and Gerok, W. (1980). Influence of dietary protein on the activity of the key-enzymes of urea-synthesis in normal persons and in patients with liver cirrhosis. *XI. Internat. Congress Gastroenterology*, June, Hamburg

14
Leukotrienes and liver injury

D. KEPPLER, C. FORSTHOVE, W. HAGMANN, S. RAPP,
C. DENZLINGER AND H. K. KOCH

The recent advances in our knowledge on biological actions and metabolism of the leukotrienes[1-3] have enabled us to study the relationship of leukotrienes to liver injury. The leukotrienes are mainly derived from arachidonate which can be liberated from phospholipids by phospholipase A_2 or by the sequential action of phospholipase C and diglyceride lipase. The peptide leukotrienes C_4, D_4, and E_4 as well as the dihydroxylated leukotriene B_4 are formed on the calcium-dependent 5-lipoxygenase pathway (Figure 14.1)[1-3].

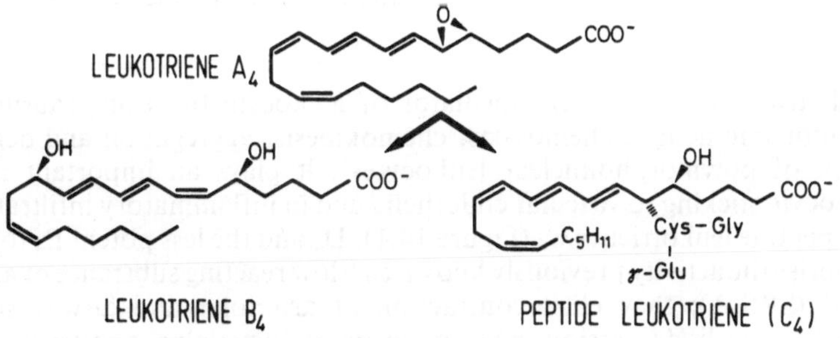

Figure 14.1 Oxidative conversion of arachidonate to 5-HPETE (5S-hydroperoxy-6-*trans*-8,11,14-*cis*-eicosatetraenoate), the epoxide leukotriene A_4 (5,6-*trans*-oxido-7,9-*trans*-11,14-*cis*-eicosatetraenoate), the dihydroxylated leukotriene B_4 (5S-12R-dihydroxy-6,14-*cis*-8,10-*trans*-eicosatetraenoate), and the initial peptide leukotriene LTC$_4$ (5S-hydroxy-6R-S-glutathionyl-7,9-*trans*-11,14-*cis*-eicosatetraenoate. 5-HPETE can also be degraded yielding 5-HETE (5S-hydroxy-6-*trans*-8,11,14-*cis*-eicosatetraenoate)

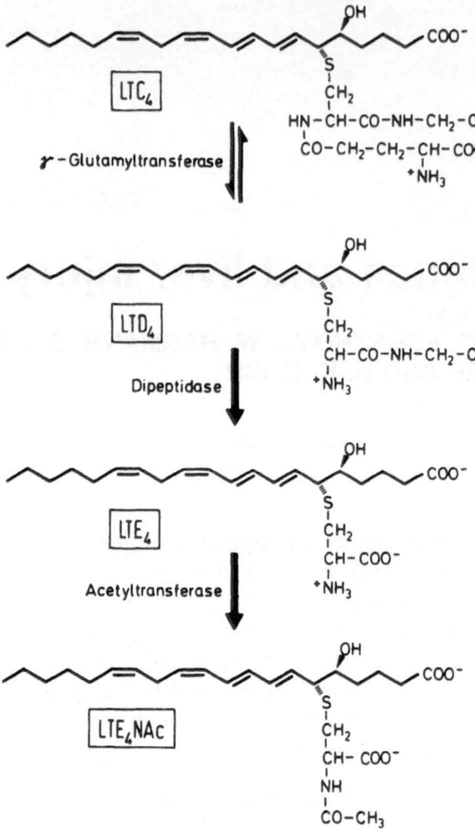

Figure 14.2 Catabolism of leukotriene C$_4$ on the mercapturic acid pathway. Leukotriene D$_4$ is more active than leukotriene C$_4$ in several biological systems, whereas leukotriene E$_4$ has lost most of the biological activity[11]. The mercapturate, N-acetyl-leukotriene E$_4$ (LTE$_4$NAc), has recently been identified as the major endogenous metabolite of peptide leukotrienes in rat bile[10]

Leukotriene B$_4$ is a potent mediator of leukocyte functions causing, via receptor interaction, chemotaxis, chemokinesis, aggregation and degranulation of polymorphonuclear leukocytes[4]; it plays an important role in leukocyte sticking to vascular endothelia and in inflammatory infiltrations[5]. The peptide leukotrienes C$_4$ (Figure 14.1), D$_4$ and the less potent E$_4$ together comprise the activity previously known as 'slow reacting substance of anaphylaxis' (SRS-A); they elicit contraction of arteriolar and airway smooth muscles, cardiodepression due to coronary arteriolar constriction and enhanced vascular permeability to macromolecules in postcapillary venules[1-3, 5]. Major sources for the generation of leukotriene B$_4$ by human cells include macrophages, monocytes and neutrophils[3], whereas mast cells, eosinophils and monocytes are active producers of leukotriene C$_4$[3, 6]. Injected leukotrienes C$_3$[7], C$_4$, or D$_4$[8] are rapidly eliminated from the vascular space, taken up predominantly by hepatocytes[9], and eliminated through bile[2, 7, 8]. Endogenous peptide leukotrienes generated *in vivo* are also detected in bile[8, 10]. Cellular ectoenzymes, γ-glutamyltransferase and a dipeptidase, catalyse the cleavage of the peptide moiety of leukotriene C_4 yielding leukotriene E_4[2, 7] (Figure 14.2).

IMPAIRMENT OF THE HEPATOBILIARY ELIMINATION OF PEPTIDE LEUKOTRIENES IN CHOLESTASIS

The rapid elimination of peptide leukotrienes represents a most important function of the hepatobiliary system in view of the powerful actions of leukotriene C_4 and D_4 at nanomolar concentrations. Injection of small doses of leukotriene C_4 or D_4 evokes shock-like symptoms with renal, pulmonary and cardiac dysfunction[12, 13]. Peptide leukotriene production and its subsequent elimination into bile has been demonstrated *in vivo* in endotoxin-shocked rats[8, 10] (Figure 14.3).

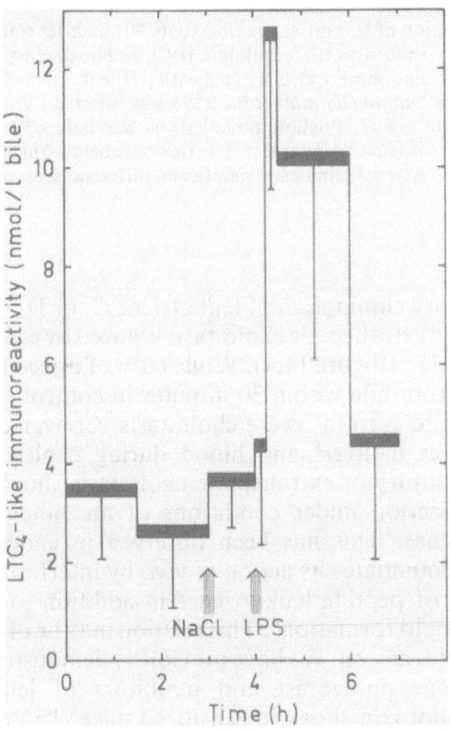

Figure 14.3 Production of peptide leukotrienes in endotoxin-treated rats. Unanaesthesized rats were injected i.v. with endotoxin (LPS) from *Salmonella minnesota* R595 at a dose of 15 mg/kg. Analyses in bile represent the formation of *N*-acetyl-leukotriene E_4 as described recently[10] (from Reference 10)

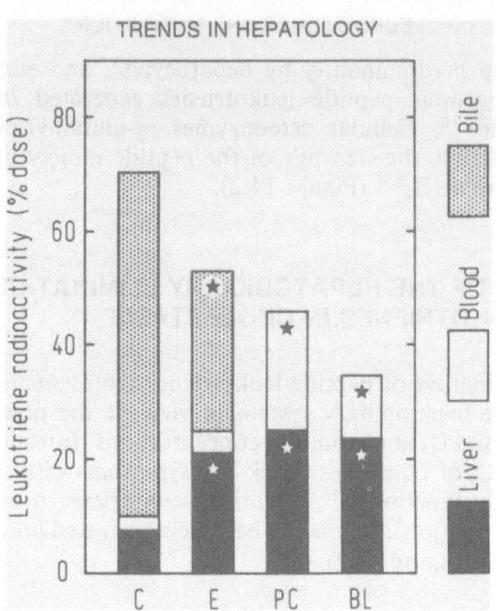

Figure 14.4 Distribution of leukotriene radioactivity 30 min after tracer injection in rats with cholestasis induced by endotoxin (E), phalloidin (PC), or bile duct ligation (BL). Control rats (C) with bile duct cannulation were also injected with [^{3}H]leukotriene C$_4$ (1 μCi or 25 pmol/kg, i.v.). Endotoxin from *Salmonella minnesota* R595 was injected i.v. at the sublethal dose of 2 mg/kg 3 h before the tracer. Phalloidin cholestasis was induced by i.v. injection of 0.7– 1.0 mg/kg, 4 h before the leukotriene tracer; bile flow was below 5 μl min^{-1} (kg body weight)$^{-1}$ under this condition. Asterisks indicate significant differences as compared to control by $p < 0.01$

The hepatobiliary elimination of leukotriene C$_4$ or D$_4$ is strongly impaired in intrahepatic and extrahepatic cholestasis induced by endotoxin[8], phalloidin and bile duct ligation (Figure 14.4). While 60% of injected tracer leukotriene C$_4$ is recovered from bile within 30 minutes in control rats, this fraction is diminished down to zero in severe cholestasis. Conversely, the leukotriene concentration rises in liver[8] and blood during cholestasis (Figure 14.4). Cholestatic liver injury or extrahepatic cholestasis should be considered as a serious complication under conditions of an enhanced production of peptide leukotrienes. This has been observed in endotoxin-shocked rats where the toxin potentiates its action *in vivo* by interfering with the hepatobiliary clearance of peptide leukotrienes in addition to stimulating leukotriene and prostanoid formation[8]. This relation may be of critical importance in other shock states as well. We have previously demonstrated that a selective peptide leukotriene antagonist and inhibitors of leukotriene synthesis prevent lethal endotoxin shock in sensitized mice[8, 14, 15].

Peptide leukotrienes themselves caused a rapid extravasation of blood plasma in bile ducts and gall bladder of the guinea pig[16]. This mechanism may contribute to cholestasis under conditions of leukotriene release into the circulation[8].

ROLE OF LEUKOTRIENES IN FULMINANT HEPATITIS

Fulminant hepatitis can be induced in experimental animals by the synergistic action of a small endotoxin dose and an inhibitor of hepatocellular ribonucleic acid synthesis (Tables 14.1 and 14.2). This was originally observed after combined administration of endotoxin and D-galactosamine[17]. The latter selectively inhibits hepatic ribonucleic acid synthesis[18], and is hepatotoxic in the absence of endotoxin[19, 20]. However, an additional injection of endotoxin induces fulminant hepatitis within 6 hours, even in the NMRI mouse strain which is relatively resistant to D-galactosamine[19, 21] (Table 14.1). Corresponding to this action of D-galactosamine (Table 14.1), α-amanitin, an

Table 14.1 Prevention of fulminant hepatitis in mice[a] by inhibitors of leukotriene synthesis and action

Treatment	Alanine aminotransferase (U/l plasma) (n)	Sorbitol dehydrogenase	
Control (NaCl)	22 (17–27)	6 (5–9)	(14)
LPS[b]	36 (26–50)	13 (9–19)	(5)
GalN[c]	29 (23–36)	6 (4–9)	(5)
LPS + GalN	343 (114–1025)	113 (35–363)	(60)
LPS + GalN + diethylcarbamazine[d]	52 (27–99)	17 (11–27)	(10)
LPS + GalN + FPL 55712[e]	81 (53–124)	24 (15–38)	(22)
LPS + GalN + BW 755C[f]	59 (36–97)	17 (10–29)	(19)
LPS + GalN + dexamethasone[g]	63 (41–97)	23 (15–36)	(5)

Results are given as the geometric mean, the numbers in parenthesis indicate the antilog SD range
[a]Female NMRI mice, 12–14 weeks of age; plasma analysed 6 h after LPS
[b]LPS (endotoxin) from *Salmonella minnesota* R595, 0.3 mg/kg, i.v. at 0 h
[c]D-Galactosamine, 3.5 mmol/kg, i.v. at 0 h
[d]0.2 mmol/kg, i.p., every 45 min between 0 and 6 h
[e]20 μmol/kg, i.p., every 30 min between 0 and 6 h
[f]0.75 mmol/kg, p.o., at 2 h before LPS + GalN
[g]5 μmol/kg, i.v., at 0 h

Table 14.2 Induction of fulminant hepatitis by the synergistic action of endotoxin and α-amanitin in NMRI mice[a], and its prevention by dexamethasone pretreatment

Treatment	Alanine aminotransferase (U/l plasma) (n)	Sorbitol dehydrogenase	
Control (NaCl or LPS[b])	22 (17–27)	6 (5–9)	(14)
α-Amanitin[c]	19 (18–21)	5 (3–10)	(4)
LPS[b] + α-amanitin[c]	294 (98–883)	88 (24–227)	(12)
LPS[b] + α-amanitin[c] + dexamethasone[d]	32 (17–58)	8 (5–15)	(8)

Results are given as the geometric mean, the numbers in parenthesis indicate the antilog SD range
[a]Female NMRI mice, 12–14 weeks of age
[b]LPS (endotoxin) from *Salmonella minnesota* R595, 1 μg/kg, i.v., 4 h before blood sampling
[c]0.2 μmol/kg, i.p., 6 h before blood sampling
[d]9 μmol/kg, i.v., 7 h before blood sampling

inhibitor of ribonucleic acid polymerase II[22], sensitized the liver to the action of a small dose of endotoxin (Table 14.2). The histological changes in liver observed 6 h after administration of endotoxin and D-galactosamine (for dose schedule see Table 14.1) were characterized by widespread zonal necroses and acidophilic single cell necroses with formation of Councilman bodies. The inflammatory infiltration was marked by the appearance of lymphocytes, monocytes and granulocytes. Leukocyte sticking was pronounced in terminal hepatic veins, venules and sinusoids. Leukostasis and inflammatory infiltration by monocytes and granulocytes was also seen in the lung. Most of the animals died between 6 and 12 h after endotoxin injection. Similar changes with comparable fulminant liver injury were observed when D-galactosamine was replaced as the inhibitor of ribonucleic acid synthesis by α-amanitin. An endotoxin dose of 1 µg/kg body weight was sufficient to induce fulminant hepatitis within 4 h when α-amanitin had been given 2 h before the lipopolysaccharide (Table 14.2).

Several inhibitors of leukotriene synthesis and action (for summary *see* Reference 23) were highly effective in reducing the histological changes in liver and in preventing severe hepatocyte injury as determined by the activity of enzymes released into blood plasma (Tables 14.1 and 14.2; Figure 14.5). This protective action was exerted by diethylcarbamazine which inhibits the synthesis of leukotriene A_4, and by FPL 55712 which is a selective receptor antagonist for peptide leukotrienes; both drugs must be injected repeatedly because of their short plasma halflife (Table 14.1). Protection by a single dose pretreatment was achieved by the arachidonate lipoxygenase inhibitor

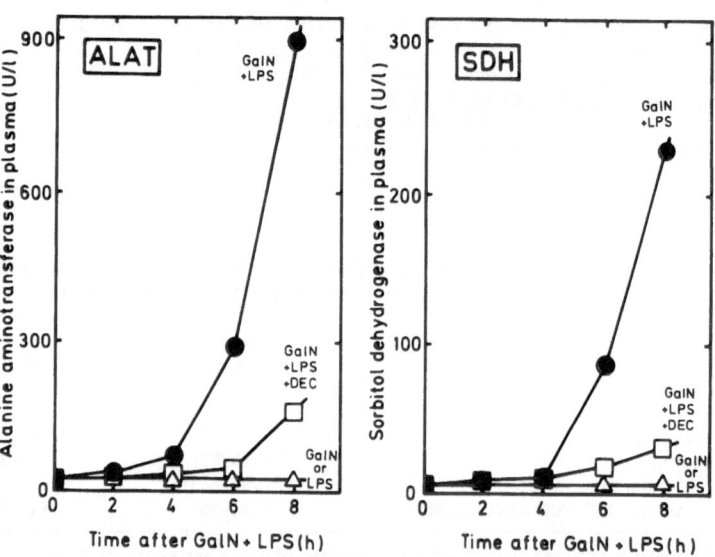

Figure 14.5   Activity of enzymes in blood plasma of NMRI mice treated with endotoxin (LPS), D-galactosamine (GalN), and diethylcarbamazine (DEC). Experimental conditions and doses were those described in Table 14.1. Blood samples were withdrawn from the aorta; plasma was assayed for alanine aminotransferase (ALAT or SGPT) and sorbitol dehydrogenase (SDH)

18. Keppler, D., Pausch, J. and Decker, K. (1974). Selective uridine triphosphate deficiency induced by D-galactosamine in liver and reversed by purimidine nucleotide precursors. Effect on ribonucleic acid synthesis. *J. Biol. Chem.*, **249**, 211–16
19. Keppler, D., Lesch, R., Reutter, W. and Decker, K. (1968). Experimental hepatitis induced by D-galactosamine. *Exp. Mol. Pathol.*, **9**, 279–90
20. Rasenack, J., Koch, H. K., Nowack, J., Lesch, R. and Decker, K. (1980). Hepatotoxicity of D-galactosamine in the isolated perfused rat liver. *Exp. Mol. Pathol.*, **32**, 264–75
21. Liehr, H., Grün, M., Seelig, H.-P., Seelig, R., Reutter, W. and Heine, W.-D. (1978). On the pathogenesis of galactosamine hepatitis. Indications of extrahepatocellular mechanisms responsible for liver cell death. *Virchows Arch. B. Cell Path.*, **26**, 331–44
22. Fiume, L. (1972). Pathogenesis of the cellular lesions induced by α-amanitin. In Farber, E. (ed.) *Pathology of Transcription and Translation.* pp. 105–22. (New York: Marcel Dekker)
23. Bach, M. K. (1984). Inhibitors of leukotriene synthesis and action. In Chakrin, L. W. and Bailey, D. M. (eds.) *The Leukotrienes, Chemistry and Biology.* pp. 163–94. (Orlando: Academic Press)
24. Higgs, G. A., Mugridge, K. G., Moncada, S. and Vane, J. R. (1984). Inhibition of tissue damage by the arachidonate lipoxygenase inhibitor BW 755C. *Proc. Natl. Acad. Sci. USA*, **81**, 2890–2
25. Blackwell, G. J., Carnuccio, R., Di Rosa, M., Flower, R. J., Langham, C. S. J., Parente, L., Persico, P., Russel-Smith, N. C. and Stone, D. (1982). Glucocorticoids induce the formation and release of anti-inflammatory and anti-phospholipase proteins into the peritoneal cavity of the rat. *Br. J. Pharmacol.*, **76**, 185–94
26. Hirata, F., Schiffmann, E., Venkatasubramanian, K., Salomon, D. and Axelrod, J. (1980). A phospholipase A_2 inhibitory protein in rabbit neutrophils induced by glucocorticoids. *Proc. Natl. Acad. Sci. USA*, **77**, 2533–6
27. Trudell, J. R., Bendix, M. and Bösterling, B. (1984). Hypoxia potentiates killing of hepatocyte monolayers by leukotrienes, hydroperoxyeicosatetraenoic acids, or calcium ionophor A23187. *Biochim. Biophys. Acta*, **803**, 338–41
28. Grases, P. J., Lesch, R., Stein, U., Heissmeyer, H. and Reutter, W. (1972). Aggravating and protecting effects of Triton and prednisolone in galactosamine induced hepatitis. *Z. Klin. Chem. Klin. Biochem.*, **10**, 539–42
29. Schiessel, C., Forsthove, C. and Keppler, D. (1984). [45]Calcium uptake during the transition from reversible to irreversible liver injury induced by D-galactosamine *in vivo*. *Hepatology*, **4**, 855–61
30. Perez, H. D., Roll, F. J., Bissell, D. M., Shak, S. and Goldstein, I. M. (1984). Production of chemotactic activity for polymorphonuclear leukocytes by cultured rat hepatocytes exposed to ethanol. *J. Clin. Invest.*, **74**, 1350–7
31. Perez, H. D., Bissell, D. M., Roll, F. J., Shak, S. and Goldstein, I. M. (1983). A possible explanation for leukocytic infiltration of the liver in acute alcoholic hepatitis: Ethanol-induced generation by hepatocytes of a lipid chemotactic factor. *Trans. Assoc. Am. Physic.*, 56–64

15
Heterogeneous turnover of plasma membrane glycoproteins in the liver

W. REUTTER

According to the work of different authors the half life of the total proteins of liver plasma membranes is two to three times longer than that of the total carbohydrates[1-4]. Since these studies were performed with unfractionated plasma membranes, there are basically two possible explanations for the shorter half life of the oligosaccharide fraction:

(1) Most of the glycoproteins have a shorter half life than those proteins not conjugated with carbohydrate.

(2) The carbohydrate moiety of glycoproteins has a higher turnover rate than the protein moiety.

Elucidation of this question was possible only by the determination of the half lives of separated protein and oligosaccharide moieties of isolated membrane glycoproteins.

When these experiments were started in 1978, isolation and enrichment procedures were known only for NAD-glycohydrolase[5] and nucleotide pyrophosphatase[6]. Later the isolation of the histocompatibility antigen was reported[7]. For our purposes, the reported isolation procedures were far too time consuming, because it was necessary to perform and reproduce half life measurements using three protein precursors and four oligosaccharide precursors at four different time points.

Wolfgang Kreisel in my laboratory developed a method for the isolation of a membrane glycoprotein, which enabled a half life determination within 1 week using a single precursor. This protein has a M_r of 110 000, and exists in its native state as a dimer. It was subsequently identified as dipeptidyl-aminopeptidase IV[8, 9].

The procedure consisted of the following steps:

(1) Solubilization of the plasma membranes with Triton X-100
(2) Affinity chromatography on concanavalin A- and wheat germ-agglutinineSepharose
(3) SDS-gel electrophoresis.

The stained protein bands were quantified by photometric comparison with calibration standards; the bands were then cut from the gel and their radioactivity measured, thus enabling the calculation of specific radioactivity.
The following half lives were determined for this glycoprotein:

Protein moiety	60–80 h
Mannose:	56 h
N-acetylglucosamine	40 h
Galactose	20 h
N-Acetylneuraminic acid	33 h
L-Fucose	12 h

From these measurements it follows that the terminal and subterminal monosaccharides of dipeptidylpeptidase IV are cleaved more rapidly than mannose and the protein moiety.

Reutilization of radioactive amino acids, and especially the sugars, was greatly reduced by adding large quantities of unlabelled precursor at 2, 6 and every 12 hours after addition of the isotope. For example the pools of GDP-fucose and CMP-N-acetylneuraminic acid (6 and 40 nmole per gram liver, respectively) can be increased to values greater than 300 nmole by the addition of 500 mg fucose or N-acetyl-mannosamine/kg. Reutilization of radioactive material is thereby largely prevented. The results of these determinations show that certain monosaccharides of dipeptidylpeptidase IV are cleaved more rapidly than, for example, mannose and the protein moiety.

The most rapid turnover of all is shown by the terminal L-fucose, followed by the subterminal D-galactose. N-Acetylglucosamine shows a half life of 40 h. Since this amino sugar occurs both subterminally and in the so-called core region (like mannose) the measured half life may be interpreted as the average of 60 h (for the core sugar) and 20 h (for the subterminal sugar). Thus, as shown by Brigitte Volk[10] the carbohydrate moiety of this glycoprotein therefore contains two regions, one which contains mannose and in which oligosaccharide turnover is relatively slow, and the other in which oligosaccharide turnover is more rapid.

The initial question can, therefore, be answered. There is indeed a membrane glycoprotein in which the carbohydrate is more rapidly degraded than the protein.

This leads to the next question. Is this hitherto unrecognized property peculiar to dipeptidylaminopeptidase, or can it be demonstrated in other membrane glycoproteins?

Rudolph Tauber and Choon-Sik Park isolated five other glycoproteins from liver plasma membranes, showing molecular weights of 60K, 80K, 120K, 140K and 160K in SDS-gel electrophoresis. Measurements of the half

Table 15.1 Heterogeneous turnover of different membrane glycoproteins

Precursor			Half life (h)			
	GP 60	GP 80	DPP IV[a]	GP 120	GP 140	GP 160
[³H]leucine	62	85	60	88	78	52
[¹⁴C]mannose	58	38	56	51	66	26
[¹⁴C]fucose	21	17	12	21	16	16
N-[³H]acetyl-mannosamine	33	31	30	27	29	26

Half-lives are calculated from four to five time points (12, 24, 36, 48 and, in the case of protein labelling, 72 h). At each time point the specific radioactivity of each isolated glycoprotein was determined. For further information see refs 8, 11

lives of these glycoproteins gave results fundamentally similar to those obtained with dipeptidylaminopeptidase IV. In all five glycoproteins, the carbohydrate moiety was degraded more rapidly than the protein[11]. Half lives varied between 52 and 88 hours when [³H]leucine was used as the precursor (Table 15.1). Among the carbohydrates, L-fucose always showed the highest turnover rate *in vivo*, with a half life of 12–21 h (Table 15.1).

It is still not possible to explain the fact that N-acetylneuraminic acid always shows a relatively long half life compared with that of the other terminal sugar, L-fucose. In this connection it should be remembered that glycoproteins possess several oligosaccharide side-chains. It is quite conceivable that these different side-chains have different rates of turnover. N-Acetylneuraminic acid could, therefore, be the terminal sugar of these less rapidly degraded oligosaccharides, whereas fucose is found as the terminal sugar of the more rapidly degraded oligosaccharides. It should be possible to resolve this question by glycopeptide mapping.

With respect to its half life, mannose occupies a special position. In glycoprotein 60K and dipeptidylaminopeptidase IV (and glycoprotein 140K?) the half life of mannose is similar to that of the protein moiety. In glycoproteins 80K and 160K, mannose has the same half life as N-acetylneuraminic acid, whereas in glycoprotein 120K, its half life lies between the two extremes. It appears that the accessibility of the oligosaccharide side chains to the mannosidases varies from glycoprotein to glycoprotein. From these findings it can be assumed that the partially separate degradation of the oligosaccharide (the so-called heterogeneous turnover) is a general property of membrane glycoproteins[11].

Which cell compartments are involved in this turnover?

Hydrolytic processes take place *in vivo* primarily in the lysosomes. Klaus Heinze and Rudolf Tauber showed that inactivation of lysosomes *in vivo* with chloroquine caused no change in the half life of protein-bound L-fucose, whereas the half life of the protein moiety more than doubled. This shows that the removal of L-fucose occurs extralysosomally, probably in the Golgi apparatus, in which neutral glycosidases have already been demonstrated.

What is the biological significance of this property of membrane glycoproteins?

At the moment, we have more hypotheses than facts. Nevertheless, Wolfgang Kreisel, now at the Medizinische Universitätsklinik in Freiburg, showed that the half life of L-fucose in dipeptidylaminopeptidase IV is increased from 12 to 28 hours in regenerating liver[12]. Christel Kronenberger and Rudolf Tauber made similar observations for the L-fucose of glycoproteins 60K and 120K. Moreover, they demonstrated that the total content of these glycoproteins in the plasma membrane is unchanged during the regeneration phase. If there had been an increase (i.e. an extended life of the total glycoprotein) an increased fucose half life would automatically have been observed. The above observation provides important evidence concerning the participation of this mechanism in the processes of accelerated growth. Since membrane recycling, a decrease of this process during the growth phase of the liver would make sense on the grounds of cellular economy.

Another important clue to the possible biological importance of this phenomenon was provided by Reinhard Büchsel. The half life of L-fucose varies, depending on the domain of the liver cell in which it is measured. The shortest half life was measured in sinusoidal and bile canicular membrane (12 h) and the longest in the lateral membrane (28 h). The different locations and functions of these membranes are very probably related to the different half lives. Since the sinusoidal plasma membrane is rich in receptors, it was proposed that the turnover of membrane glycoproteins is closely linked with receptor recycling[1]. If a receptor on the cell surface recognizes a specific ligand, e.g. a growth factor, which must be transported into the cell interior, then this is a signal for the internalization of the ligand–receptor complex

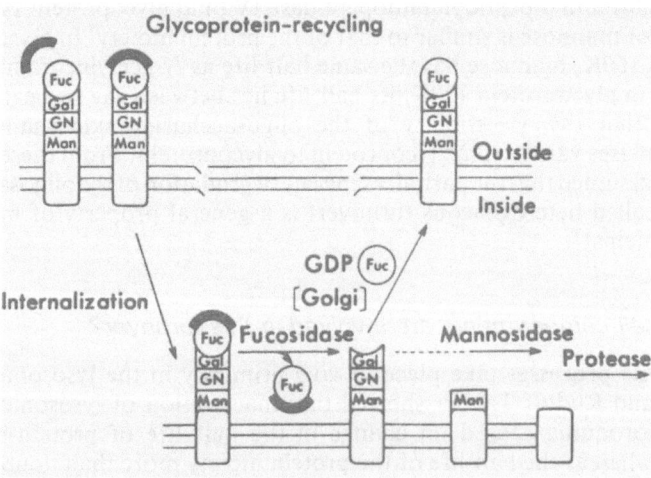

Figure 15.1 Possible biological significance of the heterogeneous turnover of membrane glycoproteins. Hypothesis 1: Glycoprotein recycling[13, 14]

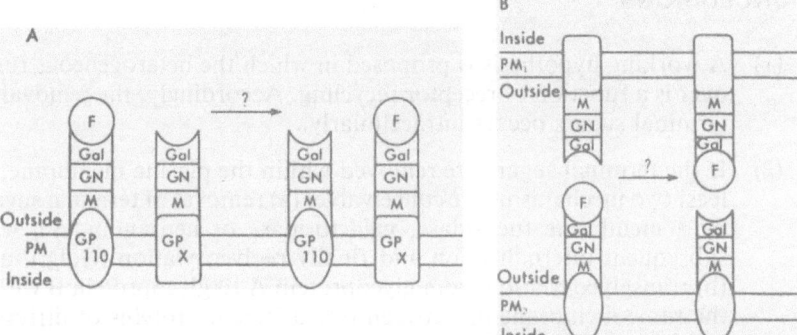

Figure 15.2 Possible biological significance of the heterogeneous turnover of membrane glycoproteins. Hypothesis 2: Transglycosylation. This hypothesis implies the existence of cell surface localized enzymes transferring mono- or oligosaccharides from a glycoprotein to another one. These glycoproteins can be localized within one cell surface (A) or at the cell surface of two different cells (B). This transglycosylation should follow a mechanism similar to glycogen branching or debranching, and therefore, would not be dependent from nucleotide sugars.

(to which, in addition, membrane fragments can be attached). In the cell interior, the terminal and subterminal sugars that carry the ligand are removed by cleavage. The ligand is thus released and can, for example, enter the cell nucleus by other mechanisms. Degradation of the receptor occurs only in the region of ligand binding. The remaining, partially deglycosylated glycoprotein can be reglycosylated in the Golgi apparatus, then returned to the plasma membrane via the vesicle[13, 14]. In this way the receptor protein can be utilized several times, because it does not need to be totally degraded every time it is internalized (Figure 15.1). Another hypothesis is given in Figure 15.2.

SUMMARY

A hitherto unknown property of membrane glycoproteins of the liver is described.

(1) The oligosaccharide moiety, especially the terminal and subterminal sugars, undergo more rapid turnover than the protein moiety and the core sugars.

(2) Extralysosomal glycosidases are responsible for this heterogeneous turnover.

(3) This heterogeneous turnover is most pronounced in the sinusoidal and bile canacular plasma membrane domains.

(4) During increased growth (regenerating liver after 2/3 resection) the half life of fucose in membrane glycoproteins is more than doubled, whereas that of the protein moiety remains unchanged.

CONCLUSIONS

(1) A working hypothesis is proposed in which the heterogeneous turn-over is a function of receptor recycling. Accordingly, the removal of terminal sugars occurs intracellularly.

(2) If the terminal sugars are removed within the plasma membrane, at least two mechanisms are conceivable: (a) removal of terminal sugars by a membrane fucosidase, galactosidase or neuraminidase, with subsequent internalization and finally reglycosylation (Golgi), and (b) transglycosylation from glycoprotein A to glycoprotein B within the same membrane or between two different proteins of different cells[2].

(3) Is this property distributed equally or unequally among all the oligo-saccharide chains of a membrane glycoprotein?

(4) Is this mechanism disturbed in tumour cells? Can this mechanism explain the different content of protein-bound fucose in, for example, hepatoma plasma membrane[15]?

(5) Is similar behaviour shown by plasma membrane glycolipids, especially gangliosides?

Table 15.2 Protein-bound carbohydrate composition of plasma membranes of hepatoma 7777 and host liver[15]

| Sugar | Content (nmol/mg protein) | |
	Morris hepatoma 7777	Host liver
L-Fucose	26.1 ± 3.7	6.1 ± 1.7
N-Acetylneuraminic acid	60.7 ± 8.7	50.1 ± 8.7
Galactose	100.3 ± 9.1	81.4 ± 8.4
Mannose	44.6 ± 4.2	35.2 ± 2.5
N-acetyl-glucosamine	127.4 ± 32.9	95.8 ± 8.8
N-acetyl-galactosamine	78.4 ± 12.9	49.8 ± 6.6

After acid hydrolysis the carbohydrates have been determined colorimetically (L-fucose, N-acetylneuraminic acid and amino sugars) and enzymatically (D-galactose and D-mannose)

References

1. Kawasaki, T. and Yamashina, J. (1971). Metabolic studies of rat liver plasma membranes using D-1-^{14}C-glucosamine. *Biochim. Biophys. Acta*, **225**, 234–8
2. Gurd, F. W. and Evans, W. H. (1973). Relative rates of degradation of mouse-liver surface-membrane proteins. *Eur. J. Biochem.*, **36**, 273–9
3. Harms, E. and Reutter, W. (1974). Half-life of N-acetylneuraminic acid in plasma membranes of rat liver and Morris hepatoma 7777. *Cancer Res.*, **34**, 3165–72
4. Tauber, R. and Reutter, W. (1978). Protein degradation in the plasma membrane of regenerating liver and Morris hepatomas. *Eur. J. Biochem.*, **83**, 37–45
5. Bock, K. W., Siekewitz, P. and Palade, G. E. (1971). Localization and turnover studies of membrane nicotinamide dinucleotide glycohydrolase in rat liver. *J. Biol. Chem.*, **246**, 188–95

 6. Decker, K. and Bischoff, E. (1972). Purification and properties of nucleotide pyrophosphatase from rat liver plasma membranes. *FEBS Lett.*, **21**, 95-8
 7. Dobberstein, B., Kvist, S. and Roberts, L. (1982). Structure and biosynthesis of histocompatibility antigens (H-2, HLA). *Philos. Trans. R. Soc. London B.*, **300**, 161-72
 8. Kreisel, W., Volk, B. A., Büchsel, R. and Reutter, W. (1980). Different half-lives of the carbohydrate and protein moieties of a 110000-dalton glycoprotein isolated from plasma membranes of rat liver, *Proc. Natl. Acad. Sci. USA*, **77**, 1828-31
 9. Kreisel, W., Heussner, R., Volk, B. A., Büchsel, R., Reutter, W. and Gerok, W. (1982). Identification of the 110000 M_r glycoprotein isolated from rat liver plasma membrane as dipeptidylaminopeptidase IV, *FEBS Lett.*, **147**, 85-8
10. Volk, B. A., Kreisel, W., Köttgen, E., Gerok, W. and Reutter, W. (1983). Heterogeneous turnover of terminal and core sugars within the carbohydrate chain of dipeptidylaminopeptidase IV isolated from rat liver plasma membrane, *FEBS Lett.*, **163**, 150-2
11. Tauber, R., Park, C.-S. and Reutter, W. (1983). Intramolecular heterogeneity of degradation of plasma membrane glycoproteins: a general characteristic. *Proc. Natl. Acad. Sci. USA*, **80**, 4026-9
12. Kreisel, W., Reutter, W. and Gerok, W. (1984). Modification of the intramolecular turnover of terminal carbohydrates of dipeptidylpeptidase IV isolated from rat liver plasma membranes during liver regeneration. *Eur. J. Biochem.*, **138**, 435-8
13. Kreisel, W., Büchsel, R., Volk, B. A., Reutter, W. and Gerok, W. (1983). Turnover of liver plasma membrane glycoproteins. In Popper, H., Reutter, W., Köttgen, E. and Gudat, F. (eds.) *Structural Carbohydrates of the Liver*. pp. 51-61. (Lancaster: MTP Press)
14. Reutter, W. and Tauber, R. (1983). Turnover of plasma membrane glycoprotein from liver and hepatoma. *GANN Monograph Cancer Res.*, **29**, 59-65
15. Vischer, P. and Reutter, W. (1978). Specific alterations of fucoprotein biosynthesis in the plasma membrane of Morris hepatoma 7777. *Eur. J. Biochem.*, **84**, 363-8

16

The structure of connexons in the open and closed state as revealed by rotary shadowed freeze-fracture replicas of rat hepatocyte gap junctions

L. LANDMANN AND L. BIANCHI

INTRODUCTION

Gap junctions, zonulae communicantes or nexuses are localized in the apposed lateral plasma membranes of adjacent hepatocytes. They are the morphological equivalent of cell-to-cell channels which mediate and regulate the passage of ions, dyes and small molecules from one hepatocyte to the next, thereby allowing intercellular communication between liver cells[1,2]. These junctions are characterized by aggregated integral membrane proteins which are exactly in register on the two adjoining plasma membranes and are linked to each other. The unit consisting of a particle pair has been termed a connexon[3,4]. Caspar et al.[4] and Makowski et al.[5] have inferred that the particles are composed of six polypeptide subunits arranged in the form of an anulus, each having an apparent molecular weight of 26 000–28 000[6,7]. The particles are thought to span the lipid bilayer and to create a channel along their central axis which in turn provides the hydrophilic pathway connecting the cytoplasm of two adjacent cells.

Unwin explained the relation of the subunits to the membrane and the hydrophilic channel in the 'open' and 'closed' state of the connexon[8–10]. According to this model (Figure 16.1) the six subunits are rod shaped, about 2.5 nm in diameter, and 7 nm long. They have a tilt with respect to the membrane and to the six-fold symmetry axis that gives the whole assembly a left-handed twist. The central channel delineated by the subunits is about 2 nm wide. The transition to the closed state is produced by a radial inwards motion of the subunits on the cytoplasmic end and a reduction of their

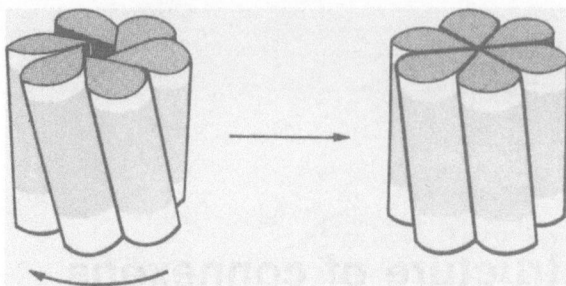

Figure 16.1 Drawing of a connexon illustrating the transition from the open (left) to the closed (right) configuration (according to Unwin and Zampighi, 1980[8]). The closure of the channel in the cytoplasmic portion of the particle (top) is achieved by subunits sliding against each other, decreasing their inclination tangentially around the channel and rotating at the extracellular pole (bottom). The shading on the side of the model indicates the region embedded in the membrane

inclination tangential to the six-fold axis. The appropriate stimulus which induces closure of the channel is an increasing concentration of free cytoplasmic Ca^{2+} or H^+ ions[2, 11]

Conventional freeze-fracture replication of gap junctions reveals arrays of 6–9 nm particles at an average spacing of 10 nm on the protoplasmic fracture face (PF) corresponding to a similar array of pits in the extracellular fracture face (EF)[12]. These particles correspond to half a connexon, i.e. to an ensemble of six subunits. Thus, the fracture face exposed in a PF shows the extracellular region of the assembly[13]. The arrangement of the particles has been shown to be variable: randomly arranged particles are believed to represent the open state, while particles arranged in a hexagonal lattice have closed channels[14]. The examination of rotary shadowed particles revealed a central depression or pore – corresponding to the extracellular portion of the channel – but failed so far to resolve further details[15, 16].

By combining the rotary shadowing freeze-fracture technique with a simple image-integration method we are able to demonstrate the subunits and their configurational change in the open and closed state of the connexon.

MATERIAL AND METHODS

Male Wistar rats weighing from 200 to 250 g were anaesthesized i.p. with Nembutal® (5 mg/100 g body weight, Abbott Laboratories). The portal vein was cannulated and the liver perfused for 45 minutes with Eagles medium gassed with O_2 or N_2, respectively. Anoxia is known to uncouple cells by indirectly causing the connexon channels to close (*see* Discussion). After perfusion with 20 ml 2.5% glutaraldehyde – 2% paraformaldehyde in 0.1 mol/l phosphate buffer, pH 7.4, the liver was excised, cut into small blocks, and immersed in the same fixative for 1 h at 0–4°C. The tissue was thoroughly washed in phosphate buffer, equilibrated in 25% glycerol, and rapidly frozen in melting nitrogen. The specimens were fractured at $-100°C$, rotary shadowed with 1 or 2 nm Pt/C at a shadowing angle of 25°, and replicated with 20 nm C in a Balzers BAF 400 D apparatus. Replicas were cleaned in Cr/H_2SO_4 and examined in a Philips EM 301 operating at 80 kV. Micrographs were taken at a primary magnification of 190 000. Images were integrated according to Markham et al.[17] by a six-fold rotation of the photographic paper for 360°/6 and its exposure at each rotational step. Controls were rotated five-fold for 360°/5 and seven-fold for 360°/7.

RESULTS

Rotary shadowed replicas of O_2-perfused livers show the random arrangement of particles typical for the open state of gap junctions (Figure 16.2). Connexons with a closed channel are regularly arranged in a hexagonal lattice as illustrated by Figure 16.3 in a N_2-perfused liver.

Figures 16.4A and 16.5A show high power views of singular particles in the open state, while Figures 16.6A and 16.7A represent particles the channel of which is closed. The replicas demonstrated in Figures 16.4 and 16.6 were shadowed with 2 nm Pt/C while those in Figures 16.5 and 16.7 received a

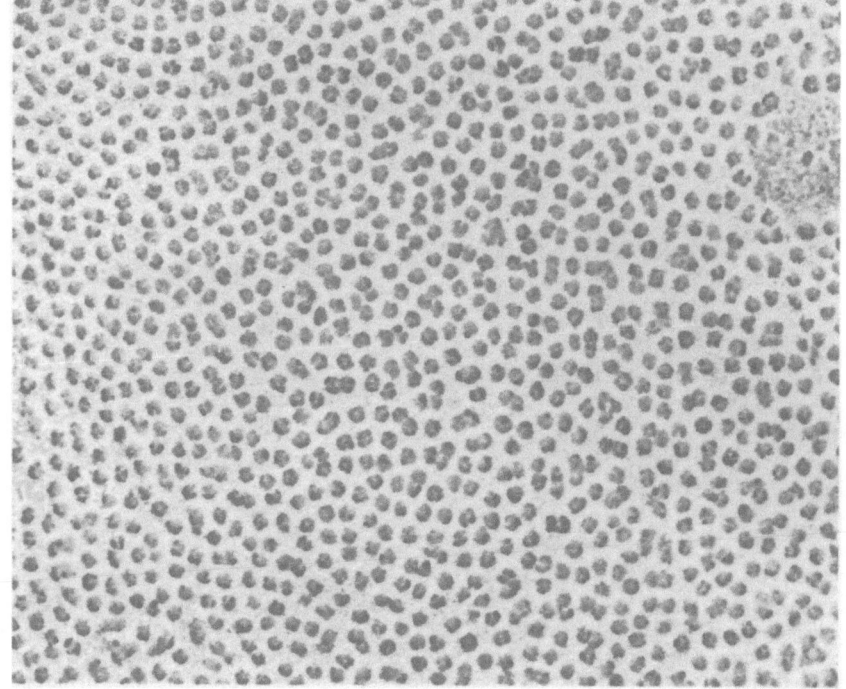

Figure 16.2 The protoplasmic fracture face of a gap junction in the open state displays a random arrangement of particles. × 315 000

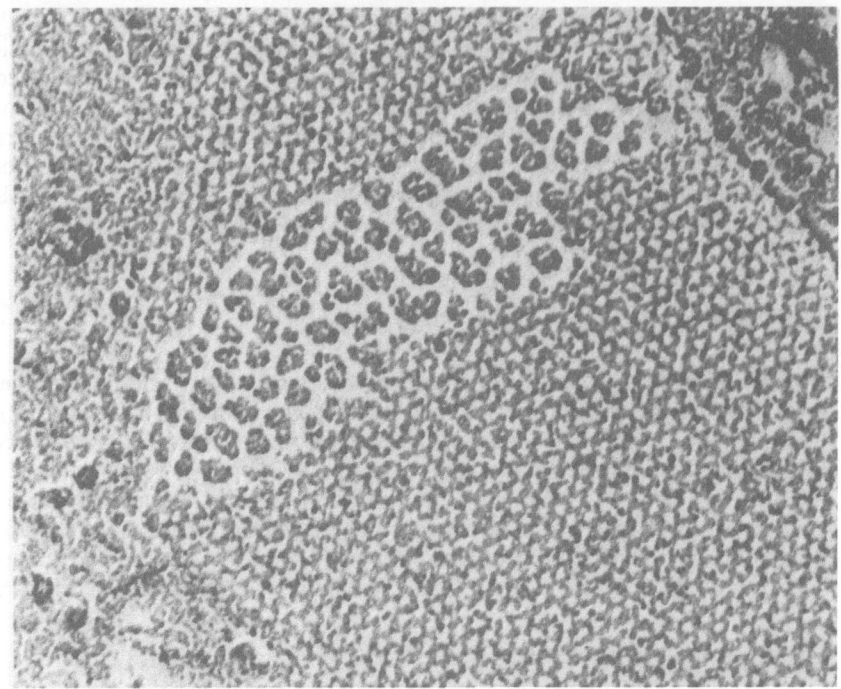

Figure 16.3   In the closed state particles of the protoplasmic fracture face and even more so pits in the extracellular fracture face reveal a regular hexagonal array. × 315 000

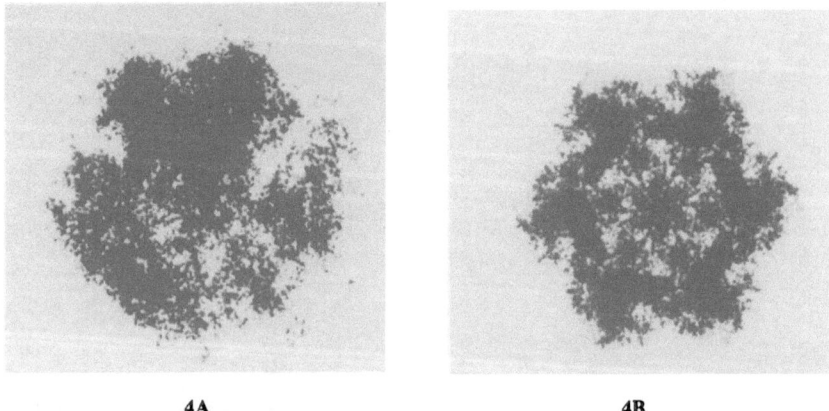

4A   4B

Figures 16.4–7   High power views of particles before (A) and after (B) rotational image-integration. × 1 875 000. Figures 16.4 and 16.5 show the open, Figures 16.6 and 16.7 the closed configuration. The evaporation of a 1 nm Pt/C layer (Figures 16.5 and 16.7) instead of the usual 2 nm (Figures 16.4 and 16.6) increases resolution of the replicas. The subunits tilted in the open state (Figures 16.4B and 16.5B) are arranged radially by transition of the particle to the closed state (Figures 16.6B and 16.7B). The extracellular portion of the connexon revealed by the fracturing process displays an open central channel in either configuration

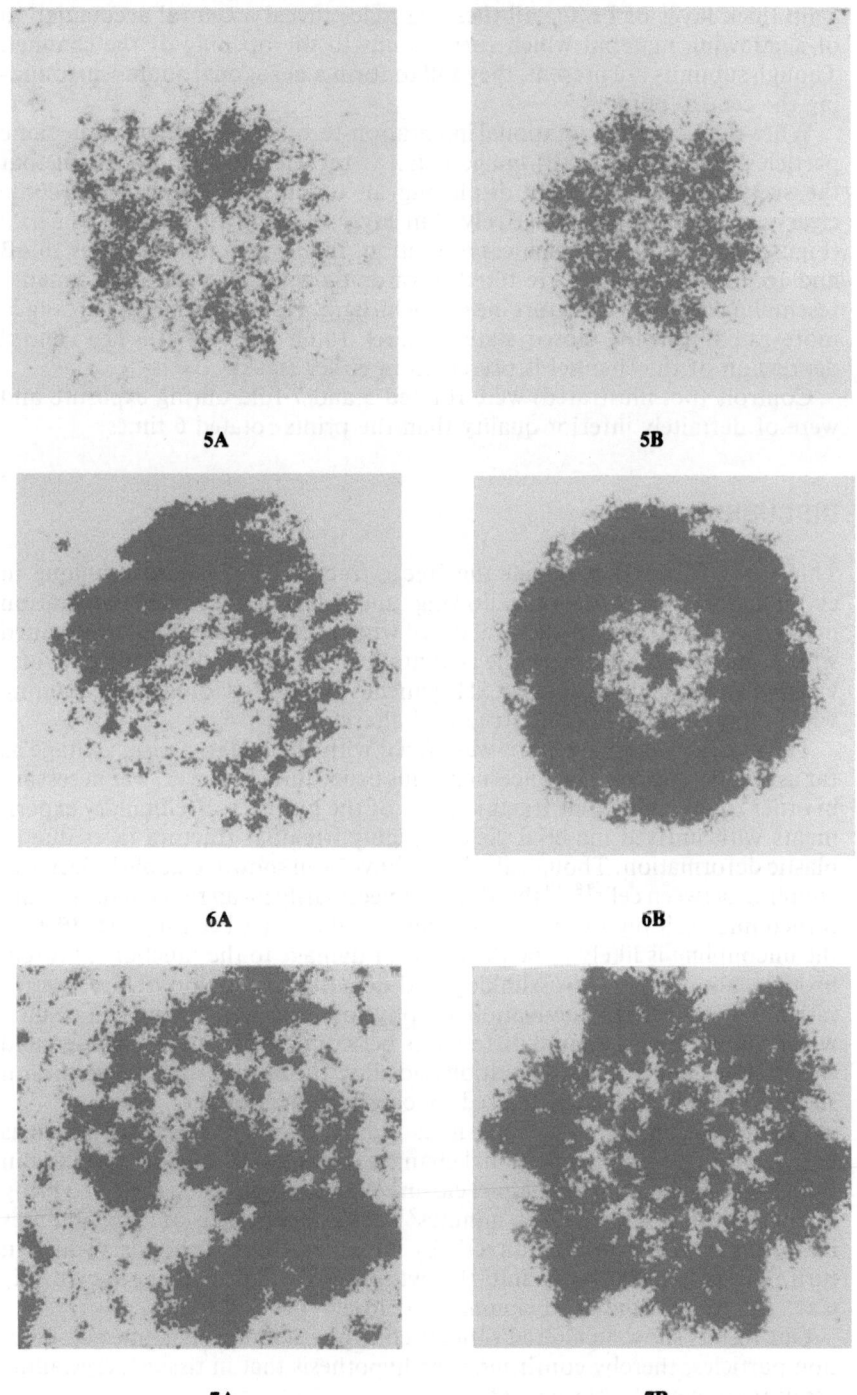

5A

5B

6A

6B

7A

7B

1 nm thick layer of Pt/C. All these particles reveal a central accumulation of shadowing material which corresponds to the opening of the channel. Though subunits are present, they fail to form a hexagonal anulus surrounding the central pore.

When the Markham rotational integration-technique is applied to the same particles (Figures 16.4–7B) image detail is revealed to such an extent that the six subunits apparently displaying an oblongate appearance become clearly recognizable. A relatively thin layer of contrast-forming material (Figures 16.5 and 16.7) enhances resolution. In the open state (Figures 16.4B and 16.5B) the subunits are tilted towards the symmetry axis in a manner resembling the vanes of a turbine or a whirligig. However, they are arranged more radially in the closed state (Figures 16.6B and 16.7B). The central depression of the channel is preserved in either state.

Controls (not illustrated) were rotated 5 and 7-fold during exposure and were of definitely inferior quality than the prints rotated 6 times.

DISCUSSION

This study demonstrates that the freeze-fracture replication technique in combination with rotary shadowing and Markham's image-integration method is able to show structural detail with a resolution until now obtained with negative staining only. The advantage of this method is that it provides views of tissue, and not of isolated organelles as required for negative staining which may have undergone structural alteration.

The examined gap junctions were fixed with aldehydes, a disadvantage as far as protein structure is concerned. This procedure, however, was necessary in order to obtain regular fracture faces of the particles. Preliminary experiments with unfixed material yielded highly irregular fracture faces due to plastic deformation. Though aldehydes have been shown to abolish electrical coupling between cells[18, 19] this does not necessarily mean that connexons are turned into their high-resistance or closed state. It has been suggested[20] that the uncoupling is likely to be the result of damage to the junctional protein brought about by the crosslinking and denaturating action of the fixative rather than the selective activation of a physiological mechanism. Our results, which show clear structural differences between connexons in the open and closed state, confirm this suggestion and allow the assumption that connexon structure is not essentially altered by chemical fixation.

Crystallization of connexons in a tightly packed hexagonal lattice is believed to reflect conformational changes within the connexons resulting in functional uncoupling or channel closure[14]. Anoxia has been shown to bring about this effect within 20–30 minutes[21]. Anoxia as well as other procedures inhibiting metabolism act indirectly by impairing the mitochondria which in turn release free Ca^{2+} ions into the cytoplasm[22]. This increase in cytosolic Ca^{2+} causes the connexon channels to close.

Our results show an altered subunit configuration in crystalline gap junction particles, thereby confirming the hypothesis that in tissue a crystalline array represents the closed state.

The data presented in this paper show that the extracellular part of gap junction connexons consists of six subunits, most probably corresponding to six polypeptides which together form a hexagon surrounding a central pore. This agrees well with connexon models based on other techniques[4, 10]. The observed configurational change of the subunits, from a tilted arrangement in the open state to an almost radial one in the closed state, supplements the Unwin-model (*loc. cit.*) describing the motion of the subunits during channel closure. In addition to the reduction of their tangential inclination around the channel (*see* Figure 16.1) and their closer position to the central axis near the cytoplasmic face of the connexon, our results imply that the subunits are rotated about their axis, provided that the protein is rigid. This somewhat contradicts the Unwin-model postulating a rearrangement of the subunits by tilting and sliding along their lines of contact[9].

Our observation that the subunits have an oblongate appearance is in agreement with other results. Unwin and Ennis[9] noted that the cross-section of the subunits tapers significantly towards the central symmetry axis. Biochemical results suggest that the junctional polypeptide representing a subunit crosses the membrane at least twice[6]. Although it is not known whether the transmembrane portion of the polypeptide chain is in the α-helix or in the β-pleated-sheet configuration, a protein traversing the membrane twice is likely to feature an elongated cross-section as postulated by our results and other morphological data.

The observation that the central channel remains open in the uncoupled state suggests that the closing mechanism is located elsewhere in the connexon. There is indeed evidence indicating that the mechanism controlling channel permeability is located near the cytoplasmic end (Unwin *loc. cit.*). Visualization of the cytoplasmic surface of gap junctions in the closed state reveals smooth surfaces with no visible pores[15, 16] and supports this view.

Acknowledgements

We thank Ms E. Weber for expert technical assistance and Mr B. Peretti for drawing Figure 16.1. This study was supported by grants from Fonds zur Förderung von Lehre und Forschung, Sandoz-Stiftung, Geigy-Jubiläums-Stiftung and Emil Barell-Stiftung.

References

1. Popper, H., Bianchi, L., Gudat, F. and Reutter, W. (1980). *Communications of Liver Cells.* (Lancaster: MTP Press)
2. Loewenstein, W. R. (1981). Junctional intercellular communication: the cell-to-cell channel. *Physiol. Rev.*, **61**, 829
3. Goodenough, D. A. (1976). *In vitro* formation of gap junction vesicles. *J. Cell Biol.*, **68**, 220
4. Caspar, D. L. D., Goodenough, D. A., Makowski, L. and Phillips, W. C. (1977). Gap junction structures. I. Correlated electron microscopy and X-ray diffraction. *J. Cell Biol.*, **74**, 605
5. Makowski, L., Caspar, D. L. D., Phillips, W. C. and Goodenough, D. (1977). Gap junction structures. II. Analysis of the X-ray diffraction data. *J. Cell Biol.*, **74**, 629
6. Nicholson, B. J., Hunkapiller, M. W., Grim, L. B., Hood, L. E. and Revel, J. P. (1981). Rat liver gap junction protein: properties and partial sequence. *Proc. Natl. Acad. Sci. USA.*, **78**, 7594

7. Hertzberg, E. L., Anderson, D. J., Friedlander, M. and Gilula, N. B. (1982). Comparative analysis of the major polypeptides from liver gap junctions and lens fiber junctions. *J. Cell Biol.*, **92**, 53

8. Unwin, P. N. T. and Ennis, P. D. (1983). Calcium-mediated changes in gap junction structure: evidence from the low angle X-ray pattern. *J. Cell Biol.*, **97**, 1459

9. Unwin, P. N. T. and Ennis, P. D. (1984). Two configurations of a channel-forming membrane protein. *Nature*, **307**, 609

10. Unwin, P. N. T. and Zampighi, G. (1980). Structure of the junction between communicating cells. *Nature*, **283**, 545

11. Spray, D. C., Stern, J. H., Harris, A. L. and Bennett, M. V. L. (1982). Gap junctional conductance: comparison of sensitivities to H and Ca ions. *Proc. Natl. Acad. Sci. USA*, **79**, 441

12. Chalcroft, J. P. and Bullivant, S. (1970). An interpretation of liver cell membrane and junction structure based on observation of freeze-fractured replicas of both sides of the fracture. *J. Cell Biol.*, **47**, 49

13. Staehelin, L. A. (1974). Structure and function of intercellular junctions. *Intern. Rev. Cytol.*, **39**, 191

14. Peracchia, C. (1977). Gap junctions. Structural changes after uncoupling procedures. *J. Cell Biol.*, **72**, 628

15. Hirokawa, N. and Heuser, J. (1982). The inside and outside of gap-junction membranes visualized by deep etching. *Cell*, **30**, 395

16. Dermietzel, R., Janssen-Timmen, U., Willecke, K. and Traub, O. (1984). Cytoplasmic and cell surface structure of purified liver gap junctions revealed by freeze-drying. *Eur. J. Cell Biol.*, **33**, 84

17. Markham, R., Frey, S. and Hills, G. J. (1963). Methods for the enhancement of image detail and accentuation of structure in electron microscopy. *Virology*, **20**, 88

18. Bennett, M. V. L. (1973). Function of electrotonic junctions in embryonic and adult tissues. *Fed. Proc..*, **32**, 65

19. Spray, D. C., Harris, A. L. and Bennett, M. V. L. (1981). Glutaraldehyde differentially affects gap junctional conductance and its pH and voltage dependence. *J. Biophys.*, **33**, 108a

20. Peracchia, C. (1980). Structural correlates of gap junction permeation. *Intern. Rev. Cytol.*, **66**, 81

21. Raviola, E., Goodenough, D. A. and Raviola, G. (1980). Structure of rapidly frozen gap junctions. *J. Cell Biol.*, **87**, 273

22. Politoff, A. L., Socolar, S. J. and Loewenstein, W. R. (1969). Permeability of a cell membrane junction. Dependence on energy metabolism. *J. Gen. Physiol.*, **53**, 498

17
Insulin and liver disease: effect of proinsulin on hepatic carbohydrate metabolism

W. CREUTZFELDT

The frequent occurrence of impaired glucose tolerance and diabetes mellitus in liver disease, especially liver cirrhosis, is of multifactorial origin[1]. Recent findings have demonstrated that the first measurable event in patients with early idiopathic haemochromatosis in the non-cirrhotic stage of the disease is hyperinsulinaemia without hyperglycaemia[2]. This hyperinsulinaemia was not a consequence of insulin hypersecretion because the response of serum C-peptide levels to glucose ingestion was normal, but rather it was due to a decreased insulin extraction by the liver even before shunting of portal blood. Obviously, decreased binding of insulin to the liver cell membranes results in decreased hepatic insulin extraction and decreased hepatic insulin effects, i.e. to reduced glucose uptake and, thus hyperglycaemia. Hyperinsulinaemia also induces down-regulation of insulin receptors in peripheral tissues and by this general insulin resistance, which is further enhanced by increased growth hormone and glucagon levels as frequently observed in liver cirrhotics. This, finally, leads to an exhaustion of the pancreatic B-cells (Figure 17.1).

However, it all starts with decreased insulin binding and extraction by the abnormal hepatocyte.

The availability of proinsulin by recombinant DNA technology has prompted comparative investigations on the effect of proinsulin and insulin on the carbohydrate metabolism of different tissues. The relative biological potency of proinsulin compared to insulin is only 1–5% in muscle and adipose tissue. Recent investigations demonstrated that proinsulin-mediated glucose disposal was 8% that of insulin. In contrast, proinsulin-mediated suppression of hepatic glucose output in healthy subjects was 12% that seen with insulin[3].

In vitro studies, performed in co-operation with the Department of Biochemistry in Göttingen, using cultured hepatocytes and the perfused rat

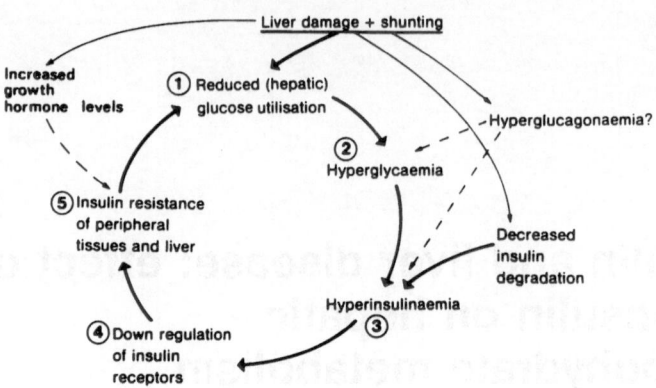

Figure 17.1 Pathogenesis of hepatogenous diabetes

liver, revealed that stimulation of glycolysis, induction of glucokinase and pyruvate kinase and the suppression of glucagon-induced phosphoenol-pyruvate carboxykinase required hundredfold higher concentrations of proinsulin than of insulin. However, the suppression of glucagon-induced glycogenolysis in the isolated perfused liver could be achieved with identical concentrations of proinsulin and insulin[4]. This preferential hepatic effect of proinsulin may become of great interest for the treatment of type II diabetes, especially in the obese patient with fatty liver – named over 30 years ago by Himsworth and later by Bearn, Billing and Sherlock as 'hepatic-sensitive-diabetics'[5]. These obese patients should profit from proinsulin because the peripheral, i.e. lipogenetic effect of insulin is a disadvantage for them and unwanted.

References

1. Creutzfeldt, W., Hartmann, H., Nauck, M. and Stöckmann, F. (1983). Liver disease and glucose homeostasis. In Bianchi, L., Gerok, W., Landmann, L., Sickinger, K. and Stalder, G. A. (eds.) *Liver in Metabolic Diseases.* pp. 221–34. (Lancaster: MTP Press)
2. Niederau, C., Berger, M., Stremmel, W., Starke, A., Strohmeyer, G., Ebert, R., Siegel, E. and Creutzfeldt, W. (1984). Hyperinsulinaemia in non-cirrhotic haemochromatosis: impaired hepatic insulin degradation? *Diabetologia,* **26**, 441–4
3. Revers, R. R., Henry, R., Schmeiser, L., Kolterman, O., Cohen, R., Bergenstal, R., Polonsky, K., Jaspan, J., Rubenstein, A., Frank, B., Galloway, J. and Olefsky, J. M. (1984). The effects of biosynthetic human proinsulin on carbohydrate metabolism. *Diabetes,* **33**, 762–70
4. Probst, I., Hartmann, H., Jungermann, K. and Creutzfeldt, W. (1985). Insulin-like action of proinsulin on rat liver carbohydrate metablism *in vitro. Diabetes.,* **34** (In press)
5. Bearn, A. G., Billing, B. and Sherlock, S. (1953). Response of the liver to insulin; hepatic vein catheterization studies in man. In *Ciba Foundation Colloquia on Endocrinology. Vol. VI: Hormonal Factors in Carbohydrate Metabolism.* pp. 250–60. (London: Churchill)

Section 3

18
Wilson's disease

I. STERNLIEB

Remarkable improvements in the accuracy of the diagnosis, and an increased range of therapeutic measures available for the treatment of Wilson's disease have dramatically changed the clinical picture and the prognosis of patients with this previously progressive and fatal disorder[1]. This inherited disturbance of copper metabolism is distributed worldwide[2]. It is characterized by copper toxicosis first affecting the liver and later the central nervous system, eyes and kidneys. Despite the presence of the genetic disorder from birth, clinically overt disease hardly ever occurs before 5 years of age. As shown in Figure 18.1, no symptoms were noted before the age of 5 years, yet 50% of

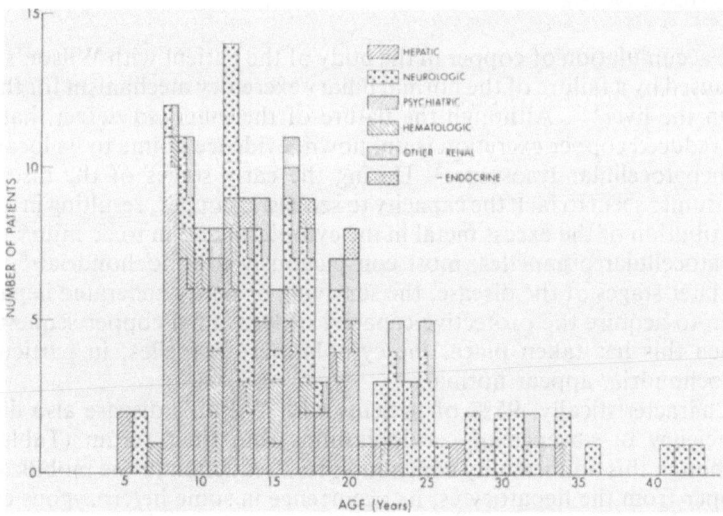

Figure 18.1 Initial mode of onset of clinical manifestations as a function of age in a group of 151 symptomatic patients with Wilson's disease (from Scheinberg and Sternlieb[2], with permission of the publisher)

this group of 151 patients manifested symptoms by the age of 15, with the majority of the remainder becoming ill during early adult life. In 42% of the total group of patients, the first sign or symptom of Wilson's disease was one or several manifestations of liver disease.

CLINICAL PRESENTATIONS OF HEPATIC WILSON'S DISEASE

The hepatic disease may be acute and self-limiting, mimicking acute hepatitis, or infectious mononucleosis, or sudden illness and a rapid progression of hepatic dysfunction may suggest fulminant hepatitis, generally associated with severe haemolysis. In most patients, however, the liver disease resembles chronic active hepatitis or progresses insidiously to cirrhosis, without overt signs of illness. In this last group of patients, hepatic insufficiency with jaundice, spider angiomas, ascites, oedema, anasarca, bleeding from oesophageal varices or other manifestations of portal hypertension develop if the patient is not treated in time. In some patients, abnormal bleeding or bruisability result from a combination of thrombocytopenia, due to hyper-splenism, and deficiencies of various clotting factors. Finally, primary or secondary amenorrhoea in girls, or gynaecomastia and delayed puberty in boys may alert the physician to the presence of liver disease.

If the correct diagnosis is delayed and no specific treatment to remove excess copper is given, deterioration of hepatic function, progression of portal hypertension, appearance of neurologic or psychiatric abnormalities and death will supervene.

PATHOGENESIS

The accumulation of copper in the body of the patient with Wilson's disease is caused by a failure of the normal biliary excretory mechanism for the metal from the liver[3-5]. Although the nature of the inherited defect that causes the reduced copper excretion is unknown, evidence points to its localization to hepatocellular lysosomes[5]. During the early stages of the disease, the lysosomes seem to lack the capacity to sequester copper, resulting in a diffuse distribution of the excess metal in the cytoplasm and in toxic injury to other hepatocellular organelles, most conspicuously to mitochondria[2,6]. During the later stages of the disease, the surviving or newly generated hepatocytes seem to acquire the protective capacity of lysosomal copper sequestration. When this has taken place, the cytoplasmic organelles, in particular the mitochondria, appear normal.

Characteristically, 95% of patients with Wilson's disease also display a deficiency or absence of ceruloplasmin from their serum (Table 18.1). Although this abnormality contributes to a reduction in the mobilization of copper from the hepatocytes, its occurrence in some heterozygous carriers, in whom no extra storage of copper occurs, indicates that this copper-protein does not play a central role in the pathogenesis of the disease. Consequently, it does not seem to be a primary product of the abnormal gene.

Table 18.1 Concentration of ceruloplasmin in serum of symptomatic patients with Wilson's disease

Ceruloplasmin (mg/dl)	Patients	
	No.	%
0–<1	113	28
1–4.9	107	26
5–9.9	98	24
10–14.9	47	11
15–19.9	28	7
20–29.3	16	4
Total	409	100

(Normal: 20–40 mg/100 ml)

HEPATIC PATHOLOGY

The structural changes observed in the livers of patients with Wilson's disease are non-specific. Yet, certain characteristic histologic patterns can be recognized. Thus, during the early stage of Wilson's disease, particularly in

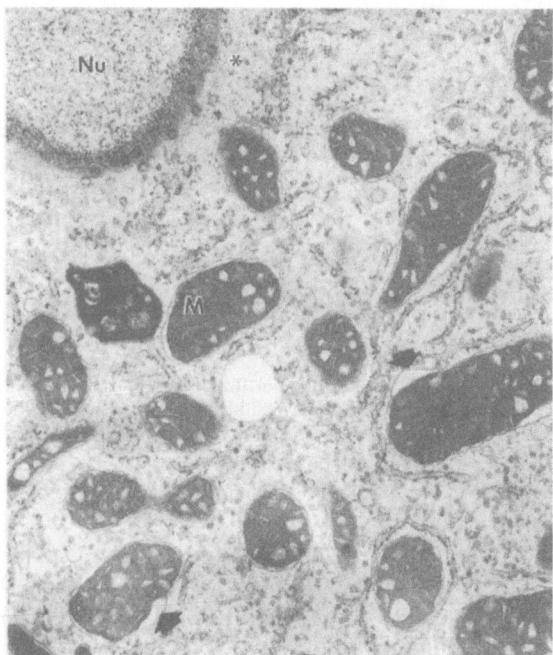

Figure 18.2 Electron micrograph showing portion of hepatocyte from a 5 year-old asymptomatic girl containing a small lipid droplet (L) and abnormal mitochondria with dense matrices, dilated cristae, prominent granules, irregularly shaped vacuoles and separated outer from inner membranes (arrows). (Nu), nucleus with prominent nuclear pores and converging perinuclear filaments (asterisk). Hepatic copper, 991 µg/g dry tissue. × 13 600

asymptomatic patients, a histologic picture of fatty infiltration of varying severity is seen. This fatty infiltration is almost always associated with characteristic mitochondrial abnormalities (Figure 18.2). Occasionally, when these abnormalities are less pronounced in certain patients with fatty infiltration, structural abnormalities of peroxisomes are present (Figure 18.3). From this initial stage, progression of liver injury may proceed with an indolent deposition of collagen or it may evolve through stages suggestive of toxic hepatitis. It may also escalate with biochemical and light microscopic characteristics indistinguishable from those of chronic active hepatitis[7]

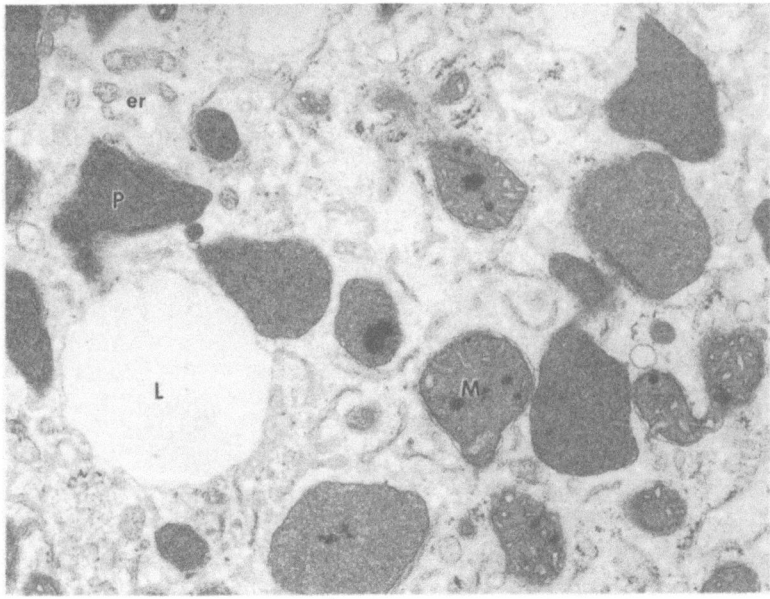

Figure 18.3 Electron micrograph showing portion of hepatocyte from an 8 year-old asymptomatic boy with Wilson's disease. The single membrane bounded peroxisomes (P) are irregularly shaped, dense and larger than the adjacent mitochondria (M); er, endoplasmic reticulum; L, lipid droplet. × 13 500

(Figure 18.4). Features of submassive necrosis with severe haemolysis, always superimposed on a background of cirrhosis, may predominate in patients with a fulminant, fatal course[8]. In the majority of patients with neurologic disease, however, a micro- or macronodular cirrhosis, without necessarily displaying significant inflammatory changes, is invariably present. At this final stage, electron dense lysosomes concentrate a large portion of the cellular copper, seemingly protecting the cytoplasm from the toxic effects of excess metal[2, 6]

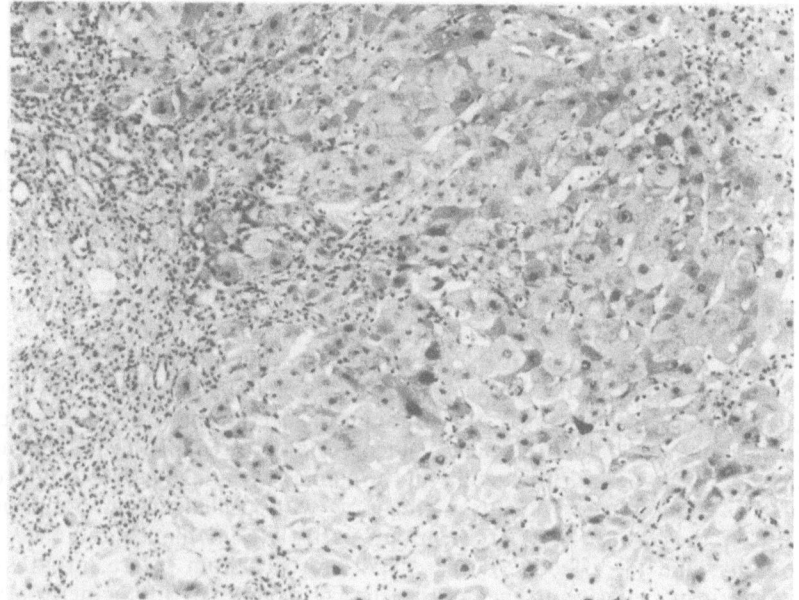

Figure 18.4 Light micrograph of histologic section of surgical liver biopsy specimen showing piecemeal necrosis, Councilman bodies and proliferation of bile ducts within bands of fibrous tissue. The patient is a 28 year-old Haitian woman diagnosed and treated for 2 years as 'chronic active hepatitis with cirrhosis'. After a diagnosis of Wilson's disease was made in her brother she was found to have Kayser-Fleischer rings; serum ceruloplasmin, 3 mg/dl; hepatic copper, 719 μg/g dry tissue; and urinary copper, 270 μg/24 h. Heamatoxylin and eosin. × 230

DIAGNOSIS

The diagnosis of Wilson's disease can almost always be established or excluded by performing a slit-lamp examination of the eyes for Kayser-Fleischer rings and a determination of the serum concentration of ceruloplasmin. Most patients with Wilson's disease display corneal rings *and* a reduction of the concentration of ceruloplasmin below 20 mg/dl. The presence of both abnormalities in the same patient indicates Wilson's disease. In the absence of Kayser-Fleischer rings, in a young, hypoceruloplasminaemic subject, the presence of an elevated hepatic copper concentration, above 250 μg/g dry tissue, is an indication of Wilson's disease. In the presence of low normal ceruloplasmin concentrations, 20–30 mg/dl, and in the absence of Kayser-Fleischer rings, demonstration of elevated hepatic copper levels with compatible histologic changes and a diagnostic radiocopper loading test may be required before the physician can commit himself to a diagnosis of Wilson's disease.

Determinations of urinary copper excretion play a secondary role in the diagnosis of Wilson's disease because of the frequency of inaccurate assays. Therefore this test should not be used as a screening procedure.

TREATMENT

Chelation therapy with D-penicillamine[9] or trientine (Trien, TETA)[10], started as soon as the diagnosis is firmly established, enables most patients with Wilson's disease to lead a normal life. Asymptomatic homozygotes remain so, provided that they are compliant with the anti-copper regimen. Sensitivity reactions to penicillamine are common, but can usually be controlled through desensitization[2]. The occasional severe toxic effects on the kidneys, bone marrow or the immune system may require the substitution of trientine. Experience with zinc therapy is limited, and, therefore, its indications are still uncertain, even though favourable clinical results have been reported in some patients with neurologic Wilson's disease[11].

Liver transplant[12] has to be considered in three groups of patients: (1) those presenting with a clinical picture of fulminant hepatitis; (2) young cirrhotic patients with laboratory findings of severe hepatic decompensation (profound hypoalbuminaemia, uncorrectable hypoprothrombinaemia, progressive hyperbilirubinaemia and uraemia) who have failed to improve after 2–3 months of adequate chelation with D-penicillamine and non-specific therapy for water rentention, electrolyte imbalance and encephalopathy; and (3) effectively treated patients in whom severe, progressive hepatic insufficiency and haemolysis, clinically similar to fulminant hepatitis, develops acutely following discontinuation of penicillamine.

We should realize, however, that even though the prognosis of the diagnosed patient has dramatically improved, numerous adolescents and young adults continue to become severely incapacitated and die of Wilson's disease not because of the complexity of the required tests, but simply because their physicians have failed to think of this diagnosis.

Acknowledgements

The technical assistance of P. S. Grushoff and N. Quintana is gratefully acknowledged. Supported in part by grants from the National Institutes of Health AM-17702, 5M01-RR50 and CA06576 and the Foundation for the Study of Wilson's Disease, Inc.

References

1. Wilson, S. A. K. (1912). Progressive lenticular degeneration: a familial nervous disease associated with cirrhosis of the liver. *Brain*, **34**, 295–509
2. Scheinberg, I. H. and Sternlieb, I. (1984). *Wilson's Disease*. 171 pp. (Philadelphia: W. B. Saunders)
3. O'Reilly, S., Weber, P. M., Oswald, M. and Shipley, L. (1971). Abnormalities of the physiology of copper in Wilson's disease. III. The excretion of copper. *Arch. Neurol.*, **25**, 28–32
4. Frommer, D. J. (1974). Defective biliary excretion of copper in Wilson's disease. *Gut*, **15**, 125–9
5. Sternlieb, I., van den Hamer, C. J. A., Morell, A. G., Alpert, S., Gregoriadis, G. and Scheinberg, I. H. (1973). Lysosomal defect of hepatic copper excretion in Wilson's disease (hepatolenticular degeneration). *Gastroenterology*, **64**, 99–105

6. Goldfischer, S. and Sternlieb, I. (1968). Changes in the distribution of hepatic copper in relation to the progression of Wilson's disease (hepatolenticular degeneration). *Am. J. Pathol.*, **53**, 883–901
7. Sternlieb, I. and Scheinberg, I. H. (1972). Chronic hepatitis as a first manifestation of Wilson's disease. *Ann. Intern. Med.*, **76**, 59–64
8. McCullough, A. J., Fleming, C. R., Thistle, J. L. *et al.* (1983). Diagnosis of Wilson's disease presenting as fulminant hepatic failure. *Gastroenterology*, **84**, 161–7
9. Walshe, J. M. (1973). Copper chelation in patients with Wilson's disease. *Q. J. Med.*, **46**, 73–83
10. Walshe, J. M. (1982). Treatment of Wilson's disease with Trientine (Triethylene tetramine) dihydrochloride. *Lancet*, **i**, 643–7
11. Hoogenraad, T. U., van den Hamer, C. J. A. and van Hattum, J. (1984). Effective treatment of Wilson's disease with oral zinc. *Br. Med. J.*, **288**, 273–6
12. Sternlieb, I. (1984). Wilson's disease: Indications for liver transplants. *Hepatology*, **4**, 15S–17S

19
Studies on the development of Mallory bodies

H. DENK, R. HAZAN, E. LACKINGER, D. L. SCHILLER
AND W. W. FRANKE

Mallory bodies (MBs) are characteristic hepatocellular cytoplasmic inclusions, predominantly, but not exclusively associated with alcoholic hepatitis (*see* references 1, 2 for review). This disease is the link between the reversible fatty liver and the irreversible liver cirrhosis of the alcoholic. The pathogenesis of alcoholic hepatitis is still unresolved. Studies on structure and mechanisms of MB formation may, however, provide not only further information on cellular alterations specifically associated with alcohol intoxication but also on basic mechanisms of liver cell injury. Studies on the development of MBs are facilitated by the existence of an animal model, the griseofulvin-treated mouse, in which MBs can be produced under standardized conditions[3]. The data presented in the following communication were mainly obtained using this model.

Morphologic, immunohistochemical and chemical analyses revealed similarities between MBs and the intermediate filament cytoskeleton of the cytokeratin type, particularly of hepatocytes, e.g. filamentous ultrastructure, resistance to solubilization in non-denaturing solvents at neutral or slightly alkaline pH values, composition of several polypeptides with molecular weights between 48 000 and 65 000 and isoelectric pH values between 5.4 and 6.4, immunoreactivity with cytokeratin antibodies, and occasional association with desmosomes[4-6]. On the other hand, several features of MBs are different from those of normal hepatocytic cytokeratins, e.g. irregular distribution of filaments, presence of fuzzy material coating MB filaments proper, immunoreactivity with antibodies to epidermal cytokeratins, additional constituent polypeptides, and derangement of cytokeratin architecture concomitant with MB development[4, 7, 8].

When isolated MBs are analysed by 1- and 2-dimensional SDS-polyacrylamide gel electrophoresis three major polypeptide bands with molecular weights of 48 000, 55 000 and 65 000 are revealed[5]. The lower molecular weight components of MBs (component 2, M_r 55 000, component 3, M_r 48 000) closely resemble, in molecular weights and isolelectric pH values, the major cytokeratin components of mouse hepatocytes, whereas component 1 (65 000 M_r) is different and apparently has no counterpart in normal mouse liver cytokeratin. However, tryptic peptide maps of components A and D of normal mouse liver cytokeratin and components 2 and 3 of MBs revealed additional compositional differences (Denk, Hazan, Lackinger, Schiller, Franke, manuscript in preparation). While a close similarity, if not identity, of tryptic products was noted between cytokeratin A and MB component 2, the peptide maps of MB component 3 were different from those of cyto-keratin D and closely resembled the pattern of proteolytic products of cytokeratin A. This indicates that most of these materials represent degra-dation products of cytokeratin A. Whether these differences in composition are related to the abnormal morphology of MB filaments remains to be elucidated.

Further analyses of MBs were performed by using monoclonal antibodies raised against MB material. Two cell lines producing antibodies with exclusive reactivity with MBs were selected. One antibody designated M_M 120-1 only reacted, in indirect immunofluorescence microscopy, with MBs in murine and human livers but not with cytokeratins from human and murine tissues. The other antibody, designated K_M 54-5, recognized murine MBs but not MBs of human origin. It did not decorate structures associated with normal hepato-cytes. However, in addition to MBs it stained some basal cells (apparently reserve cells) in the forestomach and in hair bulbs of the mouse. In immuno-blots, it reacted with keratin polypeptides of human and murine origin, indicating that this antibody recognizes epitopes of cytokeratin filaments that were not accessible in most cells *in situ* but were exposed in the course of MB formation, indicating changes in cytokeratin organization. When different stages of MB development were studied by indirect immuno-fluorescence microscopy using antibodies M_M 120-1 and K_M 54-5, differences in immunostaining were observed. M_M 120-1 recognized MBs in all stages of their development, even in the earliest stage when MBs appear as small granules closely associated with cytokeratin fibrils[6]. In contrast, K_M 54-5 did not react with MBs in such very early stages (Figure 19.1). This finding suggests that the antigen recognized by K_M 54-5 becomes accessible to interaction with the antibodies only at a later stage of MB development. The changes in cytokeratin organization indicated by this immunologic reactivity are, therefore, probably secondary phenomena. On the other hand, the epitope recognized by M_M 120-1, which has yet to be identified, may play a primary role in MB evolution and aggregation.

SUMMARY

Altered cytokeratins are major, but not the only, components of MBs. During MB development changes in cytokeratin organization occur which can be assessed by their reactivity with the monoclonal cytokeratin antibody K_M 54-5. Proteolytic degradation also takes place during MB development.

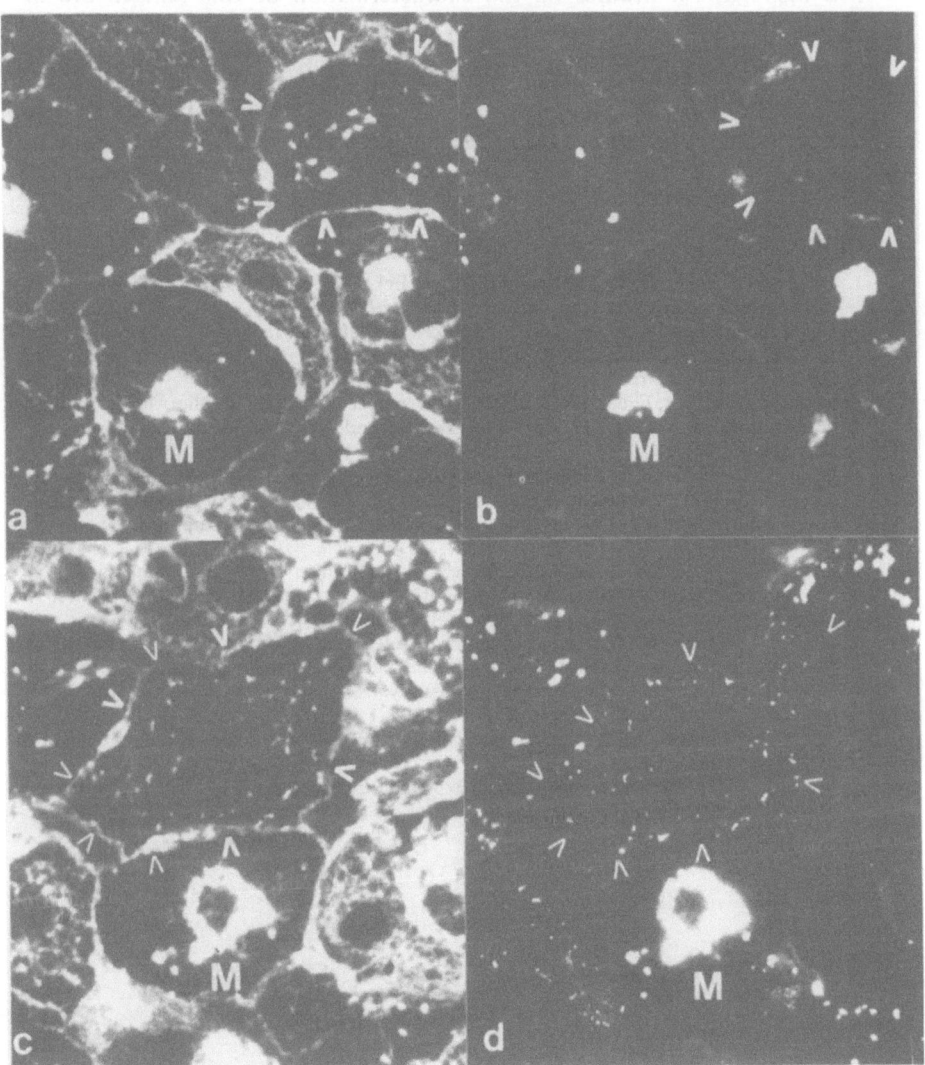

Figure 19.1 Indirect immunofluorescence microscopy of liver derived from mice fed griseo-fulvin for 2.5 months using monoclonal antibodies to Mallory body material K_M 54-5 (b) and M_M 120-1 (d), as well as antibodies to liver cytokeratin component D (a, c). Mallory bodies in different stages of development are seen. The earliest stages are granules closely associated with cytokeratin fibrils (a, c; arrow heads). K_M 54-5 and M_M 120-1 stain large Mallory bodies (M) but differ in their immunoreactivities with very early stages of Mallory bodies. K_M 54-5 does not react with Mallory in very early stages of development (b; arrow heads), whereas M_M 120-1 recognizes even the earliest and smallest Mallory body granules (d; arrow heads). × 540

Additional non-keratin components are also associated with MBs. Some of them, e.g. the component recognized by the monoclonal antibody M_M 120-1, are present in the earliest stages of MB development and may be involved in MB aggregation. Studies on the characterization of this antigen are in progress.

Acknowledgement

Supported in part by Fonds zur Förderung der wissenschaftlichen Forschung No. P 4708 (H.D.).

References

1. Denk, H., Franke, W. W., Kerjaschki, D. and Eckerstorfer, R. (1979). Mallory bodies in experimental animals and man. *Int. Rev. Exp. Pathol.*, **20**, 77
2. Denk, H. and Franke, W. W. (1982). Cytoskeletal filaments. In Arias, I. M., Popper, H., Schachter, D. and Shafritz, D. A. (eds.) *The Liver: Biology and Pathobiology*. pp. 55-71. (New York: Raven Press)
3. Denk, H., Gschnait, F. and Wolff, K. (1975). Hepatocellular hyalin (Mallory bodies) in long term griseofulvin-treated mice: a new experimental model for the study of hyalin formation. *Lab. Invest.*, **32**, 773
4. Franke, W. W., Denk, H., Schmid, E., Osborn, M. and Weber, K. (1979). Ultrastructural, biochemical, and immunological characterization of Mallory bodies in griseofulvin-treated mice. Fimbriated rods of filaments containing prekeratin-like polypeptides. *Lab. Invest.*, **40**, 207
5. Denk, H., Krepler, R., Lackinger, E., Artlieb, U. and Franke, W. W. (1982). Immunological and biochemical characterization of the keratin-related component of Mallory bodies: A pathological pattern of hepatocytic cytokeratins. *Liver*, **2**, 165
6. Denk, H., Franke, W. W., Dragosics, B. and Zeiler, I. (1981). Pathology of cytoskeleton of liver cells: demonstration of Mallory bodies (alcoholic hyalin) in murine and human hepatocytes by immunofluorescence microscopy using antibodies to cytokeratin polypeptides from hepatocytes. *Hepatology*, **1**, 9
7. Yokoo, H., Minick, O. T., Batti, F. and Kent, G. (1972). Morphologic variants of alcoholic hyalin. *Am. J. Pathol.*, **69**, 25
8. Wiggers, K. D., French, S. W., French, B. A. and Carr, B. N. (1973). The ultrastructure of Mallory body filaments. *Lab. Invest.*, **29**, 652

20
Are constitutional factors and/or HLA phenotypes in males predisposing factors for alcoholic cirrhosis?

H. THALER, H. THALER AND W. R. MAYR

The different sensitivity of the male and the female liver is well established, but in addition there are more apparent differences in the male liver. One possible explanation for these differences might be the existence of genetic peculiarities among patients with alcoholic cirrhosis. In the early 20th century, Chvostek, in Vienna, was the first to draw attention to a constitutional element which he believed to be fundamental: absent body hair, absent or extremely sparse hair on the limbs, and pubic hair of the female type i.e. with a horizontal upper border[1]. He placed special emphasis on the fact that these anomalies were of genetic origin and were not a secondary phenomenon due to alcoholism or cirrhosis. The feminine pattern of hair distribution, the so-called 'Chvostek's habitus', is a frequently seen condition, but the statistical proof of its association with alcoholic cirrhosis in man is still missing.

The purpose of our study was to investigate whether:

(1) The feminine pattern of hair distribution in male patients with alcoholic cirrhosis is a genetic characteristic.
(2) This anomaly is more frequently encountered in alcoholic rather than in posthepatitic cirrhosis.
(3) The reported discrepancies of HLA frequencies are due to genetic differences.

MATERIALS AND METHODS

From 1.10.1980 all male patients with alcoholic or posthepatitic cirrhosis admitted to our department were accepted for this study. The study[2] was concluded in October, 1982, when 100 patients with alcoholic cirrhosis and

179

Table 20.1

	Alcoholic cirrhoses	Material Posthepatitic cirrhoses	Controls
Number	100	50	50
Age	54 ± 11	60 ± 10	56 ± 18
Alcohol (g)	107 ± 57	22 ± 32	—
$\geqslant 60\,g/d$	94	6	—
$< 60\,g/d$	6	44	—
Duration (y)	23 ± 21	—	—

50 patients with posthepatitic cirrhosis (45 due to hepatitis B, 5 due to hepatitis NANB) were registered. The controls were 50 male patients, admitted over the same period who neither suffered from liver disease nor admitted to drinking alcohol habitually every day (Table 20.1).

In addition to history, physical examination, biochemical data, sonography, oesophagoscopy, liver biopsy and/or peritoneoscopy we recorded whether the trunk and the limbs were obviously hairy (masculine body hair pattern) or whether this hair was strikingly deficient or absent (feminine body hair pattern), and whether the pubic hair terminated in a horizontal boundary (feminine pubic hair pattern) or tapered upwards towards the umbilicus (masculine pubic hair pattern). Patients with the feminine type of hair distribution were carefully questioned if they had always looked this way (primary feminine hair pattern) or if the anomaly was due to a loss of hair (secondary feminine hair pattern).

Forty-five histocompatibility antigens were determined in all patients, and compared with those of 3000 controls for HLA-A, B and C, and with 160 controls for HLA-DR.

The statistical evaluation of the frequencies was carried out by the four-field Chi-squared test. In order to avoid type I errors the p-value computed from the four-field Chi-squared test was multiplied by the number of comparisons made when $p < 0.05$ had been observed for the first time in a given association (Pc). In addition the relative risk (RR) was calculated by Woolf's method.

RESULTS

Sixty-three patients with alcoholic cirrhosis displayed a feminine body hair pattern; 45 of them insisted that their body hair had not been more abundant in the past, but 18 had noted a loss of hair during their illness. Out of the 50 patients with hepatitic cirrhosis 17 had a feminine body hair pattern; in 10 of them it was primary and in 7 secondary. Among the controls this anomaly of body hair was noted in only 6 men; in none of them was it due to hair loss commencing in later life. The primary type of feminine body hair pattern was significantly commoner among patients with alcoholic cirrhosis than in patients with posthepatitic cirrhosis ($p < 0.001$) or among the controls ($p \ll 0.001$) (Table 20.2).

Table 20.2 Markers in males. Comparison of alcoholic cirrhosis, posthepatitic cirrhosis, and controls

Marker	Alcoholic cirrhosis (n = 100)		Posthepatitic cirrhosis (n = 50)		Controls (n = 50)
Absent body hair					
Primary	45	$p < 0.001$	10	$p < 0.01$	6
			$p \ll 0.001$		
Secondary	18	n.s.	7		—
Female pubic hair	70	$p < 0.002$	22	$p = 0.01$	10
Type			$p \ll 0.001$		

p from 40 field χ^2 test; n.s. = not significant

A feminine pattern of pubic hair was found in 70% of patients with alcoholic cirrhosis, 44% of the patients with hepatic cirrhosis and 20% of the controls. The difference between patients with alcoholic cirrhosis and those with hepatic cirrhosis was significant ($p < 0.002$), as was the difference between the former and the controls ($p \ll 0.001$) (Table 20.2).

The body hair abnormality showed a significant association with the feminine pubic hair pattern ($p \ll 0.001$).

The HLA phenotypes, claimed in the literature to be connected with alcoholic cirrhosis (Table 20.3), appeared to be not significant, as did all other considered parameters, although this only became apparent for the correlations between alcoholic cirrhosis and Aw31 or Bw35 after the correction of Pc. The link between posthepatitic cirrhosis B and Bw35 has been described in the literature more than once, and was also apparent among our patients.

Table 20.3 HLA-antigens possibly related to alcoholic liver disease

	A2, B8, Bw35, B40 DR2

CONCLUSIONS

In this study a feminine body hair pattern was observed in 63% and a feminine pubic hair pattern in 70% of male patients with alcoholic cirrhosis.

In 70% of these patients the anomaly was primary, i.e. inborn. The incidence of a primary feminine body hair pattern was significantly higher in patients with alcoholic cirrhosis that in patients with posthepatitic cirrhosis ($p < 0.001$) or controls ($p \ll 0.001$). Therefore, the observation by Chvostek that males with alcoholic cirrhosis frequently display peculiar genetic characteristics is correct. The livers of women[3] and of men with a primary feminine hair pattern are obviously more susceptible to alcohol than men with a masculine hair pattern.

Attempts to find evidence of some predisposing constitutional factor(s) in the HLA-system were disappointing. Conflicting statements in the literature[2] seem to be caused by type I errors.

References

1. Chvostek, F. (1922). Zur Pathogenese der Leberzirrhose. *Wien. Klin. Wochenschr.*, **35**, 381, 408
2. Thaler, H., Thaler, H. and Mayr, W. R. (1984). Constitutional factors and HLA phenotypes in males with alcoholic cirrhosis. *Liver.* (In press)
3. Péquignot, G. (1974). Les problèmes nutritionelles de la société industrielle. *Vie Méd. Can. Fr.*, **27**, 216

21
New aspects of piecemeal necrosis

V. J. DESMET

INTRODUCTION

Half a century ago, the term 'chronic hepatitis' was a synonym for cirrhosis of the liver[1]. According to Eppinger, the activity of the cirrhotic process was thought to be reflected in an irregular outline of cirrhotic nodules crowded with mononuclear inflammatory cells[2].

Since the 1950s, the concept of non-cirrhotic chronic hepatitis gradually emerged[3,4] as a result of the introduction of transaminase determinations, laparoscopy and needle liver biopsy[2].

Again, the activity of chronic hepatitis was thought be reflected in an irregular outline of the lobular parenchymal periphery, due to periportal infiltration by mononuclear inflammatory cells[5]. This intriguing feature of accumulation of lymphoid type cells around the portal tracts, associated with progressive loss and destruction of zone 1 hepatocytes, has been termed 'piecemeal necrosis'[2].

It became clear that piecemeal necrosis (PMN) occurred not only in progressive, active or aggressive chronic hepatitis of any aetiology (hepatitis virus B, hepatitis virus(es) non-A, non-B, auto-immune and drug induced) but also in primary biliary cirrhosis, primary sclerosing cholangitis, some cases of alcoholic liver disease, and cases of clinically acute hepatitis. The latter cases were considered to represent 'acute hepatitis with signs of possible transition to chronicity'[6,7]. Furthermore, distinction should be made between 'true' PMN, as observed in chronic aggressive hepatitis, and 'biliary piecemeal necrosis', characterized by cholate-stasis of zone 1 hepatocytes and sometimes a polymorphonuclear cell component, as observed in conditions of chronic cholestasis of diverse aetiology[2,8].

From the beginning, PMN has been considered to represent an immunologically based phenomenon, originally thought to be a feature of 'self-perpetuation' of the disease[2]. However, the true nature of the phenomenon, its biological meaning and prognostic significance remain a matter of intense investigation and scientific debate.

PROGNOSTIC SIGNIFICANCE OF PIECEMEAL NECROSIS

In a widely accepted classification of chronic hepatitis[5], it was proposed that PMN is a sign of worse prognosis, since it characterizes the more active or aggressive variants of chronic hepatitis, as compared to cases with a more benign and quiescent course which lack PMN and were classified as chronic persistent hepatitis. It was recognized that lobular parenchymal lesions were also important. However, in emphasizing the prognostic value of PMN, this may have been stated too shortly as 'lesions of acute hepatitis may be superimposed'[5].

Others have emphasized the importance of lobular parenchymal lesions for progression to chronicity and evolution to cirrhosis[9–11]. Severe confluent necrosis of the lytic type[12], occurring in various degrees and described as bridging hepatic necrosis[13] and multilobular necrosis[14] are recognized as accelerating the progression to cirrhosis[7, 15, 16]. However, extensive confluent lytic necrosis in the liver of patients with hepatitis has repeatedly been shown to reflect more the severity of the disease rather than its propensity for progression into a chronic course[17]. It, therefore, still holds true that PMN is the hallmark of 'perpetuation' or 'chronicity'[18], but lobular lesions such as confluent necrosis of the 'bridging' type may be superimposed, even repeatedly superimposed, and as such carry an increased risk for faster remodelling of the liver architecture into cirrhosis[1]. With the present therapeutic armamentarium, lobular parenchymal lesions may also be a better yardstick than PMN for antiviral therapy in virally induced cases of chronic hepatitis[2]. Nevertheless, PMN remains an essential requirement for the diagnosis of chronic hepatitis of the active, aggressive or progressive variety.

Discussion also centres on the prognostic value of PMN versus confluent necrosis in acute hepatitis. Some studies[19, 20] suggested that PMN has no predictive value in acute hepatitis, whereas others emphasized the importance of extensive confluent lytic necrosis bridging portal tracts and central veins[9].

Subsequent studies, however, have indicated that bridging hepatic necrosis by itself does not carry an increased risk of progression to chronic liver disease[21–23], but when associated with PMN, a chronic course frequently follows[24].

It appears that the prognostic weight of PMN in acute hepatitis depends on a number of factors, such as the extent of PMN, the aetiology of the viral hepatitis and the time when the biopsy is taken.

It looks as if PMN may be a component of the histological picture of self-healing acute hepatitis when studied in the very early stage at the height of transaminase elevation[20]. There is a lack of information on this early stage of acute hepatitis, since liver biopsies are not usually taken in the first few weeks of acute hepatitis, except in prospective studies[20]. However, in a study where the time factor and aetiology of the disease were taken into consideration, it appeared that the detection of clearcut PMN in a liver biopsy taken 1 month or more after the clinical onset of acute hepatitis – at least in viral hepatitis B and non-A, non-B – strongly suggests an evolution into chronic liver disease which actually occurred in 95% of the cases[24]. Also the extent and degree of PMN should be considered, since patients in whose biopsies only minimal or mild PMN was recognized developed chronic liver disease to a lower, although still significant extent (67%)[24].

It further appears that in acute viral hepatitis it is of the utmost importance to consider the aetiology of the disease. Indeed, acute viral hepatitis type A is often characterized by periportal inflammation and necrosis diagnosed as piecemeal necrosis, but it does not lead to chronic liver disease[24, 25].

This is a puzzling observation. If PMN has so strong a predictive value in acute viral hepatitis type B and non-A, non-B, but not in type A, one may suspect that the nature of the underlying process is fundamentally different, in spite of a superficial morphological similarity.

This indicates the need for a more careful evaluation of the histopathological features of what is considered as 'piecemeal necrosis' in different forms of hepatitis, and also urges further studies to unravel the biological meaning of this still mysterious PMN.

BIOLOGICAL MEANING OF PIECEMEAL NECROSIS

The essential morphological features of PMN comprise an intimate contact between lymphoid type cells and parenchymal cells[26, 27] at the connective tissue–parenchymal interface (periportal, periseptal), associated with progressive, step by step (piecemeal) necrosis and disappearance of hepatocytes in this area[8]. Which are the cell types accumulating in these connective tissue–parenchymal interfaces? What are the mechanisms triggering the extravasation of lymphoid cells in these territories? How is liver cell damage and necrosis brought about? Why is it usually progressive and not easily self-healing?

Although today PMN still remains a scientific challenge, at least a partial answer to some questions has evolved, as a result of numerous studies in immunology, immunohistochemistry, electronmicroscopy and cell biology. This short review will be restricted to mainly new morphological information.

Analysis of lymphoid cell types

Several techniques have been used to identify lymphocyte subsets in liver biopsy infiltrates. Some investigators eluted lymphocytes from liver biopsies and characterized them by rosette formation or other techniques[28, 29]. With the advent of monoclonal antibodies, it has become feasible to phenotype lymphocyte subsets *in situ* in cryostat sections of frozen liver specimens using immunofluorescence or immunoperoxidase techniques.

The most commonly used monoclonal antibodies include OKT_4 (and Leu 3) identifying the helper/inducer T lymphocyte subset, OKT_8 giving positive staining with a cytotoxic/suppressor subpopulation of T lymphocytes, OKM and Leu 7, identifying Killer and Natural Killer (K/NK) non-T lymphocytes, and OK_{11} identifying all T cells.

In recent years, a rapidly growing number of studies of this nature have been published[28-42]. At the risk of scotomizing some important details, the following generalizations can be made. In viral hepatitis type B, there is evidence that liver cell damage and necrosis is not due to a direct cytopathic effect of the hepatitis B virus, but results from immunological defence mechanisms on behalf of the host[43, 44]. Whereas in acute viral hepatitis type B[30] and cytomegalovirus hepatitis[40] Killer and/or Natural Killer cells seem to be involved in immunologically mediated liver cell killing, PMN in chronic active type B hepatitis is mainly characterized by a predominance of OKT_8^+ cytotoxic/suppressor T lymphocytes[30–32, 36–40].

Although the monoclonal antibody OKT_8 cannot distinguish between suppressor and cytotoxic effector T lymphocytes, it is usually assumed that the OKT_8^+ lymphocyte population represents cytotoxic T cells, and hence that the mechanism involved in immunologically mediated liver cell killing in PMN corresponds to antigen-specific, genetically restricted T lymphocyte cytotoxicity.

It is not clear which viral antigen in the liver cell plasma membrane is the target antigen for the immunological attack, but HBcAg is considered a good candidate[44, 45]. In auto-immune chronic active hepatitis, areas of PMN also contain OKT_8^+ lymphocytes, but there is also participation of K/NK cells[30], a higher proportion of OKT_4^+ helper/inducer cells (or a higher OKT_4/OKT_8 ratio)[32, 39], and admixture of immunoglobulin containing plasma cells[30].

In view of the finding of Liver Membrane Antibody (LMA) in the serum of patients whose liver biopsy is characterized by PMN, it is concluded that the mechanism of liver cell destruction operative in auto-immune CAH corresponds to antibody dependent cellular cytotoxicity, whereby the effector cells are non-T non-B Killer lymphocytes which attack the hepatocytes, hereby directed through their Fc-receptor mediated binding to LMA covering the liver cell surface[35, 44, 46]. Important in the generation of autoreactive LMA may be a defect in the suppressor T cell population[47].

A similar antibody dependent cellular cytotoxicity may be operative in the anti-e antibody positive phase of some cases of viral chronic hepatitis type B, in which LMA is also detected in the serum (although at lower level) and the OKT_4/OKT_8 ratio of lymphocytes in PMN is intermediate between that of auto-immune CAH and HBV induced, e-antigen positive CAH[32, 35, 46]. According to the latter concept, spotty or focal necrosis in chronic hepatitis B virus induced hepatitis should be due to cytotoxic T lymphocyte lysis of hepatocytes containing replicating virus, whereas the PMN component would reflect an auto-immune response to native liver membrane antigens as in auto-immune CAH, but initiated by viral replication[35, 46], and based on a disturbed immunoregulation due to defective suppressor T lymphocyte function[48].

In primary biliary cirrhosis, likewise considered to be an auto-immune disease with immunological attack on bile duct cells and hepatocytes, and also characterized by PMN, mainly OKT_4^+ helper/inducer lymphocytes and IgM containing plasma cells were found in the portal tracts, whereas the periportal areas of PMN mainly contained OKT_8^+ cytotoxic/suppressor T lymphocytes[30]. Comparable, but also more complex results were obtained in another study[42].

This leads to the tentative conclusion that in auto-immune liver disease (PBC, but mainly CAH) PMN reflects an antibody dependent cellular cytotoxicity directed by antibodies against native (self) liver cell membrane constituents[18]. In hepatitis B virus induced chronic hepatitis, the main mechanism of liver cell destruction in PMN seems to correspond to antigen specific T cell mediated lysis, possibly followed in some patients by the emergence of an auto-immune complication after seroconversion from an e-antigen positive to an e-antibody positive phase.

Analysis of antigen presenting cells

Lymphocyte reactions to antigens usually require cooperation from 'macrophages', which take up the antigen, process it in some way, and express it at their surface. Such 'antigen presentation' by macrophages is required for B and T lymphocyte reactions to occur[49]. Two lines of investigation have contributed to this problem: functional immunological studies and morphological investigation of lymphoid tissues. From immunological studies the concept has emerged that antigen-presenting accessory cells are a special class of bone marrow derived cells, different from conventional macrophages, present in tissues in small numbers, and referred to as 'dendritic cells' (dendritic cells of Steinmann) because of their irregular cytoplasmic extensions[50,51]. Such dendritic accessory cells carry, at their surface, the immune associated antigens (Ia antigens), encoded for by the I-region of the major histocompatibility complex (MHC) in the mouse, the equivalent of which in man are the HLA-D(DR) antigens or MHC class II antigens; these are required for efficient antigen presentation and triggering of lymphocytes[50,52]. Such specialized Ia positive dendritic cells were shown to be present in normal rat liver, mainly in the periphery of portal tracts and only occasionally within the liver lobules[51].

Similar HLA-DR positive dendritic cells have also been shown to be present in human connective tissue; moreover, a fraction (about 10%) of these cells also expresses the OKT_8 antigen (which is the human suppressor/cytotoxic T-cell marker), suggesting that interstitial dendritic cells in human tissues may not be a homogeneous group of cells, and – like T cells – might be composed of subsets possibly having different functions[53].

On the other hand, as a result of morphological analysis of lymphoid tissues, special types of cells with 'dendritic' morphology have been known for several years: so-called dendritic, interdigitating, fibroblastic and histocytic reticulum cells in lymphoid tissues[54] and the Langerhans cell in the skin[55]. The precise relationship between the dendritic cell of Steinmann and the other cell types (Langerhans cell, different types of reticulum cells in lymphoid tissue) is not yet clearly established[53].

An ultrastructural study on the cytological composition of PMN (performed in 1979 but delayed in publication because of the return of the first author to Eastern Europe) revealed the presence, in areas of PMN, of all the various types of reticulum cells known to occur in lymphoid tissue[56,57]. Dendritic reticulum cells (synonyms: follicular dendritic cells, dendritic reticular cells, desmodendritic cells) with the same ultrastructural characteristics as those encountered in the B regions of peripheral lymphoid tissues (lymph nodes, tonsils, spleen) were observed in the central parts of portal tracts with follicle-like aggregations of lymphocytes, indicating a similarity between the central portal areas and the B areas of lymphoid tissues. Portal lymphoid follicles with B phenotype lymphocytes were recently studied[36] in HBsAg⁺ CAH.

The origin of the dendritic reticulum cell is still under study; while some suggest a derivation from the monocyte/macrophage lineage[58], most authors adhere to a derivation from a reticulum cell of mesenchymal origin[59], more specifically the fibroblastic reticulum cell[56, 57, 60]. The dendritic reticulum cell is able to trap and retain antigen on its extensive cell processes. The antigen retention requires the presence of specific antibodies (antigen–antibody complexes). Non-antigenic materials are not trapped, except when present in very large amounts. These cells are able to trap and retain more than one antigen at the same time. The trapped immune complexes seem to play a role in stabilizing the membrane systems of the dendritic processes. The antigens trapped at the surface of dendritic reticulum cells are presented to B lymphocytes. However, the antigens trapped in the deep folds of the cell extensions are only infrequently in close contact with lymphocytes, suggesting that dendritic reticulum cells may also protect lymphocytes against an excess of immune complexes which might inhibit stimulation of lymphocytes. Dendritic reticulum cells thus act as regulators of contact between lymphocytes and antigen or immune complexes[61].

Interdigitating reticulum cells, with ultrastructural characteristics identical to those of similar cells found in lymphoid tissues, were observed in the periportal areas of piecemeal necrosis[56].

In lymphoid tissues, interdigitating reticulum cells are a characteristic component of the T regions (paracortical area of lymph nodes, periarteriolar sheets in the spleen, and the medulla and inner cortex of the thymus).

Their detection in periportal areas of PMN indicates an analogy between PMN and T regions of lymphoid tissues.

Interdigitating reticulum cells seem to be monocyte derived cells. They have a low phagocytic activity, and are thought to create a microenvironment which is necessary for the differentiation and proliferation of T lymphocytes. Their precise role in the immune response has not been elucidated. However, their occurrence in periportal areas of PMN correlates with the findings mentioned above of the predominance of T lymphocytes in areas of PMN.

It can be summarized that recent studies on antigen presenting accessory cells have emphasized the fundamental importance of this apparently heterogeneous population of cells in calling forth and modulating the immune response. The detection of dendritic and interdigitating reticulum cells, in portal tracts and areas of PMN in the liver of patients with CAH, suggests their active participation in the course of immunologically mediated chronic liver disease. Further studies should clarify their occurrence in different forms and stages of chronic liver disease. The recent availability of monoclonal antibodies reacting with dendritic reticulum cells[62] should be helpful in the better identification of these cells in PMN.

Endothelial changes and fibroplasia

Blood vessels and sinusoids should not be considered as passive conduits through which cells, antibody and complement components flow. There exists a dynamic interplay between immunocompetent cells and vascular endothelium that may be important in the initiation, the progress and the resolution of a wide range of immune responses[63].

Endothelial cells can be altered morphologically, physiologically and antigenically by their interaction with lymphocytes and monocytes, or by infection with viruses. It may be of importance in this respect that hepatitis B viral DNA was recently demonstrated in cells other than hepatocytes, e.g. endothelial cells[64].

An intriguing question in relation to PMN remains the mechanism by which circulating lymphocytes leave the blood stream to accumulate in areas of PMN[18].

In 24 different diseases, characterized by lymphocytic infiltrates, and studied by light and electron microscopy and histochemistry, special venules were identified in the inflammatory aggregates. These vessels and their endothelium exhibited striking similarities to the so-called high endothelial venules (or post-capillary or epithelioid venules) in lymphoid tissues[65], which are the preferential sites for intense lymphocyte traffic from blood to tissue. Similar functions are ascribed to the ellipsoids in the spleen[66].

Electron microscopic study of areas of PMN in CAH also revealed striking changes in sinusoidal endothelial cells[57], including swelling of the cytoplasm, disappearance of the sieve plates, protrusion of the cell body into the sinusoidal lumen, increase in micropinocytotic vesicles and the appearance of numerous dense bodies. Such 'activated' endothelial cells approach the appearance of the lining cells of high endothelial venules of lymphoid tissue which play a role in the 'homing' of lymphocytes, and resemble those observed in lichen planus[54]. It is of interest in this respect that associations between CAH and lichen planus have been reported, and the similarities between the lymphocyte–epithelial interactions in lichen planus and CAH have been emphasized[67, 68]. These endothelial changes in areas of PMN may be important for homing of lymphocytes to areas of PMN. Once outside the vessels, further migration and homing of lymphocytes may be determined by the framework of interdigitating reticulum cells[69].

In the same study[57] evidence was obtained for a progressive transformation of 'activated endothelial cells' into fibroblastic reticulum cells[57]. The fibroblastic reticulum cell is known to be a component of lymphoid tissue, presumably involved in the synthesis of reticulin fibres[54]. This transformation was associated with the deposition of basement membrane-like material and reticulin fibres in the space of Disse, leading to a 'capillarization of the sinusoids'[70].

In recent studies, focussing on the synthesis of collagen and fibronectin by non-parenchymal cells cultivated from fibrotic human liver, two types of cells were described: 'endothelial-like' and 'smooth muscle like' cells[71]. It is tempting to speculate that the 'endothelial-like' cells of the latter study are related to the endothelial-derived fibroblastic reticulum cell found in PMN[57], and that the 'smooth muscle like' cells correspond to myofibroblasts derived from perisinusoidal cells or Ito cells.

Although further investigation is required to establish these relationships, the presumed transformation of endothelial cells into fibroblastic reticulum cells would provide a link between inflammation and fibroplasia, both of which are typical characteristics of PMN.

Several described humoral factors are candidate modulators for inducing this cell transformation with the subsequent stimulation of fibre formation: lymphokines released by activated lymphocytes[72, 73] and fibrosis stimulating factors derived from injured parenchymal liver cells[74].

Major Histocompatibility Complex (MHC) antigen expression

The immune response is also regulated by the gene products of a linked set of genes on chromosome 6 (Major Histocompatibility Complex, MHC) that determine the structure of the major transplantation or histocompatibility antigens, also termed the human leukocyte antigens (HLA)[75, 76].

The HLA-A,B,C or class I antigens are glycoproteins located on the cell surface in association with β_2-microglobulin. These antigens are found on all nucleated cells as well as platelets. HLA-A and B antigens are complex integral glycoproteins of the cell membrane. Their synthesis and cell surface expression requires roughly one hour[77]. The primary immunoregulatory function of the HLA-A,B,C gene products appears to be to determine the number and specificity of cytotoxic T cells which are produced on immunization with a given antigen.

It appears that cytotoxic T cells can kill cells bearing viral antigens and foreign antigens only if these target cells also share at least one HLA-A or B antigen[76].

The capability to mount a successful immune response against a particular virus might depend on the ability to present the viral antigens in conjunction with the class I antigens of the responding host[78, 79]. The recognition by lymphocyte receptors of antigens together with molecules controlled by the MHC is referred to as MHC restriction or genetic restriction.

The murine I region and the human D/DR region of the MHC codes for gene products called the Ia antigen in the mouse and HLA-D(DR) antigens or MHC class II antigens in man.

HLA-D region gene products have a complex set of immunologic functions. These cell surface antigens are the strongest antigens in eliciting the mixed-lymphocyte-culture reaction and the graft-versus-host reaction. They also appear to influence the efficiency of the interaction between T cells and macrophages, between T cells and B cells, and perhaps between B cells and macrophages[76]. The usual sequence of events involves the display of an antigen at the surface of an antigen presenting accessory cell in close association with the HLA-D antigens. This complex of 'self' and 'non-self' is recognized by helper T cells, which then cooperate with B cells and cytotoxic T cells. Thus the HLA-D antigens are important in the afferent or priming limb of the immune response, although they also affect some aspects of the efferent or effector limb[80]. They determine the manner in which antigen presenting cells present foreign antigens to T cells, thus influencing whether or not T cells will respond, and whether the subset responding will be helper or suppressor T cells[76]. HLA-D antigens are present on the surface of B lymphocytes, some T lymphocytes, and on antigen-presenting cells, including Langerhans cells in the epidermis and Kupffer cells in the liver[76, 81].

Monoclonal antibodies against HLA-A,B,C (Class I) antigens and HLA-D(DR) (Ia antigen) (Class II antigens) have become available, allowing immunohistochemical investigation of the surface expression of these antigens on different cells in various tissues.

Studies on the distribution of MHC class I antigens in normal human liver tissue have revealed a continuous staining along all sinusoids, as well as staining of the bile duct epithelial cells[82-86]. Except in one study[87], staining of the blood vessel endothelium was also observed. The liver parenchymal cells, however, displayed no immunoreactivity for class I antigens or β_2-microglobulin. Similar results have been obtained in rats[87] and mice[88]. MHC class II antigens have been demonstrated in sinusoidal lining cells in man[84, 89, 90], rats[85], mice[91], and guinea pigs[92], on the bile duct cells in man[87], but never on the surface of hepatocytes.

A few reports are available on the distribution of MHC antigens in pathological liver tissue during liver disease. Barbatis *et al.*[82] studied the expression of HLA-A,B,C antigens usings a monoclonal antibody directed to the heavy chains of HLA Class I antigens, and found membrane staining of hepatocytes in a variety of liver diseases. Montano *et al.*[93] studied class I and class II antigens in the liver of patients with chronic hepatitis B virus infection, and demonstrated an increased expression of HLA-A,B,C antigens and a concomitant decreased expression of viral antigens at the surface of hepatocytes of patients with a low level of viral replication (anti-e antibody positive). They also noted an increased number of HLA-DR positive Kupffer and endothelial cells in the liver specimens of patients with chronic hepatitis B virus infection as compared to controls. They concluded that differences in the density of HLA and viral antigen display might influence the efficiency of lysis of hepatitis B virus infected cells by immune T lymphocytes.

Van den Oord and Desmet[94] tried to correlate MHC antigen expression patterns with the presence or absence of PMN. They studied class I and class II antigen patterns in a large series of (near) normal and pathologic liver specimens.

MHC class I antigens were observed in different patterns: a sinusoidal pattern, indicating positivity of sinusoidal lining cells, or a honeycomb pattern, reflecting positive staining of hepatocyte plasma membranes. The presence of a sinusoidal pattern correlated well with the absence of PMN. A diffuse honeycomb pattern, corresponding to class I antigen expression on liver cell membranes all over the lobule, was found to be not disease-specific. However, a focal honeycomb pattern restricted to the periportal area was found in a significantly larger number of liver specimens demonstrating PMN. Plasma membrane expression of class I antigens by hepatocytes was further shown to be restricted to the basolateral domains of the cell membrane[95].

MHC antigens class II (HLA-DR) were found on the surface and in the cytoplasm of sinusoidal lining cells. A larger number of positive sinusoidal lining cells was present in diseased livers than in normal ones, and the largest numbers were found in viral hepatitis cases, confirming previous results[93]. It has been demonstrated that specific immunologic stimuli induce greater percentages and absolute numbers of Ia positive 'macrophages' than do non-specific inflammatory stimuli[96].

In a significantly larger number of liver specimens demonstrating PMN, a more extensive expression of MHC class II antigens was observed in the periportal area and in areas of spotty necrosis. In these areas, class II antigens were found on long cytoplasmic extensions of sinusoidal lining cells which surrounded singular or small groups of hepatocytes[94].

The extent of class II antigen expression by accessory cells is regulated by agents that trigger phagocytosis, by a number of inhibitory molecules, and, more importantly, by the products of antigen-stimulated T cells[97]. Activation of helper T cells by antigen-bearing, Ia positive antigen-presenting cells is followed by production of lymphokines by these T cells which in turn induce Ia expression in the antigen-presenting cells. A quantitative correlation exists between Ia expression and accessory cell function[98].

Hence, the strong Ia expression and the observed increase in cytoplasmic extensions of sinusoidal lining cells encircling hepatocytes in periportal areas of PMN (areas with accumulating OKT_8 positive cytotoxic/suppressor T lymphocytes (*cf.* above) may be of importance for the efficient development of local defence.

Further studies will have to clarify the relationship, if any, between the 'hyperplastic' Ia positive sinusoidal lining cells and the ultrastructurally recognized interdigitating reticulum cells[56] described above.

Although the strong expression of Ia antigens in areas of PMN at first sight seem necessary for an optimal development of local immune response, adverse effects may result.

First, if reactivity to a 'self' liver membrane antigen[99] is not suppressed, an uncontrolled autoreactive T cell response could result. The consequent induction of high levels of Ia antigen display on sinusoidal lining cells and other accessory cells would further amplify this T cell proliferation and possibly result in tissue damage[97]. Second, an uncontrolled enhanced expression of Ia antigens by accessory cells could have a deleterious effect by producing severe inflammation at that site leading to tissue injury[97]. Any of these two adverse effects could be related to the progressive and, ultimately, destructive effect of PMN.

In summary, this study[94] indicates that a liver cell membrane expression of MHC class I antigens is in itself not disease-specific, and may be induced by a wide variety of agents. It also shows, however, that topographical differences may exist in the expression of both class I and class II antigens, and that a particular distribution pattern with focally enhanced display may be found in liver biopsies demonstrating PMN, apparently in the areas of PMN itself. The stronger expression of class I antigens at the surface of periportal hepatocytes, and of class II antigens at the surface of extending cytoplasmic processes of hyperplastic sinusoidal lining cells in areas of PMN, allow us to suppose that in these areas the necessary microenvironment for T lymphocyte triggering, proliferation and effector function is definitely present; whether these microenvironmental conditions in PMN are present at optimal or beyond optimal level is not yet clear.

Mode of cell death in piecemeal necrosis

The mechanism of liver cell necrosis in PMN appears to correspond to apoptosis[12, 100, 101]. Apoptosis represents a programmed or physiological cell death, whose role in cell population kinetics is equally important to that of mitosis. Apoptosis occurs in normal tissue turnover, in embryogenesis, metamorphosis and endocrine dependent tissue atrophy[102].

However, cell killing mediated by T lymphocytes also shows the morphology of apoptosis[103-108]. Under the light microscope, apoptic cells are rather inconspicuous, appearing singly or in small groups and consisting of portions of intensely staining cytoplasm, usually with a smooth contour and sometimes including in the plane of section small densely basophilic nuclear fragments; thus nuclear pyknosis is one of the features of apoptosis[102]. Apoptosis has been investigated at the ultrastructural level. The cellular alterations include loss of cell junctions, condensation of the cytoplasm and margination of chromatin clumps. Subsequently, the cell fragments into several membrane-bound, smooth surfaced 'apoptotic bodies', which undergo phagocytosis by neighbouring cells, both hepatocytes and phagocytes.

Apoptosis requires energy; these cells retain normal ATP levels, remain metabolically active, exclude sodium and retain potassium normally, and exclude trypan blue. Apoptosis requires macromolecular synthesis, and is associated with endogenous endonuclease activation. The findings are consistent with a genetic programming for cell death. This emphasizes the physiological role of apoptosis in maintaining the normal turnover in cell populations[102].

The fact that T lymphocyte mediated cell killing has the morphology of apoptosis indicates that toxic lymphokines, released from activated lymphocytes and assembling on the target cell surface[108], influence the target cell's function in such a way that the programme of apoptosis is switched on, since apoptosis represents a cellular function activated from within[102].

CONCLUSION

Exciting progress is being made in the understanding of the immunological mechanisms causing CAH and creating the histopathological features of PMN. However, numerous problems await further solution.

The phenotyping of lymphocyte subsets with the help of actually available monoclonal antibodies does not yet allow us to specify their effector function in all cases. It is said[109, 110] that OKT_4 not only recognizes helper/inducer lymphocytes, but also some inducer/suppressor cells and probably some cytotoxic T cells; OKT_8 not only stains suppressor and/or cytotoxic lymphocytes, but also some non-T non-B cells; Leu 7 does not identify all K/NK cells and does not distinguish between Killer and Natural Killer cells.

Most studies until now can only 'assume' that the OKT$_8$ positive population represents exclusively cytotoxic T lymphocytes.

Even if the advent of new monoclonal antibodies may soon allow more precise typing of lymphocyte subpopulations, other problems remain; e.g. one may wonder whether the insertion of hepatitis B viral DNA in mononuclear leukocytes[111] may not influence their responsive capacity.

Still unexplored in the local immune reaction is the modulating influence of the molecular immunoregulatory network. Several molecules, synthesized in and secreted by the liver parenchymal cells, e.g. α-fetoprotein[112], α-1-antitrypsin[113] and bile salts[114] have been shown to influence the immune responsiveness of circulating lymphocytes. Their effect could be enhanced at the site of the productor cells (hepatocytes).

Immunoregulatory factors present in normal liver and released by liver cell damage may influence the immune response in circumscribed parenchymal territories[115, 116]. This applies for the Lex (Liver extract) factor[117] and LIP (Liver immunoregulatory Protein)[118–120] which are very similar to a 'hepatokine' described as LIP (Liver-derived inhibitory protein)[121]. Such factors are thought to explain the focal restriction of inflammatory infiltrates in hepatitis[43, 44]. Perhaps the near future will bring about the purification of these molecules and monoclonal antibodies raised against them, allowing topographical localization studies with immunohistochemical techniques in order to appreciate their interference in areas of PMN.

The dendritic and interdigitating reticulum cells recently observed in PMN need further study and characterization. *When* do they occur? Are they also present in acute hepatitis and in all stages of all types of CAH? *How* do they reveal themselves? Can they be better recognized with monoclonal antibodies and enzyme-histochemical techniques? *Where* are they located in relation to other cell types? Are there contact areas of special significance? *What* is their function in PMN? Is it possible to identify the antigen–antibody complexes presumed to be located in the folds between the cell extensions of dendritic reticulum cells? Could interdigitating reticulum cells subserve a function similar to that of Ia positive 'macrophage-like/dendritic cells' in rheumatoid arthritis[122]? The endothelial changes are in a preliminary stage of exploration. Lymphocyte–endothelial interactions and possible viral induced endothelial alterations[64] in areas of PMN are unexplored.

The fibrogenic potential of the fibroblastic reticulum cell awaits definite proof, as well as its possible relationship with either endothelial or dendritic reticulum cells.

Further, their cooperation with other fibre-forming cells (perisinusoidal cells, myofibroblasts and fibroblasts) is still unknown, as are the mechanisms triggering their modulation from one cell type or functional state into another.

The changes in expression, or enhanced display, of MHC antigens class I and class II on different cell populations in the liver are in the early stages of investigation, and the mechanisms regulating these changes and their meaning are only partially understood.

The few steps advanced in recent time give hope that further progress will be achieved in the years to come.

References

1. Desmet, V. J. (1972). Chronic hepatitis including primary biliary cirrhosis. In Gall, E. A. and Mostofi, F. K. (eds.) *The Liver, International Academy of Pathology Monograph.* n. 13, pp. 286–341. (Baltimore: Williams & Wilkins)
2. Popper, H. (1983). Changing concepts of the evolution of chronic hepatitis and the role of piecemeal necrosis. *Hepatology*, **3**, 758
3. Kalk, H. (1947). Die chronischen Verlaufsformen der Hepatitis epidemica in Beziehung zu ihren anatomischen Grundlagen. *Dtsch. Med. Wochenschr.*, **23**, 308
4. Wepler, W. (1960). Die pathologische Anatomie der chronischen Hepatitis. In Wildhirt, E. (ed.) *Fortschritte der Gastroenterologie.* p. 231. (Munchen, Berlin: Urban & Schartzenberg)
5. De Groote, J., Desmet, V., Gedigk, P., Korb, G., Popper, H., Poulsen, H., Scheuer, P. J., Schmid, M., Thaler, H., Uehlinger, E. and Wepler, W. (1968). A classification of chronic hepatitis. *Lancet*, **2**, 626
6. Bianchi, L., De Groote, J., Desmet, V. J., Gedigk, P., Korb, G., Popper, H., Poulsen, H., Scheuer, P. J., Schmid, M., Thaler, H. and Wepler, W. (1971). Morphological criteria in viral hepatitis. *Lancet*, **1**, 333
7. Bianchi, L., De Groote, J., Desmet, V. J., Gedigk, P., Korb, G., Popper, H., Poulsen, H., Scheuer, P., Thaler, H. and Wepler, W. (1977). Acute and chronic hepatitis revisited. *Lancet*, **2**, 914
8. Bianchi, L. (1983). Liver biopsy interpretation in hepatitis. Part I. Presentation of critical morphologic features used in diagnosis (glossary). *Pathol. Res. Pract.*, **178**, 2
9. Boyer, J. L. and Klatskin, G. (1970). Patterns of necrosis in acute viral hepatitis. Prognostic value of bridging (subacute hepatic necrosis). *N. Engl. J. Med.*, **283**, 1063
10. Tisdale, W. A. (1966). Clinical and pathologic features of sub-acute hepatitis. *Medicine* (Baltimore), **45**, 557
11. Selmair, H., Vido, I. and Wildhirt, E. (1970). Die chronisch nekrotisierende Hepatitis. *Dtsch. Med. Wochenschr.*, **95**, 1397
12. Desmet, V. J. and De Vos, R. (1984). Structural analysis of acute liver injury. In Keppler, D., Bianchi, L. and Reutter, W. (eds.) *Mechanisms of Hepatocyte Injury and Death.* (Lancaster: MTP Press)
13. Conn, H. O. (1976). Chronic hepatitis: reducing an iatrogenic enigma to a workable puzzle. *Gastroenterology*, **70**, 1182
14. Baggenstoss, A. H., Soloway, R. D. and Summerskill, W. H. J. (1972). Chronic active liver disease: the range of histologic lesions, the response to treatment and evolution. *Hum. Pathol.*, **3**, 183
15. Desmet, V. J. (1978). Die Morphogenese der chronischen Hepatitis. *Munch. Med. Wochenschr.*, **120**, 1523
16. Scheuer, P. J. (1977). Chronic hepatitis: a problem for the pathologist. *Histopathology*, **1**, 5
17. Bianchi, L., Zimmerli-Ning, M. and Gudat, F. (1979). Viral hepatitis. In MacSween, R. N. M., Anthony, P. P. and Scheuer, P. J. (eds.) *Pathology of the Liver.* pp. 164–191. (Edinburgh: Churchill Livingstone)
18. Alexander, G. and Williams, R. (1984). Editorial. Characterization of the mononuclear cell infiltrate in Piecemeal Necrosis. *Lab. Invest.*, **50**, 247
19. Fauerholdt, L., Asnaes, S., Ranek, L., Schiodt, T. and Tygstrup, N. (1977). Significance of suspected 'chronic aggressive hepatitis' in acute hepatitis. *Gastroenterology*, **73**, 543
20. Houthoff, H. J., Niermeyer, P., Gips, C. H., Arends, A., Hofstee, N. and Vanguldener, M. (1980). Hepatic morphologic findings and viral antigens in acute hepatitis B. A longitudinal study. *Virchows Arch. (Pathol. Anat.)*, **389**, 153
21. Ware, A. J., Eigenbrodt, E. H. and Combes, B. (1975). Prognostic significance of subacute hepatic necrosis in acute hepatitis. *Gastroenterology*, **58**, 519
22. Theodor, E. and Niv, Y. (1978). The clinical course of subacute hepatic necrosis. *Am. J. Gastroenterol.*, **70**, 600
23. Schmid, M., Pirovino, M., Altorfer, J., Bansky, G., Buhler, H., Gudat, F. and Bianchi, L. (1981). Acute viral hepatitis B with bridging necrosis: a follow-up study. *Liver*, **1**, 222
24. Vanstapel, M. J., Van Steenbergen, W., De Wolf-Peeters, C., Desmyter, J., Fevery, J., De Groote, J. and Desmet, V. J. (1983). Prognostic significance of piecemeal necrosis in acute viral hepatitis. *Liver*, **3**, 46

25. Teixeira, M. R., Weller, I. V. D., Murray, A., Bamber, M., Thomas, H C., Sherlock, S. and Scheuer, P. J. (1982). The pathology of hepatitis A in man. *Liver*, **2**, 53
26. Bernau, D., Rogier, E. and Feldman, G. (1982). A quantification ultrastructural analysis of the leucocyte in contact with hepatocytes in chronic active hepatitis, with a cytochemical detection of mononuclear phagocytes. *Am. J. Pathol.*, **109**, 310
27. Kawanishi, H. (1977). Morphological association of lymphocytes with hepatocytes in chronic liver disease. *Arch. Pathol. Lab. Med.*, **101**, 286
28. Miller, D. J., Dwyer, J. M. and Klatskin, G. (1977). Identification of lymphocytes in percutaneous liver biopsy cores. Different T : B cell ratio in HBsAg-positive and -negative hepatitis. *Gastroenterology*, **72**, 1199
29. Mariani, E., Facchini, A., Miglio, F., Stefanini, F., Mazzetti, M., Leupers, T., Gasbarrini, G., Labo, G. and Astaldi, A. (1984). Analysis with OKT monoclonal antibodies of T-lymphocyte subsets present in blood and liver of patients with chronic active hepatitis. *Liver*, **4**, 22
30. Eggink, H. F., Houtoff, H. J., Huitema, S., Gips, C. H. and Poppema, S. (1982). Cellular and humoral immune reactions in chronic active liver disease. I. Lymphocyte subsets in liver biopsies of patients with untreated idiopathic autoimmune hepatitis, chronic active hepatitis B and primary biliary cirrhosis. *Clin. Exp. Immunol.*, **50**, 17
31. Eggink, H. F., Houthoff, H. J., Huitema, S., Wolters, G., Poppema, S. and Gips, C. H. (1984). Cellular and humoral immune reactions in chronic active liver disease. II. Lymphocyte subsets and viral antigens in liver biopsies of patients with acute and chronic hepatitis B. *Clin. Exp. Immunol.*, **56**, 121
32. Montano, L., Aranguibel, F., Boffill, M., Goodall, A. H., Janossy, G. and Thomas, H. C. (1983). An analysis of the composition of the inflammatory infiltrate in auto-immune and Hepatitis-B virus-induced chronic liver disease. *Hepatology*, **3**, 292
33. Sanchez-Tapias, J., Thomas, H. C. and Sherlock, S. (1977). Lymphocyte populations in liver biopsy specimens from patients with chronic liver disease. *Gut*, **18**, 472
34. Husby, G., Strickland, R. G., Caldwell, J. L. and Williams, R. C. (1975). Localization of T and B cells and alpha-fetoprotein in hepatic biopsies from patients with liver disease. *J. Clin. Invest.*, **56**, 1198
35. Thomas, H. C., Montano, L., Goodall, A., De Koning, R., Oladapo, J. and Wiedman, K. H. (1982). Immunological mechanisms in chronic hepatitis B virus infection. *Hepatology*, **2**, 1165
36. Si, L., Whiteside, T. L., Schade, R. R. and Van Thiel, D. H. (1983). Studies of lymphocyte subpopulations in the liver tissue and blood of patients with chronic active hepatitis (CAH). *J. Clin. Immunol.*, **3**, 408
37. Si, L., Whiteside, T. L., Schade, R. R. and Van Thiel, D. H. (1983). Lymphocyte subsets studied with monoclonal antibodies in liver tissues of patients with alcoholic liver disease. *Alcohol.: Clin. Exp. Res.*, **7**, 431
38. Si, L., Whiteside, T. L., Van Thiel, D. and Rabin, B. S. (1984). Lymphocyte subpopulations at the site of "Piecemeal" necrosis in end stage chronic liver diseases and rejecting liver allografts in cyclosporine-treated patients. *Lab. Invest.*, **50**, 341
39. Colucci, G., Colombo, M., Del Ninno, E. and Paronetto, F. (1983). *In situ* characterization by monoclonal antibodies of the mononuclear cell infiltrate in chronic active hepatitis. *Gastroenterology*, **85**, 1138
40. Pape, G. R., Rieber, E. P., Eisenburg, J., Hoffmann, R., Balch, C. M., Paumgartner, G. and Riethmuller, G. (1983). Involvement of the cytotoxic/suppressor T-cell subset in liver tissue injury of patients with acute and chronic liver diseases. *Gastroenterology*, **85**, 657
41. Govindarajan, S., Uchida, T. and Peters, R. L. (1983). Identification of T lymphocytes and subsets in liver biopsy cores of acute viral hepatitis. *Liver*, **3**, 13
42. van den Oord, J., Fevery, J., De Groote, J. and Desmet, V. J. (1984). Immunohistochemical characterization of inflammatory infiltrate in Primary Biliary Cirrhosis. *Liver*, **4**, 264
43. Levy, G. A. and Chisari, F. V. (1981). The immunopathogenesis of chronic HBV induced liver disease. *Springer Semin. Immunopathol.*, **3**, 439
44. Bianchi, L. (1983). Pathology and Immune Mechanisms of chronic hepatitis: a review. In *Current Concepts in Liver Pathology, 4th Annual Course*. pp. 33–81. (Columbia University)

45. Mondelli, M., Mieli-Vergani, G., Alberti, A., Vergani, D., Portmann, B., Eddleston, A. L. W. F. and Williams, R. (1982). Specificity of T-lymphocyte cytotoxicity to autologous hepatocytes in chronic hepatitis B virus infection: evidence that T cells are directed against HBV core antigen expressed on hepatocytes. *J. Immunol.*, **129**, 2773

46. Wiedmann, K. H., Bartholemew, T. C., Brown, D. J. C. and Thomas, H. C. (1984). Liver membrane antibodies detected by immunoradiometric assay in acute and chronic virus-induced and autoimmune liver disease. *Hepatology*, **4**, 199

47. Vento, S., Hegarty, J. E., Botazzo, G., Macchia, E., Williams, R. and Eddleston, A. L. W. F. (1984). Antigen specific suppressor cell function in autoimmune chronic active hepatitis. *Lancet*, **1**, 1200

48. Eddleston, A. L. W. F. and Williams, R. (1974). Inadequate antibody response to HB antigen or suppressor T-cell defect in development of active chronic hepatitis. *Lancet*, **2**, 1543

49. Unanue, E. R. and Cerottini, J.-C. (1970). The function of macrophages in the immune response. *Semin. Hematol.*, **7**, 225

50. Steinman, R. M., Witmer, M. D., Nussenzweig, M. C., Gutchinov, B. and Austyn, J. M. (1983). Studies with a monoclonal antibody to mouse dendritic cells. *Transplant. Proc.*, **XV**, 299

51. Hart, D. N. J. and Fabre, J. W. (1981). Demonstration and characterization of Ia-positive dendritic cells in the interstitial connective tissues of rat heart and other tissues, but not brain. *J. Exp. Med.*, **153**, 347

52. Dickler, H. B., Cowing, C., Ahmann, G. B. *et al.* (1979). Characterization of the accessory cells required in T lymphocyte dependent antigen-specific immune responses. In Rosenthal, A. and Unanue, E. (eds.) *Macrophage Regulation of Immunity.* p. 265. (New York: Academic Press)

53. Daar, A. S., Fuggle, S. V., Hart, D. N. J., Dalchau, R., Abdulaziz, Z., Fabre, J. W., Ting, A. and Morris, P. J. (1983). Demonstration and phenotypic characterization of HLA-DR-positive interstitial dendritic cells widely distributed in human connective tissues. *Transplant. Proc.*, **XV**, 311

54. Lennert, K., Mohri, N., Stein, H., Kaiserling, E. and Muller-Hermelink, H. K. (1978). *Malignant Lymphomas other than Hodgkin's Disease.* (Berlin, Heidelberg, New York: Springer Verlag)

55. Silberg-Sinakin, I., Baer, R. L. and Thorbecke, G. J. (1978). Langerhans cells: a review of their nature with emphasis on their immunological function. *Prog. Allergy*, **24**, 268

56. Bardadin, K. A. and Desmet, V. J. (1984). Interdigitating and dendritic reticulum cells in chronic active hepatitis. *Histopathology*, **8**, 657

57. Bardadin, K. A. and Desmet, V. J. (1985). Ultrastructural observations on sinusoidal endothelial cells in chronic active hepatitis. *Histopathology*. (In press)

58. Gerdes, J., Stein, H., Mason, D. Y. and Ziegler, A. (1983). Human dendritic reticulum cells of lymphoid follicles: their antigenic profile and their identification as multi-nucleated giant cells. *Virchows Arch. (Cell Pathol.)*, **42**, 161

59. Dijkstra, C. D., Kamperdijk, E. W. A. and Dopp, E. A. (1984). The ontogenic development of the follicular dendritic cell. *Cell Tiss. Res.*, **236**, 203

60. Heusermann, U., Zurbon, H. H., Schroeder, L. and Stutte, H. J. (1980). The origin of dendritic reticulum cell. An experimental enzyme-histochemical and electron microscopic study on the rabbit spleen. *Cell. Tiss. Res.*, **209**, 279

61. Radoux, D., Heinen, E., Kinet-Denoel, C., Tihange, E. and Simar, L. (1984). Precise localization of antigens on follicular dendritic cells. *Cell. Tiss. Res.*, **235**, 267

62. Naeiem, M., Gerdes, J., Abdulaziz, Z., Stein, H. and Mason, D. Y. (1983). Production of a monoclonal antibody reactive with human dendritic reticulum cells and its use in the immunohistological analysis of lymphoid tissue. *J. Clin. Pathol.*, **36**, 167

63. Baldwin, W. M. (1982). The symbiosis of immunocompetent and endothelial cells. *Immunol. Today*, **3**, 267

64. Blum, H. E., Stowring, L., Figus, A., Montgomery, C. K., Haase, A. T. and Vyas, G. T. (1983). Detection of hepatitis B virus DNA in hepatocytes, bile ducts epithelium, and vascular elements by *in situ* hybridization. *Proc. Natl. Acad. Sci. USA*, **80**, 6685

65. Freemont, A. J. (1983). A possible route for lymphocyte migration into diseased tissues. *J. Clin. Pathol.*, **36**, 161

TRENDS IN HEPATOLOGY

66. Buyssens, N., Paulus, G. and Bourgeois, N. (1984). Ellipsoids in the human spleen. *Virchows Arch. (Pathol. Anat.)*, **403**, 27
67. Rebora, A. (1981). Lichen planus and the liver. *Lancet*, **2**, 805
68. Rebora, A. and Rongioletti, F. (1984). Lichen planus and chronic active hepatitis. A retrospective study. *Acta Derm. Venereol.* (Stockholm), **64**, 52
69. Brelinska, R. and Pilgrim, C. (1983). Macrophages and interdigitating cells; their relationship to migrating lymphocytes in the white pulp of rat spleen. *Cell Tiss. Res.*, **233**, 671
70. Schaffner, F. and Popper, H. (1963). Capillarization of hepatic sinusoids in man. *Gastroenterology*, **44**, 239
71. Voss, B., Rautenberg, J., Pott, G., Brehmer, U., Allam, S., Lehman, R. and Bassewitz, D. B. (1982). Nonparenchymal cells cultivated from explants of fibrotic liver resemble endothelial and smooth muscle cells from blood vessel walls. *Hepatology*, **2**, 19
72. Allison, A. C., Clark, I. A. and Davies, P. (1977). Cellular interactions in fibrogenesis. *Ann. Rheum. Dis.* (Suppl.), **36**, 8
73. Surrenti, C., Casini, A., Nieri, S., Salvadori, G., Calabro, A., Ambu, S., Banchetti, E. and Ceccatelli, P. (1984). Mononuclear cell-mediated activation of fibroblast collagen synthesis in chronic active hepatitis. In Gentilini, P. and Dianzani, M. U. (eds.) *Liver Cirrhosis. Frontiers of Gastrointestinal Research*. Vol. 8, pp. 117-27. (Basel: Karger)
74. Fallon, A. and McGee, J. O'D. (1984). Collagen stimulating factors in human and experimental hepatic fibrogenesis. *J. Clin. Pathol.*, **37**, 542
75. Benacerraf, B. (1981). Role of MHC gene products in immune regulation. *Science*, **212**, 1229
76. McDevitt, H. O. (1980). Current concepts in immunology. Regulation of the immune response by the Major Histocompatibility system. *N. Engl. J. Med.*, **303**, 1514
77. Krangel, M. S., Orr, H. T. and Strominger, J. L. (1980). Structure, function and biosynthesis of the major human histocompatibility antigens (HLA-A and HLA-B). *Scand. J. Immunol.*, **11**, 561
78. Ploegh, H. L., Orr, H. T. and Strominger, J. L. (1981). Major Histocompatibility Antigens: the human (HLA-A, -B, -C) and murine (H-2K, H-2D) Class I molecules. *Cell*, **24**, 287
79. Zinkernagel, R. M. and Doherty, P. C. (1974). Restriction of *in vitro* T cell-mediated cytotoxicity in lymphocytic choriomeningitis within a syngeneic or semiallegeneic system. *Nature*, **248**, 701
80. Thomas, H. C., Shipton, U. and Montano, L. (1982). The HLA system: its relevance to the pathogenesis of liver disease. In Popper, H. and Schaffner, F. (eds.) *Progress in Liver Diseases*. Vol. 7, pp. 517-27. (New York: Grune and Stratton)
81. Winchester, R. J. and Kunkel, H. G. (1979). The human Ia system. *Adv. Immunol.*, **18**, 221
82. Barbatis, C., Woods, J., Morton, J. A., Fleming, K. A., McMichael, A. and McGee, J. O'D. (1981). Immunohistochemical analysis of HLA(A,B,C) antigens in liver disease using a monoclonal antibody. *Gut*, **22**, 985
83. Fleming, K. A., McMichael, A., Morton, J. A., Woods, J. and McGee, J. O'D. (1981). Distribution of HLA class I antigens in normal human tissues and in mammary cancer. *J. Clin. Pathol.*, **34**, 779
84. Koyama, K., Fukunishi, T., Barcos, M., Tanigaki, N. and Pressman, D. (1979). Human Ia-like antigen in non-lymphoid organs. *Immunology*, **38**, 333
85. Lautenschlager, I., Nyman, N., Vaananen, H., Lehto, V. P., Virtanen, I. and Hayry, P. (1983). Antigenic and immunogenic components in rat liver. *Scand. J. Immunol.*, **17**, 61
86. McGee, J. O'D., Morton, J. A., Barbatis, C., Bradley, J. F., Flemin, K. A., Goate, A. M. and Burns, J. (1982). Monoclonal antibodies to Mallory bodies/intermediate filaments and HLA (class I) antigens in human liver disease. In McMichael, A. J. and Fabre, J. W. (eds.) *Monoclonal Antibodies in Clinical Medicine*. pp. 431-55. (London, New York: Academic Press)
87. Lautenschlager, I., Taskinen, E., Inkinen, K., Lehto, V. P., Virtanen, I. and Hayry, P. (1984). Distribution of the major histocompatibility complex antigens on different cellular components of human liver. *Cell. Immunol.*, **85**, 191
88. Parr, E. L. (1979). Diversity of expression of H-2 antigens on mouse liver cells demonstrated by immunoferritin labeling. *Transplantation*, **27**, 45
89. Forsum, U., Klareskog, L. and Peterson, P. A. (1979). Distribution of Ia-antigen-like molecules on non-lymphoid tissues. *Scand. J. Immunol.*, **9**, 343

90. Natali, P. G., De Martino, C., Quaranta, V., Nicotra, M. R., Frezza, F., Pellegrino, M. A. and Ferrone, S. (1981). Expression of Ia-like antigens in normal human non-lymphoid tissues. *Transplantation*, **31**, 75

91. Natali, P. G., De Martino, C., Pellegrino, M. A. and Ferrone, S. (1981). Analysis of the expression of I-A^k-like antigens in murine fetal and adult tissues with the monoclonal antibody 10-2.16. *Scand. J. Immunol.*, **13**, 541

92. Wiman, K., Curman, B., Forsum, U., Klareskog, L., Malmnas-Tjernlund, U., Rask, L., Tragardh, L. and Peterson, P. A. (1978). Occurrence of Ia antigens on tissues of non-lymphoid origin. *Nature*, **276**, 711

93. Montano, L., Miescher, G. C., Goodall, A. L., Wiedmann, K. H., Janossy, G. and Thomas, H. C. (1982). Hepatitis B virus and HLA antigen display in the liver during chronic hepatitis B virus infection. *Hepatology*, **2**, 557

94. van den Oord, J. and Desmet, V. J. (1984). Distribution patterns of Major Histocompatibility Antigens in normal and pathologic liver tissue. *Hepato-gastroenterology*, **14**, 244–54

95. De Vos, R., van den Oord, J., De Wolf-Peeters, C. and Desmet, V. J. (1984). Immuno-electron microscopic demonstration of HLA-A,B,C antigens on human hepatocytes in liver disease. *Abstracts, 19th EASL meeting*, Berne

96. Beller, D. I., Kiely, S.-M. and Unanue, E. R. (1980). Regulation of macrophage populations. I. Preferential induction of Ia rich peritoneal exudate by immunologic stimuli. *J. Immunol.*, **124**, 1426

97. Unanue, E. R., Beller, D. I., Lu, C. Y. and Allen, P. M. (1984). Opinion: Antigen presentation: comments on its regulation and mechanism. *J. Immunol.*, **132**, 1

98. Beller, D. I. (1984). Functional significance of the regulation of macrophage Ia expression. *Eur. J. Immunol.*, **14**, 138

99. Meyer zum Buschenfelde, K.-H. and Manns, M. (1984). Mechanisms of autoimmune liver disease. *Semin. Liver Dis.*, **4**, 26

100. Bhathal, P. S., Powell, L. W. and Mackay, I. R. (1982). Apoptosis in autoimmune chronic active hepatitis (CAH). *Hepatology*, **2**, 154

101. Kerr, J. F. R., Cooksley, W. G. E., Searle, J., Halliday, J. W., Holder, L., Roberts, I., Burnett, W. and Powell, L. W. (1979). Hypothesis. The nature of piecemeal necrosis in chronic active hepatitis. *Lancet*, **2**, 827

102. Wyllie, A. H. (1981). Cell death: a new classification separating apoptosis from necrosis. In Bowen, I. D. and Lockshin, R. A. (eds.) *Cell Death in Biology and Pathology*. pp. 9–34. (London: Chapman and Hall)

103. Russell, S. W., Rosenau, W. and Lee, J. C. (1972). Cytolysis induced by human lymphotoxin. Cinematographic and electron microscopic observations. *Am. J. Pathol.*, **69**, 103

104. Battersby, C., Egerton, W. S., Balderson, G., Kerr, J. F. and Burnett, W. (1974). Another look at rejection in pig liver homografts. *Surgery (St. Louis)*, **76**, 617

105. Slavin, R. E. and Woodruff, J. M. (1974). The pathology of bone marrow transplantation. *Pathol. Annu.*, **9**, 291

106. Sanderson, C. J. (1976). The mechanism of T cell mediated cytotoxicity. II. Morphological studies of cell death by time-lapse microcinematography. *Proc. R. Soc. Lond. (Biol.)*, **192**, 241

107. Matter, A. (1979). Microcinematographic and electron microscopic analysis of target cell lysis induced by cytotoxic T lymphocytes. *Immunology*, **36**, 179

108. Ross, M. W., Yamamoto, R. S. and Granger, G. A. (1981). The role of the LT system in cell destruction *in vitro*. In Bowen, I. D. and Lockshin, R. A. (eds.) *Cell Death in Biology and Pathology*. pp. 361–77. (London, New York: Chapman and Hall)

109. Eggink, H. F., Houthoff, H. J. and Poppema, S. (1984). T-cell subsets in liver diseases. Letter to the editor. *Gastroenterology*, **86**, 780

110. Pape, G. R. (1984). Letter to the Editor (reply). *Gastroenterology*, **86**, 781

111. Pontisso, P., Poon, M. C., Tiollais, P. and Brechot, C. (1984). Detection of hepatitis B virus DNA in mononuclear blood cells. *Br. Med. J.*, **288**, 1563

112. Murgita, R. A. and Tomasi, T. B. (1975). Suppression of the immune response by α-fetoprotein. II. The effect of mouse α-fetoprotein on mixed lymphocyte reactivity and mitogen-induced lymphocyte transformation. *J. Exp. Med.*, **141**, 440

113. Breit, S. N., Robinson, J. P., Lockhurst, E., Clark, P. and Penny, R. (1982). Immunoregulation by alpha-1-antitrypsin. *J. Clin. Lab. Immunol.*, **7**, 127
114. Keane, R. M., Gadacz, T. R., Munster, A. M., Birmingham, W. and Winchurch, R. A. (1984). Impairment of human lymphocyte function by bile salts. *Surgery*, **95**, 439
115. Chisari, F. (1982). Regulation of lymphocyte function and viral transformation by hepatic bioregulatory molecules. *Hepatology*, **2**, 97
116. Edgington, T. S. (1983). Immune responses and liver disease, perhaps, but what about target organ defenses? *Hepatology*, **3**, 767
117. Chisari, F. V. (1978). Regulation of human lymphocyte function by a soluble extract from normal human liver. *J. Immunol.*, **121**, 1279
118. Schrempf-Decker, G. E., Baron, D. P., Brattig, N. W., Bockhorn, H. and Berg, P. A. (1983). Biological and immunological characterization of a human liver immunoregulatory protein. *Hepatology*, **3**, 939
119. Brattig, N. W. and Berg, P. A. (1983). Immunosuppressive serum factors in viral hepatitis. I. Characterization of serum inhibition factor(s) as lymphocyte antiactivator(s). *Hepatology*, **3**, 638
120. Brattig, N. W., Schrempf-Decker, G. E., Brockl, C. W. and Berg, P. A. (1983). Immunosuppressive serum factors in viral hepatitis. II. Further characterization of serum inhibition factor as an albumin-associated molecule. *Hepatology*, **3**, 647
121. Grol, M. and Schumacher, K. (1983). Purification and biochemical characterization of human liver-derived inhibitory protein LIP. *J. Immunol.*, **130**, 323
122. Klareskog, L., Forsum, U., Scheynius, A., Kabelitz, D. and Wigzell, H. (1982). Evidence in support of a self-perpetuating HLA-DR-dependent delayed-type cell reaction in rheumatoid arthritis. *Proc. Natl. Acad. Sci. USA*, **79**, 3632

22
The morphology of hepatitis A in man

M. SCHMID AND J. REGLI

Literature dealing with the morphology of hepatitis A infection in man is limited. Apart from the investigations of Teixeira *et al.*, from the Royal Free Hospital in London[1], and several Japanese Groups [2-5] there are few systematic studies on the histology of hepatitis A.

Virus A hepatitis in chimpanzees, especially in the early biopsy, is characterized by periportal liver cell necrosis, whereas the perivenular area of the lobule remains well preserved[6,7]. Whilst Japanese authors also found periportal necrosis in man[4,5,8], Teixeira *et al.* could not conclusively confirm these histological findings. Biopsies taken from a series of 17 patients suffering from hepatitis A were predominantly performed in a later phase of the disease[1].

In this study we looked at liver biopsies taken, from 34 patients with hepatitis A, at different stages of the disease. The purpose of this paper is to check whether there are characteristic lesions in liver biopsies in man comparable with those recorded in chimpanzees[7].

PATIENTS AND METHODS

Liver biopsies were taken from a series of 34 patients suffering from acute virus A hepatitis, and satisfying the following criteria:

(1) A history of illness of acute onset with fever, jaundice and abnormal liver function tests, e.g. high transaminases;
(2) No previous exposure to hepatotoxins;
(3) No evidence of previous liver disease;
(4) Sera taken at the time of biopsy positive for IgM anti-HAV and negative for anti-HBs and anti-HBc of the IgM class.

IgM anti-HAV was detected by direct radioimmunoassay (Abbott Laboratories). HBs-Ag, anti-HBc and IgG anti-HAV were tested by radio-immunoassay (Austria, Abbott Laboratories). Anti-HBc of the IgM class was determined using the ELISA[9] method.

Clinical presentation and follow-up

The mean age of the 28 male and 6 female patients was 41 years (range 25–55 years). Clinical jaundice had been noticed a few days after the onset of symptoms, i.e. after a rise of transaminases. In 13 patients, regardless of age, the disease followed a prolonged course with normalization of transaminases after 6 months (range 6–18 months)[10]. In 6 out of 13 patients, two peaks of transaminases had occurred.

Liver biopsy samples were taken within the first 10 days after onset of symptoms in 7 patients, within the first 20 days of disease in 21 patients, and between 21 and 120 days in 13 cases. Clinical recovery was achieved in all cases within 18 months.

RESULTS

Histology

The biopsy material was fixed in 4% neutral formalin solution. Paraffin wax sections were stained by standard methods including haematoxylin and eosin, chromatotrope aniline blue and Prussian blue. In three cases, a second biopsy was taken because of a second attack of jaundice and rise in trans-aminases.

Histologic lesions: lobular distribution of liver cell necrosis, inflammatory infiltration, cholestasis, clusters of iron storing macrophages and Kupffer cells were assessed in a semi-quantitative manner using a scale of 0–3.

Periportal liver cell necrosis

Alteration and liver cell necrosis in the periportal area of lobules was indeed one of the most impressive features seen in the majority of our cases, whilst the pericentral area was diffused (Figure 22.1). Single cells or groups of hepatocytes undergo coagulation – or lytic necrosis.

Periportal necroses were observed in 24 out of 34 cases. Although in the early biopsies, obtained within the first 10 days of a rise of transaminases (AST), necrosis of periportal hepatocytes was recorded in every case, peri-portal liver cell necrosis was also present in later biopsies (taken within 21–120 days). Marked periportal necrosis was observed in cases with a prolonged course of the disease, especially in those cases showing a second rise of transaminases and serum bilirubin, e.g. in 'relapsing hepatitis A' (Table 22.1).

Inflammatory infiltration of the portal tracts spilling over into the lobular periphery was recorded as a constant phenomenon accompanying periportal

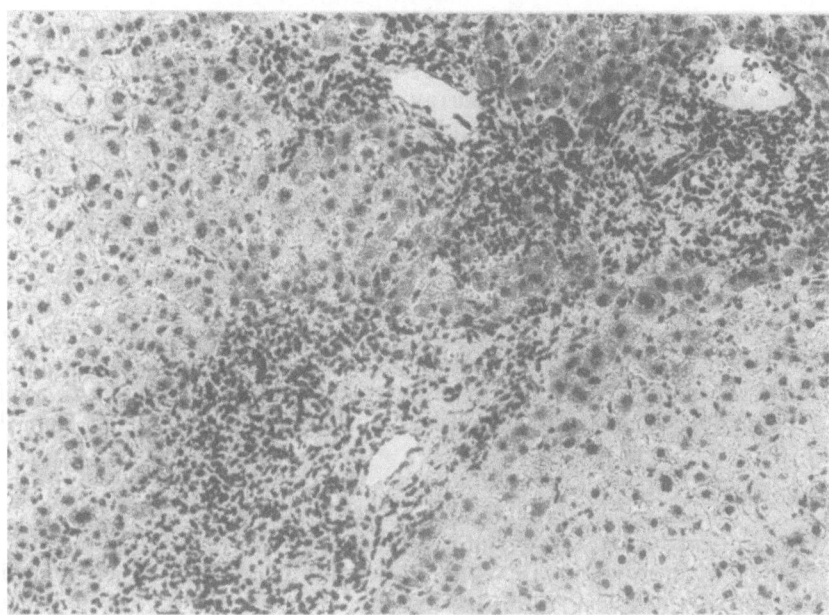

Figure 22.1 Patient No. 3. Marked chronic inflammatory infiltration spilling over into the periportal area of lobules accompanied by pronounced piecemeal necrosis. The limiting plate of parenchyma has been destroyed and isolated liver cells are seen within the infiltrate. Haematoxylin and eosin ×210

liver cell necrosis, mimicking the picture of piecemeal necrosis[11]. Very large periportal necrosis may lead to porto–portal bridging, as seen in seven biopsies in our series. The infiltrating cells were mainly lymphocytes and histiocytes, in two cases lymphofollicle formation occurred.

Plasma cells could be found in all except three biopsies, especially in the periphery of portal tracts often spilling over into the parenchyma. PAS-positive macrophages and Kupffer cells in the portal tracts, as well as in the parenchyma, were recognized as a constant and early phenomenon.

Table 22.1 Periportal necrosis in relation to time biopsy taken from onset of disease

Histology	Number of biopsies	Interval of onset to biopsy (days)			Second peak of transaminases
		0–10	*0–20*	*21–120*	
Mild or absent (grades 0–1)	10	0	4	6	0
Severe (grades 2–3)	24	7	17	7	3
Porto-portal bridging	7	3	1	3	3

Spotty necrosis

Spotty necrosis is a common feature of all three forms of viral hepatitis[12]. In hepatitis B, a conspicuous disarray of liver cell plates and very pronounced ballooning, especially of perivenular hepatocytes can very often be seen[7, 12]. The outlines of swollen liver cells became unsharp. The same histological picture, mimicking virus-B hepatitis, could be demonstrated in 12 of our hepatitis-A cases, but exclusively in biopsies taken during a later phase (after day 20 following the onset of disease).

Confluent necroses were recorded in four cases (centro–portal bridging in three, and sublobular necrosis in one case).

Outstanding pericentral lesions could only be seen in two biopsies of pure cholestatic hepatitis. Besides the typical lesions of cholestasis, many multinucleated giant liver cells were present. Multinucleated giant cells in adults are also described in seronegative hepatitis by Schmid et al.[13] and Thaler[14].

Bile duct lesions

Bile duct epithelium in most biopsies showed minor irregularities, such as pyknotic nuclei, eosinophilia and mild tortuosity, although in two biopsies obtained within the first 20 days, severe bile duct lesions with segmental swollen, multilayered and eosinophilic epithelium were seen, as described by Poulsen and Christoffersen in chronic active hepatitis[15]. In contrast to the 'Poulsen-lesion', often seen in prolonged non-A, non-B hepatitis characteristically embedded in a dense lymphocytic infiltrate[13], inflammatory infiltration in hepatitis A biopsies is rather sparse.

Iron storage in Kupffer cells and macrophages

In agreement with Teixeira et al.[1] in all except three biopsies, Kupffer cells in hepatitis A contained much stainable iron, and many clusters of iron storing macrophages could be demonstrated. Obviously in relation to the liver cell necrosis, iron positive macrophages, in early stages, with predominant portal necrosis may be found in periportal areas and within portal tracts, whereas perivenular areas remain iron-free (Figure 22.2). Widespread liver cell necroses are accompanied by spotty distributed iron-containing macrophages and Kupffer cells. In contrast to hepatitis A in acute B or non-A, non-B hepatitis, there can be found little or no iron stored in Kupffer cells and macrophages.

DISCUSSION

Spotty liver cell necrosis is a common feature of each of the three forms of viral hepatitis. Although there is no specific light microscopic picture of each of them, there are certain morphological trends more or less attributable to the different aetiological forms. Whilst in acute virus B hepatitis, a picture with marked disarray of liver cell plates, pronounced polymorphism and

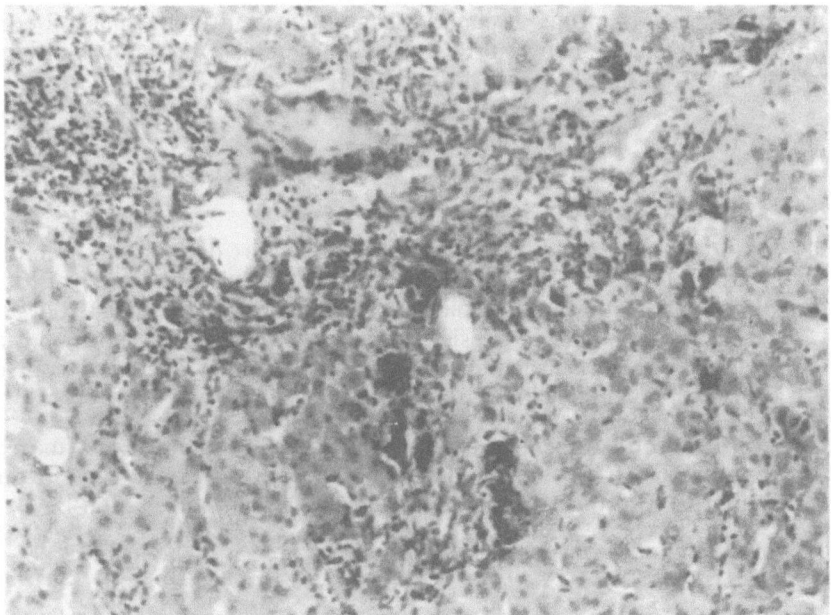

Figure 22.2 Same patient. Clusters of iron storing macrophages in portal tracts as well as in the periphery of liver lobules. Iron stain × 210

ballooning of liver cells, especially in the pericentral area, and wide-spread liver cell necrosis can be observed in the majority of cases[7, 12], in virus A hepatitis periportal necrosis is a predominant feature[1, 4, 8].

In our investigations, periportal liver cell necrosis was observed in all biopsies taken in the first 10 days and in cases showing a prolonged course of the disease, especially when biopsies were performed during a second attack of the disease[10]. In agreement with Teixeira *et al.*, we conclude that the periportal lesions may precede panlobular changes[1]. Our findings resemble those of Japanese authors[2, 4, 5, 8] and the histological changes found in chimpanzees[7]. Periportal necrosis in virus A hepatitis can be regarded as an example of piecemeal necrosis with a good prognosis, since transition into chronic active hepatitis has never been observed in this disease[16], although cases of long duration, over 6–18 months, have been described in the literature[10, 17].

Clusters of iron positive macrophages, in early stages, with predominant periportal necrosis obviously in relation to the liver cell necrosis, were observed in periportal areas and in portal tracts, whereas in pericentral areas stainable iron was lacking. In contrast, in biopsies with wide-spread liver cell necrosis, macrophages and iron storing Kupffer cells were distributed over the whole lobule.

In our studies, parallelism of the extent of liver cell damage and the level of transaminases (AST) was the only reliable correlation between bio-chemical and histological findings. Whereas far less a parallelism between the morphological symptoms of cholestasis and hyperbilirubinaemia has been observed, correlation between the level of transaminases and portal inflammatory infiltration was found to be poor.

CONCLUSION

(1) Although there is no specific histological picture of hepatitis A, in our studies periportal liver cell necrosis, mimicking piecemeal necrosis, is a prominent feature in early biopsies obtained within the first 10 days of onset. In later phase biopsies, piecemeal necroses with porto–portal bridging were recorded in cases with a prolonged clinical course, especially in cases with two peaks of transaminases.

(2) Marked iron storage in Kupffer cells, as well as in clusters of macrophages, is a frequent phenomenon in hepatitis A, in contrast to the minor iron storage seen in acute hepatitis B and non-A, non-B.

(3) For diagnostic purposes, biopsies do not appear to be helpful.

References

1. Teixeira, M. R. Jr., Weller, I. V. D., Murray, A., Bamber, M., Thomas, H. C., Sherlock, S. and Scheuer, P. J. (1982). The pathology of hepatitis A in man. *Liver*, **2**, 53-60
2. Abe, H., Ikejri, N., Sata, M., Setoyama, H. and Tanikawa, K. (1981). Histological findings of the liver in viral hepatitis type A. A comparison with viral hepatitis type B. *Acta Hepatol. Jpn.*, **22**, 22-31
3. Sakamoto *et al.* (1981). Clinical studies on sporadic acute hepatitis A. *Acta Hepatol. Jpn.*, **22**, 487
4. Tanaka *et al.* (1981). Morphological findings of acute hepatitis A. *Acta Hepatol. Jpn.*, **22**, 494
5. Tanikawa, K. (1979). Acute viral hepatitis. Type A hepatitis. Its epidemiology, clinical pictures and pathologic changes of the liver. *Gastroenterol. Jpn.*, **14**, 168
6. Dienstag, J. L., Popper, H., Feinstone, S. M., Alter, H. J. and Purcell, R. H. (1976). The pathology of viral hepatitis types A and B in chimpanzees. A comparison. *Am. J. Pathol.*, **85**, 131-48
7. Popper, H., Dienstag, J. L., Feinstone, St. M., Alter, H. J. and Purcell, R. H. (1980). The pathology of viral hepatitis in chimpanzees. *Virch. Arch. A Path. Anat. Histol.*, **387**, 91-1006
8. Abe, H., Benninger, P. R., Ikejiri, N., Setoyama, H., Sata, M. and Tanikawa, K. (1982). Light microscopic findings of liver biopsy specimens from patients with hepatitis type A and comparison with type B. *Gastroenterology*, **82**, 938-47
9. Roggendorf, M., Deinhardt, F., Frösner, G. G. *et al.* (1981). Immunoglobulin M antibodies to hepatitis B core antigen: Evaluation of enzyme immunoassay for diagnosis of hepatitis B virus infection. *J. Clin. Microbiol.*, **13**, 618-26
10. Roten, A., Altorfer, J., Frösner, G. G., Pirovino, M., Grob, P. J. and Schmid, M. (1983). Verlaufsspektrum der Hepatitis A. *Schweiz. Med. Woschrs.*, **113**, 694-700
11. Schmid, M. (1966). *Die chronische Hepatitis. Vergleichende Klinische und Bioptische Untersuchungen.* (Springer Verlag)
12. International Group (1971). Morphological criteria in viral hepatitis. *Lancet*, **i**, 333-7
13. Schmid, M., Pirovino, M., Altorfer, J., Gudat, F. and Bianchi, L. (1982). Acute hepatitis non-A, non-B; are there any specific light microscopic features? *Liver*, **2**, 61-7
14. Thaler, H. (1982). Post infantile giant cell hepatitis. *Liver*, **2**, 393-403

15. Poulsen, H. and Christoffersen, P. (1976). Abnormal bile duct epithelium in liver biopsies with histological signs of viral hepatitis. *Acta Pathol. Microbiol. Scand.*, **76**, 383
16. Vanstapel, M. J., van Steenbergen, W., de Wolf-Peeters, C., Desmet, J., Fevery, J., de Groote, J. and Desmet, V. J. (1983). Prognostic significance of piecemeal necrosis in acute viral hepatitis. *Liver*, **3**, 46–57
17. Meier, E., Richter, K. and Frühmorgen, P. (1982). Vorübergehend-chronische Hepatitis nach akuter Virushepatitis A. *Dtsch. Med. Woschrs.*, **107**, 46–50

23
Epstein–Barr virus in chronic hepatitis

F. SCHAFFNER

INTRODUCTION

Involvement of the liver in Pfeiffer's 'glandular fever'[1] was recognized soon after the term 'infectious mononucleosis' was coined in 1920[2]. Jaundice was noted in isolated patients in the 1920s[3,4]. During and after World War II, with the advent of liver biopsy and heterophile antibody testing, details of the epidemiology, transmission of the disease and the involvement of the liver were uncovered. Anicteric[5] and even subclinical cases of hepatitis were described, some in epidemics[6]. The hepatic abnormalities were long lasting in about 10% or more of cases[6,7], and even one case of cirrhosis was reported[8]. Histologically, the portal tracts and sinusoids were the sites of lymphocytic infiltration[9,10], the extent of lymphocytosis correlating with abnormal results of various hepatic tests[10]. After Henle, et al.[11] related the virus found in Burkitt's lymphoma, by Epstein et al.[12], to infectious mononucleosis, immunologic tests were rapidly developed to define the status of Epstein–Barr virus (EBV) infection[13]. EBV as well as the other human herpes viruses can be easily recognized by electron microscopy, but they cannot be distinguished from one another by appearance alone[14]. EBV can readily be transmitted by transfusions[15-17], haemodialysis[18] and intimate or sexual contact including male homosexual contact[19].

The outbreak of the epidemic of the acquired immunodeficiency syndrome (AIDS), itself probably due to human T cell leukaemia virus III, with a high incidence of hepatitis B (HBV), herpes II and cytomegalo (CMV) virus infections made clear that multiple simultaneous viral infections were possible. Surveys conducted in patients with AIDS[19], male homosexuals without AIDS and multiple transfused haemophiliacs[18] revealed that the Epstein–Barr virus was almost as common as HBV, and more often encountered than CMV. These associations prompted the search amongst a large group of patients with various forms of chronic hepatitis for evidence of EBV activity using serologic and electron microscopic methods, as well as attempting to correlate the findings with clinical and histologic features.

MATERIALS AND METHODS

A group of 86 patients with various forms of chronic hepatitis, but no history of infectious mononucleosis, were screened for antibody to EB virus viral capsid antigen (EBV-VCA) using an immunofluorescent assay. The number, sex, and biopsies of the patients and the presence of CMV and HBV markers is listed in Table 23.1. Those with titres of EBV-VCA equal to or above 1:640 were further studied, when possible, to determine the titre of EBV-VCA in the IgM fraction, the titre of antibody to early antigen (EBV-EA) as well as its pattern of immunofluorescent staining, and the titre of antibody to the EB nuclear antigen (EBNA). All the determinations were done by immuno-fluorescent assays in a laboratory specializing in immunologic testing far distant from the site of examination of the patients and without knowledge of the clinical problems. A group of six patients with a history of recent or remote infectious mononucleosis without liver disease, 14 with various liver diseases and 20 patients with primary biliary cirrhosis (PBC) followed during the same period of time as those with chronic hepatitis were used for comparisons.

A clinical assessment was made of all patients, and liver biopsies were available, or were done, on 62 of the 86 patients. Biopsy specimens from 15 of those with high EBV-VCA titres were subjected to transmission electron microscopic examination.

Table 23.1 Number and sex of patients studied, biopsies, those tested for CMV and those with hepatitis B markers. Of the 86 patients with chronic hepatitis, 12 were i.v. drug abusers, 20 male homosexuals, 5 homosexual i.v. drug abusers, 16 post transfusion, 8 health professionals, 10 auto-immune and 15 with no apparent risk factors

Male	Female	Biopsies	CMV + /N	HB + /e + /N
63	23	62	13/58	46/14/86
	PBC			
5	15	20	—	0/20
	History of mononucleosis			
14	6	8	1/8	8/3/20

RESULTS

The titres of EBV-VCA were 1:640 or more in half of the i.v. drug abusers, and in almost half the patients with post transfusion chronic hepatitis. Since most of the former had hepatitis B markers and most of the latter did not, the presence of hepatitis B virus was not a factor. None of the patients with autoimmune hepatitis had high EBV-VCA titres but most did have cirrhosis

Table 23.2   EBV-VCA titres in various histologic forms of chronic hepatitis

	1:640 or more	1:320	1:160 or less
CPH or less (23)	9	7	7
CAH (14)	3	6	5
Cirrhosis (28)	10	8	10*

*Includes 8 autoimmune

on biopsy. Therefore, cirrhosis itself was not caused by EBV. However, patients with EBV-VCA titres of 1:640 or greater were more often seen in patients with cirrhosis if autoimmune disease was not included (Table 23.2). Male homosexuality itself was not as great a risk factor for a high EBV-VCA titre as was a needle or blood route of exposure. Chronic liver disease *per se* was not a risk factor, since the patients with auto-immune disease and those with primary biliary cirrhosis had very few high EBV-VCA titres.

When the IgM-VCA, early antigen and nuclear antigen antibodies to EBV were tested in patients with initially high VCA titres only a few patients were found to have IgM antibody, most had early antigen with a diffuse staining pattern while EBNA titres varied considerably (Table 23.3). The six patients with a history of infectious mononucleosis had high VCA titres seen early and with a restricted pattern of early antigen (Table 23.4).

Table 23.3   EBV-VCA IgM, early antigen (EA) with restricted (R) or diffuse (D) distribution, and nuclear antigen NA in 17 patients with EBV-VCA titres of 1:640 or greater when first tested

EBV-VCA		EBV-VCA-IgM	
1:640 or more	12	1:10 or less	15
1:160 or less	5	1:40 or more	2
EBV-EA		EBNA	
1:20 or less	5	1:10 or less	7
1:40 or more	12	1:40 or more	6
D pattern	10		
R pattern	1		

Table 23.4   EBV antibodies in 6 patients with a history of infectious mononucleosis with liver involvement

	VCA	VCA-IgM	EA	NA
Acute (1)	1:5120–640	<1:10	1:1280R	<1:160
Convalescent (2)	1:5420–640	1:10	1:40	<1:5
	1:160	1:10	1:160R	<1:5
Old (3)	1:160	–	1:20R	1:80
	1:160	<1:10	1:40D	1:40
	1:160	<1:10	1:40D	1:40

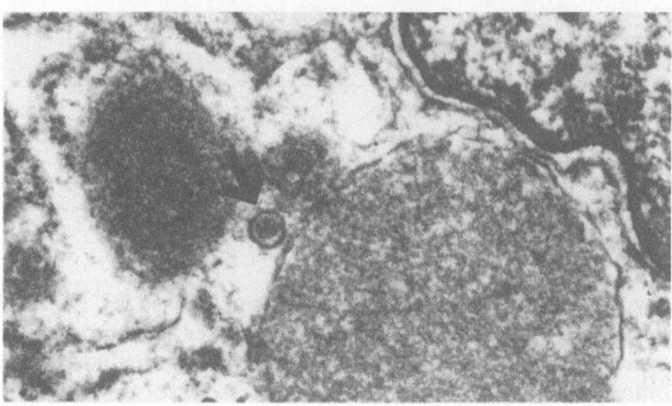

Figure 23.1 Electron micrograph of a portion of a lymphocyte in a liver biopsy specimen from a patient with chronic hepatitis and an EBV-VCA titre of 1:640. The arrow points to a herpes-viridae particle in the cytoplasm (× 39 000)

The electron microscopic studies of liver biopsy specimens revealed viral particles resembling herpesviridae in lymphocytes in six (Figure 23.1) and in hepatocytes in two patients (Figure 23.2). The particles appeared to be forming in hepatocellular nuclei (Figure 23.3).

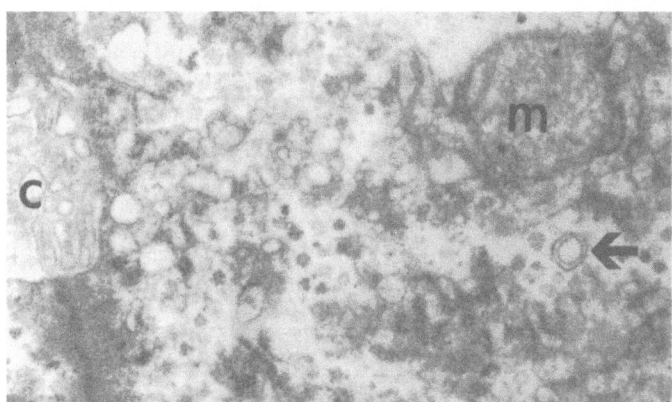

Figure 23.2 Electron micrograph of hepatocyte with empty herpesviridae particle (arrow) in the cytoplasm in a patient with chronic hepatitis and an EBV-VCA titre of 1:640 (× 28 000)

DISCUSSION

More than 75% of people studied in surveys showed antibodies to EBV-VCA[20, 21]. However, titres of 1:640 or greater were found in only about 4% of persons[20]. This last finding was similar to the 5% rate in the PBC patients, and contrasted with the over 36% rate in patients with chronic hepatitis.

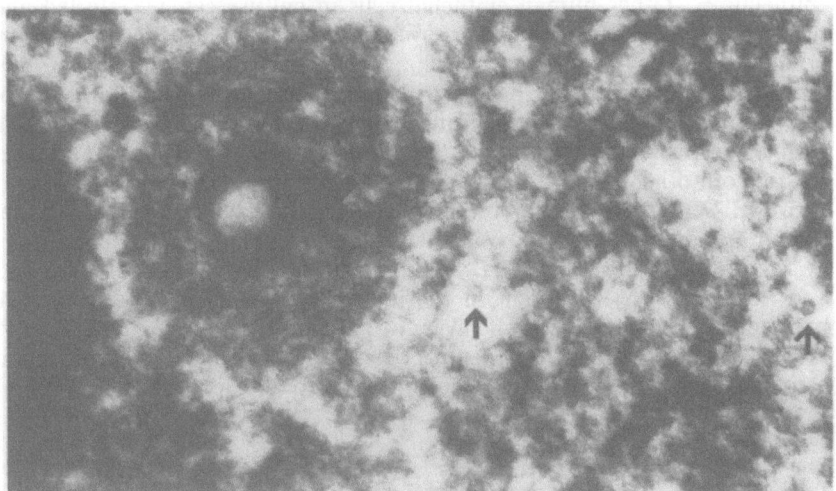

Figure 23.3 Portion of a hepatocellular nucleus containing hepatitis B core particles (small arrow) and a larger double ring particle which appears to be in formation (big arrow) in a patient with chronic active hepatitis B and EBV-VCA titre greater than 1 : 640 (× 90 000)

Infection with EBV is often not associated with clinical features of mono-nucleosis[6, 22] and many infected persons may not have heterophile anti-bodies[22]. Therefore, lack of a history of mononucleosis in a patient with chronic hepatitis does not mean that EBV can be dismissed as a factor in the disease.

This study was actually started to look for the possible involvement of the cytomegalovirus (CMV) in chronic hepatitis. The virus can produce a mild hepatitis when present by itself[23]. It has been found in AIDS[17, 19] but the number of patients with chronic hepatitis in this series with high CMV antibody titres or with IgM-CMV antibody was small (just over 20%), and, therefore, this phase of investigation was not continued. Nevertheless, in the individual patient both EBV and CMV should be looked for when appro-priate therapy becomes available.

EBV infection may be unique in that once the virus gains access to the body it infects different cells with different results (Table 23.5). B lymphocytes when initially infected proliferate and are transformed to active γ-globulin and early antigen producing cells[24, 25]. This response to the infection triggers proliferation and activity of suppressor T lymphocytes which reduce B lymphocyte activity and proliferation[26, 27]. This lymphocyte interaction leads to recovery from infectious mononucleosis. The transformation of the B lymphocyte by the virus causes it to become 'immortalized'[25]. However, the T lymphocyte immunity does not destroy the virus but rather keeps it in the B lymphocyte forever under normal circumstances. Thus the 'EB virus is harboured in peripheral lymphocytes . . . as a non-productive, unexpressed infection'[24]. While EBV may reside in and transform B lymphocytes, the main site of viral replication and shedding is the oropharyngeal mucosal epithelium[25]. Other human epithelial cells in culture can be infected and support viral replication[28-30]. Direct evidence that replication of EBV can occur in hepatocytes of man is lacking. The electron microscopic studies reported here suggest that herpesviridae particles can be found in hepato-cellular nuclei in patients with chronic hepatitis with no evidence of infection with other members of the herpes family of viruses except EBV. This does not rule out other viral infections. Particles are seen in the livers of patients with AIDS that are similar to, but smaller, than herpesviridae particles (unpublished observations). Whether these are HTLV-III virus particles awaits further study. Since AIDS was present in only six of the 86 patients and risk factors were absent in the majority, the particles (also seen in lymphocytes) which were in the livers of patients with only high EBV-VCA are assumed to be EBV. Endogenous reactivation of EBV can occur, and is associated with increased titres of antibodies to all the viral markers[31].

Table 23.5 Sites and consequence of EBV infection

B-lymphocyte	
Activation	γ-globulin up, lymphocytosis, early antigen
Immortalization	viral perpetuation without replication
T-cell stimulation	viral containment, recovery from mononucleosis
Neoplasia	Burkitt and other lymphomas
Nasopharyngeal epithelium	viral replication and shedding, carrier state, neoplasia
Hepatocyte	viral replication (?) acute and chronic (?) hepatitis, cancer (?)

Chronic hepatitis has many causes and a broad clinical–pathological spectrum. That more than one aetiology can be present simultaneously was demonstrated most clearly in a superinfection of chronic hepatitis B with delta agent[32]. The combination of infection with B and delta viruses makes the chronic hepatitis worse. Infection with hepatitis A virus in human[33] or chimpanzee[34] B virus carriers may or may not lead to more severe acute disease, but whether it makes chronic disease more active is not known. EBV superinfection, coinfection of reactivation in chronic hepatitis from any other cause seems to make the transformation of chronic hepatitis to cirrhosis more likely.

Since EBV is ubiquitous over the entire world, and since infection or reactivation can occur in many different settings, EBV infection may be an important determinant in the outcome in patients with any kind of chronic hepatitis. In addition, a relationship of EBV infection to carcinogenesis in the liver may be possible since the virus appears to be oncogenic in other cells in which it is found.

References

1. Pfeiffer, E. (1889). Drüsenfieber. *Jahrb. f. Kinderh.*, n.s. **29**, 257–64
2. Sprunt, T. P. and Evans, F. A. (1920). Mononuclear leucocytosis in reaction to acute infections ('infectious mononucleosis'). *Johns Hopkins Hosp. Bull.*, **31**, 410–17
3. Downey, H. and McKinlay, C. A. (1923). Acute lymphadenosis compared with acute lymphatic leukemia. *Arch. Intern. Med.*, **32**, 82–112
4. Mackey, R. P. and Wakefield, E. G. (1926). The occurrence of abnormal leukocytes in the blood of a patient with jaundice (infectious mononucleosis – glandular fever). *Ann. Clin. Med.*, **4**, 727–30
5. Cohn, C. and Lidman, B. I. (1946). Hepatitis without jaundice in infectious mononucleosis. *J. Clin. Invest.*, **25**, 145–51
6. Watson, J., Johnson, P., Kahn, J. and Stone, F. M. (1951). Subclinical infectious mononucleosis with hepatitis. Epidemic in a class of one hundred two medical students; a two-year study. *Arch. Intern. Med.*, **88**, 618–26
7. Bennett, H. D., Frankel, J. J., Bedinger, P. and Baker, L. A. (1950). Infectious mononucleosis with hepatitis. *Arch. Intern. Med.*, **86**, 391–401
8. Leibowitz, S. and Brody, H. (1950). Cirrhosis of the liver following infectious mononucleosis. *Am. J. Med.*, **8**, 675–85
9. Kilham, L. and Steigman, A. (1942). Infectious mononucleosis. *Lancet*, **2**, 452–4
10. Kilpatrick, Z. M. (1966). Structural and functional abnormalities of liver in infectious mononucleosis. *Arch. Intern. Med.*, **117**, 47–53
11. Henle, G., Henle, W. and Diehl, V. (1968). Relation of Burkitt's tumor-associated herpes-type virus to infectious mononucleosis. *Proc. Nat. Acad. Sci. USA*, **59**, 94–101
12. Epstein, M. A., Barr, Y. M. and Achong, B. G. (1965). Studies with Burkitt's lymphoma. *Wistar Inst. Symp. Monogr.*, **4**, 69–82
13. Henle, W., Henle, G. and Horwitz, C. A. (1974). Epstein–Barr virus specific diagnostic tests in infectious mononucleosis. *Hum. Pathol.*, **5**, 551–65
14. Pagano, J. S. and Lemon, S. M. (1981). The Herpesviruses. In Braude, A. I., Davis, C. E. and Fierer, J. (eds.) *Medical Microbiology and Infectious Diseases*. pp. 541–9. (Philadelphia: Saunders)
15. Gerber, P., Walsh, J. H., Rosenblum, E. N. and Purcell, R. H. (1969). Association of EB-virus infection with the post-perfusion syndrome. *Lancet*, **1**, 593–6
16. Turner, A. R., MacDonald, N. and Cooper, B. A. (1972). Transmission of infectious mononucleosis by transfusion of pre-illness plasma. *Ann. Intern. Med.*, **77**, 751–3
17. Cheeseman, S. H., Sullivan, J. L., Brettler, D. B. and Levine, P. H. (1984). Analysis of cytomegalovirus and Epstein–Barr virus antibody responses in treated hemophiliacs. Implications for the study of acquired immune deficiency syndrome. *J. Am. Med. Assoc.*, **252**, 83–5
18. Corey, L., Stamm, W. E., Feorino, P. M., Bryan, J. A., Weseley, S., Gregg, M. B. and Solangi, K. (1975). HBsAg-negative hepatitis in a hemodialysis unit. Relation to Epstein–Barr virus. *N. Engl. J. Med.*, **293**, 1273–8
19. Quinnan, G. V. Jr., Masur, H., Rook, A. H., Armstrong, G., Frederick, W. R., Epstein, J., Manischewitz, J. F., Macher, A. M., Jackson, L., Ames, J., Smith, H. A., Parker, M., Pearson, G. R., Parillo, J., Mitchell, C. and Strauss, S. E. (1984). Herpesvirus infections in the acquired immune deficiency syndrome. *J. Am. Med. Assoc.*, **252**, 72–7
20. Porter, D. D., Wimberly, I. and Benyesh-Melnick, M. (1969). Prevalence of antibodies to EB virus and other herpes viruses. *J. Am. Med. Assoc.*, **208**, 1675–9
21. Niederman, J. C., Evans, A. S., Subrahmanyan, L. and McCollum, R. W. (1979). Prevalence, incidence and persistence of EB virus antibody in young adults. *N. Engl. J. Med.*, **282**, 361–5
22. Evans, A. S., Niederman, J. C. and McCollum, R. W. (1968). Seroepidemiologic studies of infectious mononucleosis with EB virus. *N. Engl. J. Med.*, **279**, 1123–7
23. Snover, D. C. and Horwitz, C. A. (1984). Liver disease in cytomegalovirus mononucleosis: A light microscopical and immunoperoxidase study of six cases. *Hepatology*, **4**, 408–12
24. Rickinson, A. B., Jarvis, J. E., Crawford, D. H. and Epstein, M. A. (1974). Observations on the type of infection by Epstein–Barr virus in peripheral lymphoid cells of patients with infectious mononucleosis. *Int. J. Cancer*, **14**, 704–15
25. Miller, G. (1984). Epstein–Barr virus – immortalization and replication. *N. Engl. J. Med.*, **310**, 1255–6

26. Tosata, G., Magrath, I., Koski, I., Dooley, N. and Blaese, M. (1979). Activation of suppressor T-cells during Epstein–Barr-virus-induced infectious mononucleosis. *N. Engl. J. Med.*, **301**, 1133–7
27. Rickinson, A. B., Moss, D. J. and Pope, J. H. (1979). Long-term T-cell mediated immunity to Epstein–Barr virus in man. II. Components necessary for regression in virus-infected leukocyte cultures. *Int. J. Cancer*, **23**, 610–17
28. Sixbey, J. W., Vesterinen, E. H., Nedrud, J. G., Raab-Traub, N., Walton, L. A. and Pagano, J. S. (1983). Replication of Epstein–Barr virus in normal human epithelial cells infected *in vitro*. *Nature*, **306**, 480–3
29. Shapiro, I. M. and Volsky, D. J. (1983). Infection of normal human epithelial cells by Epstein–Barr virus. *Science*, **219**, 1225–8
30. Sixbey, J. W., Nedrud, J. G., Raab-Traub, N., Hanes, R. A. and Pagano, P. S. (1984). Epstein–Barr virus replication in oropharyngeal epithelial cells. *N. Engl. J. Med.*, **310**, 1225–30
31. Sumoya, C. V. (1975). Endogenous reactivation of Epstein–Barr virus infections. *J. Infect. Dis.*, **131**, 403–8
32. Rizzetto, M., Verme, G., Recchia, S. *et al.* (1983). Chronic hepatitis in carriers of hepatitis B surface antigen, with intrahepatic expression of delta antigen. An active and progressive disease unresponsive to immunosuppressive treatment. *Ann. Intern. Med.*, **98**, 437–41
33. Zachoral, R., Roggendorf, M. and Deinhardt, F. (1983). Hepatitis A infection in chronic carriers of hepatitis B virus. *Hepatology*, **3**, 528–31
34. Tsiquaya, K. N., Harrison, T. J., Portmann, B., Hu, S. and Zuckerman, A. J. (1984). Acute hepatitis A infection in hepatitis B chimpanzee carriers. *Hepatology*, **4**, 504–9

Index

Fibroblastic reticulum cells 188
'activated endothelial cells' and 189
Fibronectic, synthesis in liver cells,
dexamethasone effects 99, 100
Finger clubbing, primary biliary cirrhosis
84
Fischer, lithocholic acid isolation 13–14
FPL 55712, leukotriene receptor antagonist
142, 143
Free fatty acids, hepatic uptake, driving
forces 46–7
Freeze-fracture replicas
hepatocyte gap junctions 155–62
rotary shadowing 155–62

GABA
blood-brain barrier crossing, liver failure
121
coma induction 120
gut-derived, liver metabolic role 121
properties 120
receptors
hyperammonaemia 123, 124
interaction, neural inhibition 120
D-Galactosamine
endotoxin synergy, fulminant hepatitis
141–2
ribonucleic acid synthesis inhibition
141–2
Gallbladder
bile acid levels, diurnal rhythm 75–6
endoscopic papillotomy 73–9
Gallstones
dissolution 5, 7, 14, 18–19, 31–2, 33–4
T-tube infusion 34
primary biliary cirrhosis 84
see also Cholesterol gallstones
Gap junctions, hepatocyte 155–62
crystalline particles, subunit configuration
160–1
Gas chromatography, bile acids 7–8
Glandular fever, hepatic involvement
209–16
Glomerulonephritis, primary biliary
cirrhosis 84
Glucokinase, hepatocyte 96
Glutamate receptors, hyperammonaemia
123, 124
Glutamine cycle, intracellular hepatic 94
Glycoproteins, plasma membrane
half-life calculation 147–9
heterogenous turnover 147–53
Golgi apparatus, glycoprotein heterogenous
turnover 149
G-6PD, Kupffer cells 96–7
Graft-versus-host syndrome 81
Granulomas, immune complexes, primary
biliary cirrhosis 82

Grundy and Metzger, indicator dilution
techniques 12
Guanoxan, impaired oxidation, poor
metabolizers 103

Haemochromatosis, idiopathic,
hyperinsulinaemia 163
Hashimoto's thyroiditis, primary biliary
cirrhosis 82
Haslewood, G. A. D. 6
HDL, catabolism 95, 96
'Hepatic-sensitive diabetics' 164
Heaton, enterohepatic circulation studies 12
Hepatitis
acute, piecemeal necrosis 184
autoimmune
chronic active, lymphocytes 186
EBV-VCA titres 210
chronic 183–200
Epstein–Barr virus 209–16
chronic active
autoimmune, lymphocytes 186
dendritic reticulum cells 187–8
lichen planus association 189
urea cycle enzymes 133
fulminant, leukotriene role 141–4
Hepatitis A 201–7
bile duct lesions 204
clinical presentation 202
Kupffer cell and macrophage iron storage
204, 205
periportal cell necrosis 201, 202–3, 205
piecemeal necrosis 185
relapsing, periportal cell necrosis 202
spotty necrosis 204
Hepatitis B
HLA associations 191
immunological defence damage 186
spotty necrosis 204
Hepatitis B virus, AIDS 209
'Hepatitis Memoranda' xxi
Hepatitis, non-A non-B
acute 184–5
'Poulsen lesion' 204
Hepatobiliary disease, bile acids
metabolism 14–18, 61–6
toxicity 64
turnover 62–4
Hepatocarcinogens, chemical 109–18
Hepatocytes
fatty infiltration, Wilson's disease 169–70
gap junctions, freeze-fracture replicas
155–62
glucokinase levels 96
Kupffer cell metabolic cooperation 97
oleate uptake kinetics 43–4
Hepatology Raid Literature Review xxi
Hexokinase, Kupffer cells 96